Nutrition Handbook

Nutrition Handbook

Edited by **Alison Craft**

FOSTER ACADEMICS

New Jersey

Published by Foster Academics,
61 Van Reypen Street,
Jersey City, NJ 07306, USA
www.fosteracademics.com

Nutrition Handbook
Edited by Alison Craft

International Standard Book Number: 978-1-63242-299-6 (Hardback)

Printed in China.

Contents

Preface

Every living being needs to eat to survive. But for healthy growth and development, eating a healthy balanced diet is necessary. That is what comes under the purview of nutrition. It encompasses, the need, plan and the actual nutrients that one needs to include in their diet for proper growth and a healthy life. It answers all the whats, hows, and whys of food and their merits to the body.

What is unique about nutrition is that even in the ancient times scholars and researchers knew about the importance of nutrition, nutritious food and their healthy implications on the body. In modern times, dieticians, and nutritionists urge people to follow a healthy life suitably supported by nutrients rich food. These important elements of the food are extremely important for health and to prevent many health related risks, like sugar level, heart, liver and kidney problems. Deficiency of nutrients leads to poor health, low energy levels, weak bones, low immunity and to many other more serious ailments.

Not just deficiency even excess consumption of any nutrients leads to different problems like high blood pressure, obesity, hair loss, brittle nails, heart problems and so on. Even in the plants kingdom, nutrition has immense importance. Our green friends depend on sunlight, air, soil, water and fertilizers.

With the advances in molecular biology, biochemistry and genetics, the science of nutrition has become more focused to understand the biochemical sequences that breaks and converts, through metabolism, the nutrients present in our bodies to simpler substances.

Research has proved that intake of nutritious meals and practicing long-term habits of healthy eating have a positive effect on cognitive and spatial memory capacity. In fact when a pregnant mother follows a nutritious diet, her child inherits a system.

This book traces the evolution of nutrition through different stages of mankind and its growing importance in today's jet setting lifestyle.

I wish to thank all the contributing authors, my publisher and my family for their constant support.

Editor

1

Personalized Lifestyle Medicine: Relevance for Nutrition and Lifestyle Recommendations

Deanna M. Minich and Jeffrey S. Bland

Personalized Lifestyle Medicine Institute, 800 Fifth Avenue, Suite 4100, Seattle, WA 98104, USA

Correspondence should be addressed to Deanna M. Minich; deannaminich@plminstitute.org

Academic Editors: E. Kirk, C. Palacios, E. van den Heuvel, and B. Venn

Public health recommendations for lifestyle modification, including diet and physical activity, have been widely disseminated for the prevention and treatment of disease. These guidelines are intended for the overall population without significant consideration for the individual with respect to one's genes and environment. Personalized lifestyle medicine is a newly developed term that refers to an approach to medicine in which an individual's health metrics from point-of-care diagnostics are used to develop lifestyle medicine-oriented therapeutic strategies for improving individual health outcomes in managing chronic disease. Examples of the application of personalized lifestyle medicine to patient care include the identification of genetic variants through laboratory tests and/or functional biomarkers for the purpose of designing patient-specific prescriptions for diet, exercise, stress, and environment. Personalized lifestyle medicine can provide solutions to chronic health problems by harnessing innovative and evolving technologies based on recent discoveries in genomics, epigenetics, systems biology, life and behavioral sciences, and diagnostics and clinical medicine. A comprehensive, personalized approach to medicine is required to promote the safety of therapeutics and reduce the cost of chronic disease. Personalized lifestyle medicine may provide a novel means of addressing a patient's health by empowering them with information they need to regain control of their health.

1. Introduction

Chronic conditions such as type 2 diabetes, cardiovascular disease, metabolic syndrome, and obesity are, in varying degrees, associated with unhealthy lifestyle and behavior, including tobacco use, nutritional excesses, lack of physical activity, and heightened exposure to stress (Figure 1). Egger et al. [1] reported that most (about 60%–70%) health care visits in industrialized countries are correlated with these lifestyle-induced, preventable diseases. Therefore, due to the exorbitant cost and lack of resources to deal with the rising tide of illness, the importance of lifestyle factors in the origin and progression of disease can no longer be ignored. In fact, Dysinger [2] documented that in 2012, the American Medical Association issued a call to action for physicians to "acquire and apply the 15 clinical competencies of lifestyle medicine, and offer evidence-based lifestyle medicine interventions as the first and primary mode of preventing and, when appropriate, treating chronic disease within clinical medicine."

In 2010, Lianov and Johnson [3] published an article in the *Journal of the American Medical Association* that strongly advocated physician education and training in lifestyle medicine: "Physician educators at both the undergraduate and graduate medical education levels should consider incorporating the relevant lifestyle medicine competencies into education and training programs." The need for education in lifestyle medicine is so profound that prominent universities like Harvard, Stanford, and Yale have implemented the inclusion of lifestyle medicine into their curriculum, ranging from postgraduate courses to the development of separate institutes devoted to the cause. Additionally, the *American Journal of Lifestyle Medicine* is a peer-reviewed journal that was launched in 2007 for the purpose of educating practitioners on how to incorporate lifestyle medicine into clinical practice.

Lifestyle medicine is not a new or alternative medical discipline. The value of food as medicine was acknowledged several centuries ago by Hippocrates. Despite the fact that

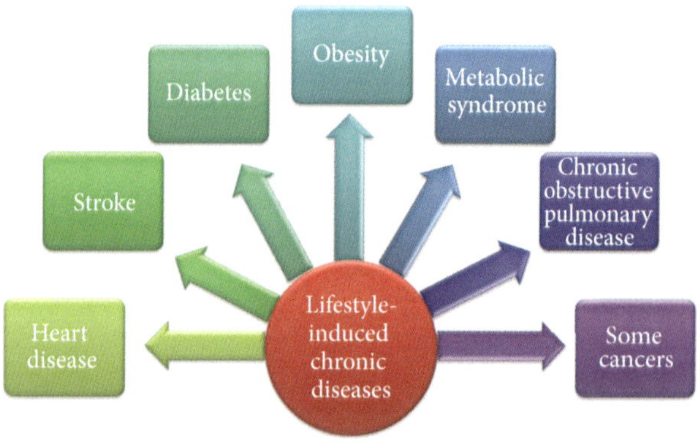

Figure 1: Lifestyle-induced chronic disease.

lifestyle recommendations have been recognized in ancient healing traditions over centuries, there are several modern-day definitions of lifestyle medicine that have been proposed. Dysinger [2] states it succinctly that lifestyle medicine is "the application of simple, natural healing approaches to chronic disease and prevention." In his textbook on lifestyle medicine, Egger refers to lifestyle medicine as "the application of environmental, behavioural, medical and motivational principles to the management of lifestyle-related health problems in a clinical setting [4]." The Lifestyle Medicine Competency Development Panel defines it as "the evidence-based practice of helping individuals and families adopt and sustain healthy behaviors that affect health and quality of life [2]." Dean Ornish, touted as the most well-recognized pioneer in lifestyle medicine, states that it is composed of nutrition, physical activity, stress reduction and rest, and social support systems [3].

For the purposes of this review, lifestyle medicine is considered in the broadest sense as follows:

(i) *nutrition,* as it relates to dietary supplements, medical foods, and functional foods;

(ii) *physical activity* as defined by the entire spectrum of movement, from anaerobic to aerobic, and from mild to vigorous in intensity;

(iii) *sress management and behavioral modification,* as needed, and all the aspects that modulate behavior such as mind-body medicine, psychosocial influences, and social networks;

(iv) *environmental exposure* to contaminants found in air, food, water, and radiation, due to the ubiquitous nature of toxins and their compounding concentration in the environment, leading to the well-recognized increasing toxin burden in physiological systems that relates directly to chronic disease.

Aspects of lifestyle medicine are as follows:

(i) whole foods and dietary patterns;

(ii) specific food-derived bioactives;

(iii) liquids and hydration;

(iv) dietary supplements;

(v) medical foods;

(vi) functional foods;

(vii) physical activities (aerobic or anaerobic);

(viii) mental fitness;

(ix) emotional regulation;

(x) mind-body medicine modalities for stress modulation;

(xi) social networks and support groups;

(xii) rest and sleep;

(xiii) environmental exposures (air, food, water or radiation).

Perhaps most importantly, lifestyle medicine is intended to be patient focused, enabling and requiring patients to be intimately involved in their health trajectory with the accompaniment of healthcare professionals. The system of mainstream medicine is designed for the "typical" patient with lab biomarkers within specific ranges; however, there is a subset of patients who tend to be outliers in this distribution of the population. In fact, these outliers may occur more frequently than is perhaps acknowledged, and, at the same time, they may experience increased difficulty with navigating the healthcare system. Even genetic variants with low penetrance can have significant effects in one's physiology, resulting in low tolerance to certain environmental influences. Furthermore, laboratory values in the low or high normal range may signify the onset of subclinical pathological syndromes, and, ultimately, these individuals may become excellent candidates for what personalized lifestyle medicine has to offer (Figure 2).

In conjunction with being a compelling solution to the chronic disease epidemic and allowing the patient to have control of their health, lifestyle medicine therapies have been shown to be cost effective. Herman et al. [5] assessed both lifestyle intervention and metformin against placebo intervention in the prevention of type 2 diabetes in individuals with impaired glucose intolerance. Lifestyle delayed the onset of type 2 diabetes by 11 years and metformin by 3 years compared with placebo. Additionally, the cost per quality-adjusted life-years (QALYs) was much lower for the lifestyle intervention relative to the implementation of metformin therapy (cost per QALY: $1,100 versus $31,300, resp.). Thus, lifestyle costs less and performs better in one of the largest, growing chronic diseases in developed countries, type 2 diabetes.

2. Public Health Recommendations for Nutrition and Lifestyle

Several opinion leader organizations have published lifestyle medicine recommendations consisting primarily of diet and physical activity benchmarks for the general public for the purpose of either prevention or as part of a treatment for diseases. For example, in 2010, the U.S. Department of Agriculture and the U.S. Department of Health and Human

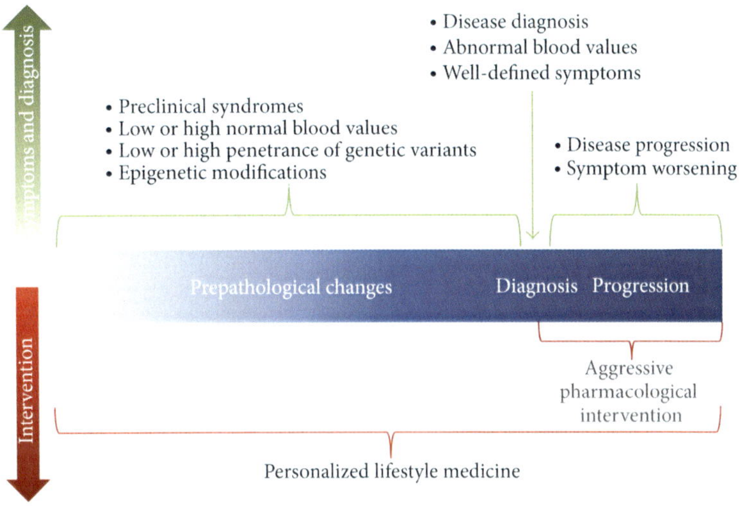

FIGURE 2: The trajectory of disease and role for personalized lifestyle medicine.

Services published extensive guidelines for the American population on what constitutes a healthy dietary pattern, supporting the widespread incorporation of nutrient-dense foods and beverages in proper amounts into the average American diet to assist in maintenance of body weight [6]. For those individuals interested in specific measures for cardiovascular disease risk reduction, the American Heart Association Nutrition Committee published a paper on both diet and lifestyle recommendations [7]. Together with highlighting the benefits of eating a diet rich in vegetables and fruits, as well as eating oily fish twice per week, they discuss lifestyle habits such as smoking cessation and the importance of physical activity in maintaining ideal body weight. According to Kushi et al. [8], the American Cancer Society nutrition and physical activity guidelines are consistent with those defined by the American Heart Association and the 2010 Dietary Guidelines for Americans, in addition to those established by the American Diabetes Association and the 2008 Physical Activity Guidelines for Americans.

Lifestyle Medicine Recommendations by National Opinion Leader Organizations. For the U.S. Department of Agriculture and the U.S. Department of Health and Human Services [6], the lifestyle medicine recommendations for general population are as follows.

Balancing Calories to Manage Weight.

(i) Prevent and/or reduce overweight and obesity through improved eating and physical activity behaviors.

(ii) Control total calorie intake to manage body weight. For people who are overweight or obese, this will mean consuming fewer calories from foods and beverages.

(iii) Increase physical activity and reduce time spent in sedentary behaviors.

(iv) Maintain appropriate calorie balance during each stage of life—childhood, adolescence, adulthood, pregnancy and breastfeeding, and older age.

Foods and Food Components to Reduce.

(i) Reduce daily sodium intake to less than 2,300 milligrams (mg) and further reduce intake to 1,500 mg among persons who are 51 and older and those of any age who are African American or have hypertension, diabetes, or chronic kidney disease. The 1,500 mg recommendation applies to about half of the US population, including children, and the majority of adults.

(ii) Consume less than 10 percent of calories from saturated fatty acids by replacing them with monounsaturated and polyunsaturated fatty acids.

(iii) Consume less than 300 mg per day of dietary cholesterol.

(iv) Keep trans fatty acid consumption as low as possible by limiting foods that contain synthetic sources of trans fats, such as partially hydrogenated oils, and by limiting other solid fats.

(v) Reduce the intake of calories from solid fats and added sugars.

(vi) Limit the consumption of foods that contain refined grains, especially refined grain foods that contain solid fats, added sugars, and sodium.

(vii) If alcohol is consumed, it should be consumed in moderation—up to one drink per day for women and two drinks per day for men—and only by adults of legal drinking age.

Foods and Nutrients to Increase. Individuals should meet the following recommendations as part of a healthy eating pattern while staying within their calorie needs.

(i) Increase vegetable and fruit intake.
(ii) Eat a variety of vegetables, especially dark-green and red and orange vegetables and beans and peas.
(iii) Consume at least half of all grains as whole grains. Increase whole-grain intake by replacing refined grains with whole grains.
(iv) Increase intake of fat-free or low-fat milk and milk products, such as milk, yogurt, cheese, or fortified soy beverages.
(v) Choose a variety of protein foods, which include seafood, lean meat and poultry, eggs, beans and peas, soy products, and unsalted nuts and seeds.
(vi) Increase the amount and variety of seafood consumed by choosing seafood in place of some meat and poultry.
(vii) Replace protein foods that are higher in solid fats with choices that are lower in solid fats and calories and/or are sources of oils.
(viii) Use oils to replace solid fats where possible.
(ix) Choose foods that provide more potassium, dietary fiber, calcium, and vitamin D, which are nutrients of concern in American diets. These foods include vegetables, fruits, whole grains, and milk and milk products.

For the American Heart Association Recommendations for Cardiovascular Risk Reduction [7], the lifestyle medicine recommendations for general population are as follows.

(i) Balance calorie intake and physical activity to achieve or maintain a healthy body weight.
(ii) Consume a diet rich in vegetables and fruits.
(iii) Choose whole-grain, high-fiber foods.
(iv) Consume fish, especially oily fish, at least twice a week.
(v) Limit your intake of saturated fat to 7% of energy, trans fat to 1% of energy, and cholesterol to 300 mg per day by
  (a) choosing lean meats and vegetable alternatives;
  (b) selecting fat-free (skim), 1%-fat, and low-fat dairy products;
  (c) minimizing intake of partially hydrogenated fats.
(vi) Minimize your intake of beverages and foods with added sugars.
(vii) Choose and prepare foods with little or no salt.
(viii) If you consume alcohol, do so in moderation.
(ix) When you eat food that is prepared outside home, follow the AHA Diet and Lifestyle Recommendations.

For the American Cancer Society Guidelines on Nutrition and Physical Activity for Cancer Prevention [8], the lifestyle medicine recommendations for general population are as follows.

(i) Achieve and maintain a healthy weight throughout life.
(ii) Be as lean as possible throughout life without being underweight.
(iii) Avoid excess weight gain at all ages. For those who are currently overweight or obese, losing even a small amount of weight has health benefits and is a good place to start.
(iv) Engage in regular physical activity and limit consumption of high-calorie foods and beverages as key strategies for maintaining a healthy weight.
(v) Adopt a physically active lifestyle.
(vi) Adults should engage in at least 150 minutes of moderate intensity or 75 minutes of vigorous intensity activity each week, or an equivalent combination, preferably spread throughout the week.
(vii) Children and adolescents should engage in at least 1 hour of moderate or vigorous intensity activity each day, with vigorous intensity activity occurring at least 3 days each week.
(viii) Limit sedentary behavior such as sitting, lying down, watching television, or other forms of screen-based entertainment.
(ix) Doing some physical activity above usual activities, no matter what one's level of activity, can have many health benefits.
(x) Consume a healthy diet, with an emphasis on plant foods.
(xi) Choose foods and beverages in amounts that help achieve and maintain a healthy weight.
(xii) Limit consumption of processed meat and red meat.
(xiii) Eat at least 2.5 cups of vegetables and fruits each day.
(xiv) Choose whole grains instead of refined grain products.
(xv) If you drink alcoholic beverages, limit consumption.
(xvi) Drink no more than 1 drink per day for women or 2 per day for men.

For the American Diabetes Association [9], the lifestyle medicine recommendations for general population are as follows.

Energy Balance, Overweight, and Obesity.

(i) In overweight and obese insulin-resistant individuals, modest weight loss has been shown to improve insulin resistance. Thus, weight loss is recommended for all such individuals who have or are at risk for diabetes.
(ii) For weight loss, either low-carbohydrate or low-fat calorie-restricted diets may be effective in the short term (up to 1 year).
(iii) For patients on low-carbohydrate diets, monitor lipid profiles, renal function, and protein intake (in those with nephropathy), and adjust hypoglycemic therapy as needed.

(iv) Physical activity and behavior modification are important components of weight loss programs and are most helpful in maintenance of weight loss.

(v) Weight loss medications may be considered in the treatment of overweight and obese individuals with type 2 diabetes and can help achieve a 5%–10% weight loss when combined with lifestyle modification.

(vi) Bariatric surgery may be considered for some individuals with type 2 diabetes and BMI 35 kg/m^2 and can result in marked improvements in glycemia. The long-term benefits and risks of bariatric surgery in individuals with prediabetes or diabetes continue to be studied.

Preventing Diabetes (Primary Prevention).

(i) Among individuals at high risk for developing type 2 diabetes, structured programs that emphasize lifestyle changes that include moderate weight loss (7% body weight) and regular physical activity (150 min/week), with dietary strategies including reduced calories and reduced intake of dietary fat, can reduce the risk for developing diabetes and are therefore recommended.

(ii) Individuals at high risk for type 2 diabetes should be encouraged to achieve the USDA recommendation for dietary fiber (14 g fiber/1,000 kcal) and foods containing whole grains (one-half of grain intake).

(iii) There is not sufficient, consistent information to conclude that low-glycemic load diets reduce the risk for diabetes. Nevertheless, low-glycemic index foods that are rich in fiber and other important nutrients are to be encouraged.

(iv) Observational studies report that moderate alcohol intake may reduce the risk for diabetes, but the data do not support recommending alcohol consumption to individuals at risk of diabetes.

(v) No nutrition recommendation can be made for preventing type 1 diabetes.

(vi) Although there are insufficient data at present to warrant any specific recommendations for prevention of type 2 diabetes in youth, it is reasonable to apply approaches demonstrated to be effective in adults, as long as nutritional needs for normal growth and development are maintained.

3. The Emergence of Science to Support Personalized Nutrition Interventions

Based on this cursory review of national guidelines, it would seem that major health organizations are disseminating essentially similar nutrition and lifestyle recommendations to the public for the purpose of disease prevention. However, it is worthwhile to question whether these standardized public health positioning statements are sufficient to meet the diversity of the average individual, including addressing the multitude of variables such as age, lifecycle, gender, medical history, family history, vitamin and mineral status, ethnic background(s), lifestyle habits, genetics, single nucleotide polymorphisms (SNPs), mutations, and epigenetics. The following are the patient characteristics to consider in establishing a personalized lifestyle medicine therapeutic protocol:

(i) age,

(ii) lifecycle,

(iii) gender,

(iv) past medical history,

(v) family history,

(vi) ethnic background and ancestry,

(vii) lifestyle habits (e.g., smoking, activity, and stress reduction practices),

(viii) nutritional status (e.g., macronutrients, micronutrients, phytonutrients, and vitamins),

(ix) medication use,

(x) dietary supplement use,

(xi) physical location and frequency of travel,

(xii) home and environment,

(xiii) genetics and mutations,

(xiv) single nucleotide polymorphisms (SNPs),

(xv) epigenetic patterns.

Xie et al. [10] illustrate the complexity of the individual by suggesting the role of metabonomics in personalized nutrition. Metabonomics, or assessment of metabolic responses based on nutrient sufficiency or deficiency, is a way to characterize the metabolic phenotype of individual and predict their corresponding interactions with gut microbiota, environment, and behavior. In addition, Xie et al. [10] discuss advances in the role of phytochemical modulation of cellular physiology and propose phytochemical profiling, or phytoprofiling, to assist in the facilitation of determining phytonutrient requirements with more effective interventions with plant-derived compounds. Hence, the needs of the individual can be complex and require in-depth assessment before interventions can be confidently applied.

In much the same way, determining how the food intake as part of a dietary intervention meets the needs of an individual can be equally daunting. The challenge in understanding the integration of the many facets of the individual with the diversity of food constituents is supported by Jacobs and Tapsell [11] who state that reducing dietary recommendations to individual nutrients without considering the whole food and its multitude of constituents, including phytonutrients, may not be accounting for "food synergy." Certainly, it would seem that the mere presence and interplay of complex constituents in food would be important to acknowledge in the formulation of dietary recommendations. Improved quantitation of phytochemicals, secondary metabolites, bacterial species, and micronutrients would be useful in positioning of plant foods for their antioxidant, anti-inflammatory, and anticancer properties. Along similar lines, Minich and Bland

[12] discussed the importance of phytochemicals from cinnamon, hops, green tea, berberine, ginseng, quercetin, and resveratrol, in the modulation of the intracellular signals related to metabolic processes specific to insulin sensitivity, referred to as selective kinase response modulators, since these phytochemicals amplify signals through the cell selectively via protein kinases and to the degree required to restore intracellular function. Therefore, dietary recommendations for a variety of high phytonutrient-dense foods might be beneficial as part of individually tailored advice due to the specific roles of these compounds in various organ systems and how they impact intracellular physiology.

The recognition of the complexity of both an individual and a food may relate to the plethora of conflicting research studies on dietary components and food consumption, whether saturated fat, cholesterol, eggs, coconut oil, or caffeine. It is difficult for nutrition researchers to take into account the complexity of how a food interacts with the multitude of variables in a single individual, including, but not limited to, genotypic or epigenetic stratification, two aspects closely associated with an individual's requirements. Part of the reason for this omission may be due to the lack of adequate diagnostics, difficulty with interpretation, or the paucity of long-term, prospective studies to demonstrate how to clinically integrate this information with therapeutics.

Despite the opportunities that lie ahead for developing a sophisticated interface between technology, metrics, and nutritional interventions, several instances of personalized nutrition approaches have begun to emerge in the literature, suggesting that the introduction of personalized lifestyle medicine is perhaps timely and appropriate at this point in the evolution of medicine.

(i) *Iron Need and Iron Transport Polymorphisms.* Most individuals with hereditary hemochromatosis could theoretically be evaluated for mutant genotypes that are associated with primary iron overload and increased transferrin saturation and/or serum ferritin levels for better and faster treatment [13].

(ii) *Zinc Need and Polymorphisms.* Select polymorphisms in interleukin-6 and metallothionein may alter one's need for dietary zinc [14].

(iii) *Vitamin D Requirement for Diabetics with Polymorphisms in the Vitamin D Receptor.* Variations in the vitamin D receptor may influence vitamin D requirement and utilization in individuals with type 2 diabetes [15].

(iv) *The Influence of Polymorphisms on Coenzyme Q10 (CoQ10) Need for Energy Production and Its Role in Cerebellar Ataxia.* Genetic variants in the biosynthesis, reduction, and metabolism have been shown to be correlated with plasma CoQ10 levels [16]. CoQ10 deficiency genes were sequenced in patients with unexplained ataxia. CABC1/ADCK3 mutations were identified in symptomatic patients along with decreased muscle concentrations of CoQ10 [17].

(v) *Folate, MTHFR Polymorphisms, and Depression.* A number of studies have demonstrated the association between low serum folate levels and incidence of depression with a higher frequency of genetic variations in the methylene tetrahydrofolate reductase (MTHFR) enzyme in depressed versus nondepressed individuals [18]. It has been suggested that MTHFR genotyping may be helpful in determining which patients would benefit from L-methylfolate supplementation to override the limitation of reduced conversion of folic acid to this biologically active form due to the polymorphism in MTHFR [18].

(vi) *B Vitamin Gene Variants and Risk to Smoking-Induced Lung Cancer.* Identification of polymorphisms in B vitamin metabolism, particularly folate, has been associated with lung cancer risk, thereby potentially providing an individualized strategy to nutritional interventions for smokers [19].

(vii) *Antioxidants and Polymorphisms in Glutathione S-Transferases (GST).* Propensity towards increased oxidative stress and inflammation can be partially determined by GST genotype. Of all the nutritional factors measured, serum vitamin C was the most consistent nutrient associated with genetic variants of GST [20].

(viii) *Bitter Tasting and Body Composition Differences.* The individual's ability to taste bitter compounds is highly variable and depends on structural and genetic differences in 25 human bitter receptors, termed T2Rs [21]. Since there appears to be a relationship between bitter tasting ability and body mass index (BMI) [22], assessment of a patient's ability to taste bitter may be a useful individualized tool for understanding modifications in metabolism and determining whether inclusion of bitter compounds in the diet or through supplemental means is warranted.

Here are additional examples of clinical conditions for personalized lifestyle medicine interventions:

(i) salt restriction for subtype of hypertension;

(ii) dietary cholesterol restriction for subtype of hypercholesterolemia;

(iii) dietary saturated fatty acid intake for apoE4;

(iv) gluten restriction for grain intolerance;

(v) fructose restriction for fructose intolerance;

(vi) lactose restriction for lactose intolerance;

(vii) fava bean restriction for favism;

(viii) carbohydrate restriction for glycogen storage disease;

(ix) folate supplementation of MTHFR polymorphisms;

(x) lutein supplementation for risk to macular degeneration;

(xi) vitamin A supplementation for poor converters of beta-carotene;

(xii) vitamin D supplementation for individuals who are not capable of efficient or sufficient hydroxylation;

(xiii) sulfate supplementation for individuals who not capable of efficient or sufficient sulfation;

(xiv) CoQ10 supplementation for statin-induced myopathy;

(xv) dietary biogenic amine restriction for poor metabolizers (phenylethylamine);

(xvi) increased long chain omega 3 fatty acids for poor delta 3 dehydrogenase and elongase activities;

(xvii) carnitine supplementation for poor acyl-carnitine biosynthesis;

(xviii) biotin supplementation for specific bone and heart related functions;

(xix) glycine supplementation for reduced detoxification capability;

(xx) arginine supplementation for reduced eNOS activity;

(xxi) N-acetylcysteine supplementation for poor glutathione biosynthesis;

(xxii) branched chain amino acid supplementation for individuals with sarcopenia;

(xxiii) magnesium supplementation for antihypertensive meds;

(xxiv) iron restriction for hemochromatosis;

(xxv) iron supplementation for iron "wasters";

(xxvi) selenium supplementation for reduced GSH peroxidase activities;

(xxvii) DHEA for steroidogenesis deficiencies;

(xxviii) graded aerobic exercise for those with exercise intolerance;

(xxix) ketogenic diets for epilepsy;

(xxx) higher protein diets for later stage insulin resistance;

(xxxi) low protein diets for chronic renal disease.

3.1. Dietary Soy (Isoflavones) and Cancer. Presently, one of the most controversial areas in nutrition research is whether dietary soy intake confers a beneficial or detrimental effect in individuals with a propensity towards estrogen-sensitive cancers due to the phytoestrogenic activity of soy isoflavones. Many of the positive epidemiological studies investigating soy (isoflavone) intake and breast cancer have focused on the Asian population, and, therefore, there has been some concern as to whether (a) American women respond similarly to soy and (b) whether the type of soy consumed in different countries is comparable. In a recent review article assessing soy intake in women with breast cancer, Magee and Rowland [23] suggest that the latest research indicates that dietary soy may have differential effects, depending on tumor type. Furthermore, there may be significant interactions between polymorphisms in genes associated with breast cancer, particularly MDM2 and CYP1B1, and dietary soy isoflavone intake. Another aspect of this evolving research is the role of soy isoflavones on epigenetic mechanisms, which is becoming elucidated. From their review of the literature, they conclude: "Recent research suggests that women who are at increased risk of breast cancer due to polymorphisms in genes associated with the disease may especially benefit from high soy isoflavone intake." Therefore, although the research remains inconclusive, it would seem that more data are required to better assess how a patient's genotype and SNPs could be determined with respect to whether or not they should eat soy products.

3.2. Food Intolerances. It has been observed that food intolerances and/or sensitivities are at an all-time high. There seems to be heightened vigilance in the general patient community about the intake of several foods and their corresponding constituents which may cause physiological symptoms within hours after consumption, including sulfites, lactose, cow's milk casein, phenylethylamine (PEA) in chocolate, histamine in fish, and gluten. More than twenty years ago, Hunter [24] proposed that food intolerances were indications that there was an underlying fermentation disorder within the gastrointestinal tract which resulted in the production of metabolites that could not properly be detoxified by liver enzymes in certain individuals with hepatic enzyme polymorphisms. Using a functional assessment to evaluate intestinal microflora, Valeur et al. [25] correlated food hypersensitivity and abdominal symptoms with higher proportions of n-butyric acid. In-depth studies are required to examine the interrelationship between food intolerances, the immune system, enzyme deficiency or inadequacy, and detoxification of colonic bacteria-generated metabolites.

Despite the etiology, the fact is that the existing overarching dietary recommendations are simply not practical and applicable for the growing segment of individuals with reactions to common foods. One instance is the worldwide increased prevalence of gluten spectrum disorders and celiac disease over the last 50 years and an increase in the rate of diagnosis of celiac disease in the last decade [26]. Individuals with these disorders, especially celiac disease, must abstain completely from gluten-containing foods to experience symptom relief, especially from grains where there is a predominance of gluten. However, several dietary recommendations advocate the consumption of relatively copious amounts of grains, especially the previous USDA Food Guide Pyramid (which has been subsequently replaced with MyPlate). Moreover, there are indications that gluten intolerance and celiac disease may be associated with neurological disorders such as multiple sclerosis [27–30], ataxia [26–38], dementia [39–41], seizure disorder [41], cognitive impairment [42], and neuropathy [43].

3.3. Omega-3 Fatty Acids and APOE. Another somewhat conflicting area of nutrition is that of omega-3 fatty acids, which are touted for their anti-inflammatory effects; however, their effects on plasma lipids have been inconsistent. The American Heart Association Nutrition Committee statement on omega-3 fatty acids [44] concluded from epidemiological and clinical trial research that intake of these essential dietary fats reduced the incidence of cardiovascular disease (CVD), with EPA + DHA supplementation ranging between 0.5 and 1.8 g/day (as fish or supplements) to reduce cardiac and all-cause mortality, specifically. These findings translate into the final recommendation of including at least two servings of fish per week (particularly fatty fish) in addition to the inclusion of vegetable oil and food sources of alpha-linolenic acid. High daily doses (up to four grams) of omega-3 fatty acids are indicated in hypertriglyceridemia.

In the context of these recommendations, consider the emerging literature on the APOE genotype modification of response to EPA and DHA effects on plasma lipid levels [45]. Liang et al. [45] determined APOE genotype status, plasma EPA and DHA levels, plasma lipids and lipoprotein subclass particles in 2340 participants, and reported significant gene-EPA/DHA interactions with HDL-C and lipoproteins. In a smaller, prospective clinical trial with 38 healthy, normolipidemic men who had been assessed for APOE genotype, Olano-Martin et al. [46] evaluated supplementation of EPA-rich oil (3.3 g EPA/day) and DHA-rich oil (3.7 g DHA/day). A significant interaction between DHA supplementation and E4 carriers was noted through the observed increase in total cholesterol, most likely due to the 10% rise in LDL-C. Consequently, it may be worthwhile for healthcare practitioners to determine APOE status before advocating high-dose supplementation, particularly of DHA, to E4 carriers.

3.4. Sodium Restriction and Hypertension. Salt restriction is a common dietary recommendation for individuals with hypertension despite the fact that there are well-known heterogenous responses to dietary salt intake. Varying degrees of salt sensitivity exist with modest reductions of intake in some individuals resulting in an immediate decrease in blood pressure while others are salt resistant. The question has been raised as to whether dietary sodium restriction is universally beneficial [47]. It has been suggested that there is a need to distinguish between individuals who would respond to sodium restriction versus those who do not, but there are no available symptomatic assessments or standardized genotypic analyses to provide the clinician with data they need to tailor the dietary recommendation to reduce sodium to their patients. Specific gene variants associated with salt sensitivity have been identified; however, translation to the clinical setting is lacking. Common genetic variants of the kallikrein-kinin system have been explored with relationship to salt sensitivity [48]. It was determined that genetic variants of the bradykinin receptor B2 gene (BDKRB2) and the endothelin converting enzyme 1 gene (ECE1) were significantly associated with salt sensitivity in 1,906 Han Chinese subjects [48]. In addition to the genetic variants, Rebholz et al. [49] has indicated that salt sensitivity of blood pressure may be influenced by environmental factors such as degree of physical activity, yet another factor to consider in a personalized approach to blood pressure reduction.

3.5. Dietary Cholesterol and Hypercholesterolemia. Limitations on dietary cholesterol have been proposed by the American Heart Association of no more than 300 milligrams daily for healthy Americans due to the perception that its intake is associated with increased risk for coronary heart disease (CHD) [50]. On the contrary, other countries, such as Canada, Australia, New Zealand, Korea, and India, have not established upper limits for dietary cholesterol intake. Fernandez [50] and Kratz [51] have questioned whether such a dietary restriction should be imposed as a general guideline considering that current epidemiological evidence does not support the correlation between dietary cholesterol and increased CHD risk. About one-quarter of the population is sensitive to dietary cholesterol and responds with increased plasma LDL; however, this elevation is accompanied by a compensatory rise in HDL-cholesterol, resulting in no significant change in the LDL/HDL cholesterol ratio, a marker of CHD risk. Moreover, as Fernandez [50] states, dietary cholesterol may be instrumental in reducing another CHD risk factor, levels of small, dense LDL particles. Further, a recent meta-analysis of prospective cohort studies by Rong et al. [52] investigating the dose-response relationship between egg consumption and risk of CHD and stroke reported no evidence of an association between higher consumption of eggs (up to one egg daily) and CHD or stroke. However, there was a subgroup of diabetic patients that responded with increased risk due to higher egg consumption.

4. Personalized Lifestyle Recommendations: Application to Physical Activity

With respect to lifestyle recommendations, there is increasing evidence and advocacy from science, industry, and government leaders that the national guidelines of increasing overall physical activity, preferably to a minimum of 150 minutes of moderate activity per week, may require some degree of personalization [53]. There are multiple questions that arise from this general activity recommendation, including the following.

(a) Are all forms of activity equal for every person?

(b) Could maximum benefit be achieved through moderate versus high-level exertion?

(c) Are there differences between individual and group responses to activity?

(d) What is the optimal duration and intensity for various genotypes and phenotypes?

(e) Should there be multimodal interventions or the implementation of a single activity only?

Some publications have begun to appear on exercise genomics and its potential application [54]. The identification of specific genetic variants in the functionality of skeletal muscle metabolism and strength may be useful for promotion of better exercise tolerance in clinical conditions such as McArdle disease. In a recent study by Williams and Thompson [55], type and intensity of exercise were examined in two large cohorts of runners ($n = 33\,060$) and walkers ($n = 15\,945$) with relationship to coronary heart disease (CHD) risk factors. They concluded that moderate walking and vigorous running led to similar risk reductions for major chronic diseases. Moreover, a review of recent findings in exercise genomics includes Rankinen et al. [56] who identified that nine specific SNPs largely accounted for the heritability of submaximal heart rate training response. Ahmetov et al. [57] have suggested that the endurance athlete may exhibit a cluster of genetic factors within metabolic pathways related to proportion of slow-twitch muscle fibers and maximal oxygen consumption that may translate into an "elite phenotype".

Additionally, it may be worthwhile to examine how combinations of lifestyle medicine factors, such as gene variants, exercise, and disease state, may interact to provide more information to the patient. Hagberg et al. [58] documented the gene-exercise interactions with relation to improved insulin sensitivity, the MTHFR gene correlation with carotid stiffness in unfit individuals, and associations between the C-reactive protein gene with training-induced alterations in left ventricular mass. Hence, an individual's genetics may play a significant role in their response to exercise as has been discussed in the recent publications on exercise genomics [58]. Also, there may be individualized responses not only to physical activity due to one's genotype, but also compounded interactions between serum lipids, exercise, and SNPs.

5. Personalized Lifestyle Recommendations: Application to Stress and Behavior

Although stressors have been estimated to be a major contributor to chronic disease development and propagation, there is less emphasis on stress modulation within public health recommendations compared with those of diet and exercise. The ability of a patient to modify their behavior and reaction to stressors is a crucial aspect to consider in the context of personalized lifestyle medicine. It is conceivably difficult to successfully implement lifestyle changes in diet or activity unless there is an underlying adjustment in behavior and locus of control as it relates to stressors. Therefore, taking the essential behavioral aspects of lifestyle medicine into account is much needed to fortify the physical changes that are required for health. An example of a successful comprehensive lifestyle medicine intervention utilizing stress management and group support meetings is reflected in the several decades of clinical research employing this multifaceted regimen into different patient groups by Dean Ornish [59].

Similar to nutrition and exercise, there is a role for personalization in one's approach to stress, which can be encompassed in the diversity of modalities that an individual can choose from to modify their behavior to help them cope with stress, including mind-body medicine practices which are known to balance the parasympathetic and sympathetic nervous systems such as the Relaxation Response developed by Herbert Benson, Mindfulness-Based Stress Reduction (MBSR) from Jon Kabat-Zinn, meditation, yoga, and diaphragmatic breathing. While the basic physiological mechanisms of these practices have been postulated for years, the underlying biological and genetic pathways mediating these effects have not been well researched. Studies in the area of mind-body medicine are gradually becoming more molecular focused.

For instance, Dusek et al. [60] compared gene expression patterns between subjects with long-term relaxation response training and those who were novices. Between the two groups, there was a statistically significant difference in expression of 2,209 genes related to cellular metabolism, oxidative phosphorylation, generation of reactive oxygen species, and response to oxidative stress. Furthermore, Black et al. [61] found that a yogic meditation for 12 minutes daily for 8 weeks prescribed to 39 caregivers resulted in significant changes in genome-wide transcriptional profiles; 68 genes were differentially expressed after adjusting for confounding variables with upregulated genes including immunoglobulin-related transcripts and downregulated transcripts for proinflammatory cytokines.

Certain individuals may be epigenetically and genetically more inclined to respond to stress. Animal studies have indicated that there are epigenetic alterations in specific brain regions in response to licking and grooming behaviors of pups by rat mothers. Specifically, Zhang et al. [62] reported that decreased frequency of pup licking and grooming resulted in increased methylation of the exon 17 glucocorticoid receptor promoter in the hippocampus, leading to increased hypothalamic-pituitary-adrenal (HPA) responses to stress. Similarly, in humans, children subjected to abuse have decreased hippocampal expression of the glucocorticoid receptor and heightened stress responses. Therefore, parental influences during offspring development are instrumental in forming an imprint for the future adult in regulation of the stress response. The early stressed offspring must learn to adapt to environmental challenges and maintain stability through change, a measurable characteristic referred to by Karatoreos and McEwen [63] as "resilience." Glucocorticoids can continue to modify the structure and function of neural circuits throughout an individual's lifetime, a process referred to as allostasis, or the process in which the individual regains stability. It has been suggested that through the influence of allostatic modulators, the brain can become more plastic and potentially mitigate the negative influence of a childhood experience [63].

In addition to epigenetic effects and continual allostatic adjustments, a number of genetic variants have been reported to cause altered responses to stress and mood disorders including genes of the serotonin transporter and endocannabinoid CB1 receptors [64]. For instance, polymorphisms in the catechol-O-methyltransferase enzyme have been implicated in human mental illness with the presence of certain SNPs resulting in increased susceptibility to posttraumatic stress disorder (PTSD) [65]. Additionally, Petersen et al. [66] found that there is a predictive interaction between serotonin transporter gene polymorphisms and anxious/depressed symptoms in adolescents, with a stronger relationship noted in late compared with early adolescence. The presence of polymorphisms and the resulting behavior can modify symptoms, such as in dermatological disorders like atopic dermatitis, which can be aggravated by anxiety [67]. One variant of the serotonin transporter gene has been shown to be associated with high-anxiety traits and correspondingly increased atopic dermatitis [67].

Table 1: Differentiation among medical systems.

Preventative medicine	Lifestyle medicine	Personalized medicine	Functional medicine	Personalized lifestyle medicine
(i) Public health recommendations from opinion leader organizations (ii) Generalized guidelines (iii) Focused on prevention rather than treatment	(i) Could be preventive or therapeutic guidelines (ii) Encompasses a broad set of therapies related to one's living and behavioral patterns (iii) Practiced by wide range of medical professionals	(i) Focused on therapeutic strategies involving individualized pharmaceutical prescriptions for improved safety and efficacy (ii) Genomics as foundational tool (iii) Investigational and research driven (iv) Practiced by physicians (v) Patient-centered treatment	(i) Operational system developed to assess a patient's etiology and to devise a treatment protocol to address underlying causes (ii) Composed of multiple heuristics to lead the process of the therapeutic encounter (iii) Involves training and certification (iv) Focus on disease origin	(i) Next generation of medicine (ii) Tailored lifestyle medicine prescriptions directed to the individual based on diagnostics, including genomics and epigenetic information (iii) Uses functional medicine as the underlying operating system but requires the integration of other medical systems (iv) Patient-centered outcomes

6. Personalized Lifestyle Recommendations: Application to Environment and Toxin Load

Another important aspect to consider in personalized lifestyle medicine recommendations is to consider the influence of human exposure to environmental toxins on health, especially since 90% of the risks of chronic disease are due to nongenetic factors [68]. It would seem that the environment of the individual would have much influence on one's ability to develop health or disease [68–70]. Thus, the concept of the "exposome" as defined by Rappaport [68] to be the totality of exposures accrued by an individual over their life span could be relevant in compiling a personalized approach to one's health. There are at least two sources of toxicants to quantify: the influx of exogenous sources of toxic chemicals from air, food, water, drugs, and radiation; and internally generated metabolites from processes such as inflammation, lipid peroxidation, oxidative stress, disease states, infections, and microflora.

Increased exposure to external pollutants is strongly associated with the incidence of chronic disease. Several studies have documented the correlation between air pollution and increased cardiovascular morbidity and mortality [71]. Gong et al. [71] used gene-expression profiling to show the interrelationship between diesel exhaust particles and oxidized phospholipids in upregulating pathways implicated in atherosclerosis. Furthermore, compelling evidence is emerging for the role of persistent organic pollutants (POPs), such as polychlorinated biphenyls, dioxins, and pesticides, in chronic diseases such as type 2 diabetes [72–75] by impacting beta-cell function [72], insulin signaling and secretion [73], and mitochondrial function [74], as well as in the development of obesity by influencing adipocyte differentiation and neural circuits that control eating behavior (these toxicants have also thus been termed "obesogens") [76]. Porta et al. [77] analyzed serum concentrations of 19 POPs in 919 people in Spain and found that more than half of the population studied had concentrations in the top quartile of ≥1 POPs.

Moreover, an individual's ability to metabolize environmental intoxicants, independent of origin, via the liver through the cytochrome P450 family of enzymes, in addition to the accessibility of secondary detoxification pathways including conjugation with glucuronic acid, sulfate, glutathione, amino acids such as taurine and glycine, acetic acid, and methyl groups, must be evaluated through indirect or direct genotypic means for a better understanding of the robustness of their excretion of these toxicants. Drug response variability due to SNPs in the hepatic cytochrome P450 oxidase family of enzymes has been well defined for several decades, although new SNPs continue to be identified [78]. Furthermore, the conjugation pathways mentioned earlier may have genetic variants resulting in altered activity. Sirivarasai et al. [79] demonstrated that increased serum lead levels confers higher C-reactive protein and systolic blood pressure levels; however, there are varying degrees of these biological responses based on the different polymorphisms in GST.

7. Transition into a Global System of Personalized Lifestyle Medicine

Several systems and medical delineations have been conceptualized in the past decades (Table 1). Personalized lifestyle medicine presents a system of medicine which merges technological advances with the traditional foundation of lifestyle through the psychosocial-behavioral interface (Figure 3). It would seem that with the advent of personalized medicine and the emergence of diagnostics to assess one's genotype and moment-by-moment biomarkers that dietary and lifestyle recommendations will inevitably become individualized to the patient. There have been differing views expressed on whether or not offering personalized nutritional advice based on an individual's genes and SNPs is welcomed by the public at large [80]. As Görman et al. [80] suggest, the evidence for sufficient guidance based on genes and even epigenetics is rather limited and gaps in knowledge need to be overcome; however, the merit in this approach, when scientific data are available, is that it may result in improved compliance and support the individuality and inherent choices to be made by the patient. Nielsen and El-Sohemy [81] used surveys

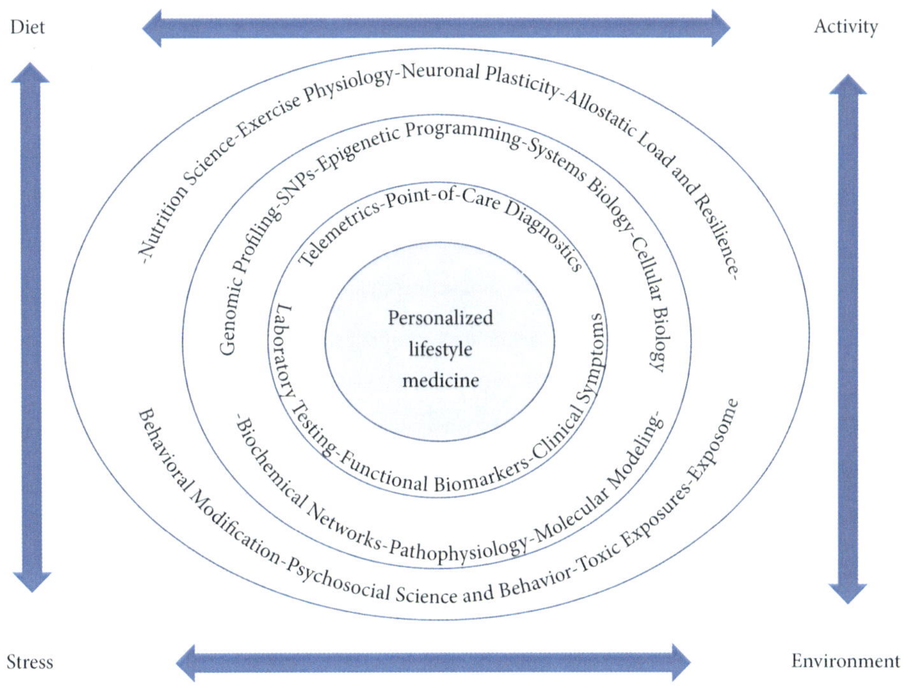

FIGURE 3: What is personalized lifestyle medicine?

to assess awareness of genotype testing and genotype-based personalized dietary advice or general dietary advice in 149 individuals between the ages of 20 and 35 years. They concluded that a majority of these individuals found dietary recommendations based on genetics to be more useful than general dietary advice.

The delivery of personalized advice requires accurate measurements on one's physiology through genomic analysis and molecular diagnostics. Tailored biomarkers, molecular imaging, rapid assessments through point-of-care devices, telemedicine, and individualized therapeutic treatments are gradually replacing the standardized, "one size fits all" form of medicine, ultimately providing the best form of care, reducing costs, and enhancing safety by limiting side effects. To date, there have been a number of functional biomarkers introduced into the clinical setting which illustrate the progression of personalized medicine, including the following.

(1) The addition of high-sensitivity C-reactive protein as part of a laboratory panel to assess inflammation, particularly as part of the diagnosis of cardiovascular disease and even periodontal disease, is the first. Several polymorphisms have been identified that correlate with increased levels of the inflammatory cytokine, interleukin-6 [82].

(2) The utilization of the liver enzyme marker, gamma-glutamyl transferase (GGT), as not just a marker of alcoholism, but an indicator of xenobiotic exposure and increased usage of hepatic glutathione, even at high normal levels, which can be of concern for individuals with polymorphisms in GST, is the second.

(3) Investigation of homocysteine levels as a potential risk factor for CVD in addition to its elevation as a possible indicator of methylation inefficiency due to genetic variants in MTHFR is the last.

As increasing recognition for the use of biomarkers as indirect or direct indicators of not just symptoms, but the underlying causes related to an individual's genotypic profile, there will be greater emphasis on a personalized approach to health. Additionally, with the advent of technologies to assist in these types of laboratory measures in becoming mainstream, lifestyle medicine areas, including diet, physical activity, stress responses, and environmental factors, will begin to merge with the outcomes of these tests, resulting in clinicallyapplied personalized lifestyle medicine approaches to most favorably address a patient's condition. In so doing, the patient will be able to regain control of their health and feel empowered in their decisions concerning their outcomes.

For several years before disease onset, a patient may have subclinical manifestations of a disease, indicated by low and/or high normal laboratory values, and the presence of ill-defined symptoms which do not classically qualify for a determined diagnosis. Personalized lifestyle medicine can be integral throughout a patient's life, from prevention to preclinical symptoms to disease manifestation and progression.

Personalized lifestyle medicine encompasses a broad array of disciplines in order to effectively prevent and treat disease, including the interface of technological advances with modern medicine discoveries for eventual dissemination into clinical medicine approaches.

References

[1] G. J. Egger, A. F. Binns, and S. R. Rossner, "The emergence of "lifestyle medicine" as a structured approach for management of chronic disease," *Medical Journal of Australia*, vol. 190, no. 3, pp. 143–145, 2009.

[2] W. S. Dysinger, "Lifestyle medicine competencies for primary care physicians," *Virtual Mentor*, vol. 15, no. 4, pp. 306–310, 2013.

[3] L. Lianov and M. Johnson, "Physician competencies for prescribing lifestyle medicine," *Journal of the American Medical Association*, vol. 304, no. 2, pp. 202–203, 2010.

[4] G. Egger, A. Binns, and S. Rossner, *Lifestyle Medicine*, McGraw-Hill, Sydney, Australia, 2008.

[5] W. H. Herman, T. J. Hoerger, M. Brandle et al., "The cost-effectiveness of lifestyle modification or metformin in preventing type 2 diabetes in adults with impaired glucose tolerance," *Annals of Internal Medicine*, vol. 142, no. 5, pp. 323–332, 2005.

[6] U.S. Department of Agriculture and U.S. Department of Health and Human Services, *Dietary Guidelines For Americans*, U.S. Government Printing Office, Washington, DC, USA, 7th edition, 2010.

[7] American Heart Association Nutrition Committee, A. H. Lichtenstein, L. J. Appel et al., "Diet and lifestyle recommendations revision 2006: a scientific statement from the American heart association nutrition committee," *Circulation*, vol. 114, no. 1, pp. 82–96, 2006.

[8] L. H. Kushi, C. Doyle, M. McCullough et al., "American cancer society guidelines on nutrition and physical activity for cancer prevention: reducing the risk of cancer with healthy food choices and physical activity," *CA Cancer Journal for Clinicians*, vol. 62, no. 1, pp. 30–67, 2012.

[9] American Diabetes Association, J. P. Bantle, J. Wylie-Rosett et al., "Nutrition recommendations and interventions for diabetes: a position statement of the American Diabetes Association," *Diabetes Care*, vol. 31, supplement 1, pp. S61–S78, 2008.

[10] G. Xie, X. Li, H. Li, and W. Jia, "Toward personalized nutrition: comprehensive phytoprofiling and metabotyping," *Journal of Proteomic Research*, vol. 12, no. 4, pp. 1547–1559, 2013.

[11] D. R. Jacobs and L. C. Tapsell, "Food synergy: the key to a healthy diet," *Proceedings of the Nutrition Society*, vol. 72, no. 2, pp. 200–206, 2013.

[12] D. M. Minich and J. S. Bland, "Dietary management of the metabolic syndrome beyond macronutrients," *Nutrition Reviews*, vol. 66, no. 8, pp. 429–444, 2008.

[13] P. C. Santos, J. E. Krieger, and A. C. Pereira, "Molecular diagnostic and pathogenesis of hereditary hemochromatosis," *International Journal of Molecular Sciences*, vol. 13, no. 2, pp. 1497–1511, 2012.

[14] E. Mocchegiani, R. Giacconi, L. Costarelli et al., "Zinc deficiency and IL-6 -174G/C polymorphism in old people from different European countries: effect of zinc supplementation. ZINCAGE study," *Experimental Gerontology*, vol. 43, no. 5, pp. 433–444, 2008.

[15] T. R. Neyestani, A. Djazayery, S. Shab-Bidar et al., "Vitamin D receptor Fok-I polymorphism modulates diabetic host response to vitamin D intake: need for a nutrigenetic approach," *Diabetes Care*, vol. 36, no. 3, pp. 550–556, 2013.

[16] A. Fischer, C. Schmelzer, G. Rimbach, P. Niklowitz, T. Menke, and F. Döring, "Association between genetic variants in the Coenzyme Q10metabolism and Coenzyme Q10status in humans," *BMC Research Notes*, vol. 4, article 245, 2011.

[17] R. Horvath, B. Czermin, S. Gulati et al., "Adult-onset cerebellar ataxia due to mutations in CABC1/ADCK3," *Journal of Neurology, Neurosurgery and Psychiatry*, vol. 83, no. 2, pp. 174–178, 2012.

[18] M. H. Lizer, R. L. Bogdan, and R. S. Kidd, "Comparison of the frequency of the methylenetetrahydrofolate reductase (MTHFR) C677T polymorphism in depressed versus nondepressed patients," *Journal of Psychiatric Practice*, vol. 17, no. 6, pp. 404–409, 2011.

[19] M. D. Swartz, C. B. Peterson, P. J. Lupo et al., "Investigating multiple candidate genes and nutrients in the folate metabolism pathway to detect genetic and nutritional risk factors for lung cancer," *Plos One*, vol. 8, no. 1, article e53475, 2013.

[20] G. Block, N. Shaikh, C. D. Jensen, V. Volberg, and N. Holland, "Serum vitamin C and other biomarkers differ by genotype of phase 2 enzyme genes GSTM1 and GSTT," *The American Journal of Clinical Nutrition*, vol. 94, no. 3, pp. 929–937, 2011.

[21] K. Maehashi and L. Huang, "Bitter peptides and bitter taste receptors," *Cellular and Molecular Life Sciences*, vol. 66, no. 10, pp. 1661–1671, 2009.

[22] E. Feeney, S. O'Brien, A. Scannell, A. Markey, and E. R. Gibney, "Genetic variation in taste perception: does it have a role in healthy eating?" *Proceedings of the Nutrition Society*, vol. 70, no. 1, pp. 135–143, 2011.

[23] P. J. Magee and I. Rowland, "Soy products in the management of breast cancer," *Current Opinion in Clinical Nutrition & Metabolic Care*, vol. 15, no. 6, pp. 586–591, 2012.

[24] J. O. Hunter, "Food allergy—or enterometabolic disorder?" *The Lancet*, vol. 338, no. 8765, pp. 495–496, 1991.

[25] J. Valeur, M. H. Morken, E. Norin, T. Midtvedt, and A. Berstad, "Intestinal fermentation in patients with self-reported food hypersensitivity: painful, but protective?" *Clinical and Experimental Gastroenterology*, vol. 3, no. 1, pp. 65–70, 2010.

[26] A. Rubio-Tapia, I. D. Hill, C. P. Kelly, A. H. Calderwood, and J. A. Murray, "ACG clinical guidelines: diagnosis and management of celiac disease," *The American Journal of Gastroenterology*, vol. 108, pp. 656–676, 2013.

[27] H. Z. Batur-Caglayan, C. Irkec, I. Yildirim-Capraz, N. Atalay-Akyurek, and S. Dumlu, "A case of multiple sclerosis and celiac disease," *Case Reports in Neurological Medicine*, vol. 2013, Article ID 576921, 3 pages, 2013.

[28] A. B. Haghighi, N. Ansari, M. Mokhtari, B. Geramizadeh, and K. B. Lankarani, "Multiple sclerosis and gluten sensitivity," *Clinical Neurology and Neurosurgery*, vol. 109, no. 8, pp. 651–653, 2007.

[29] C. D. P. Tengah, R. J. Lock, D. J. Unsworth, and A. J. Wills, "Multiple sclerosis and occult gluten sensitivity," *Neurology*, vol. 62, no. 12, pp. 2326–2327, 2004.

[30] L. Rodrigo, C. Hernández-Lahoz, D. Fuentes, N. Alvarez, A. López-Vázquez, and S. González, "Prevalence of celiac disease in multiple sclerosis," *BMC Neurology*, vol. 11, article 31, 2011.

[31] M. Hadjivassiliou, R. A. Grünewald, A. K. Chattopadhyay et al., "Clinical, radiological, neurophysiological, and neuropathological characteristics of gluten ataxia," *The Lancet*, vol. 352, no. 9140, pp. 1582–1585, 1998.

[32] M. T. Pellecchia, R. Scala, A. Perretti et al., "Cerebellar ataxia associated with subclinical celiac disease responding to gluten-free diet," *Neurology*, vol. 53, no. 7, pp. 1606–1608, 1999.

[33] K. Bürk, S. Bösch, C. A. Müller et al., "Sporadic cerebellar ataxia associated with gluten sensitivity," *Brain*, vol. 124, part 5, pp. 1013–1019, 2001.

[34] A. J. Wills and D. J. Unsworth, "The neurology of gluten sensitivity: separating the wheat from the chaff," *Current Opinion in Neurology*, vol. 15, no. 5, pp. 519–523, 2002.

[35] M. Hadjivassiliou, G. A. B. Davies-Jones, D. S. Sanders, and R. A. Grünewald, "Dietary treatment of gluten ataxia," *Journal of Neurology, Neurosurgery and Psychiatry*, vol. 74, no. 9, pp. 1221–1224, 2003.

[36] M. Hadjivassiliou, D. S. Sanders, N. Woodroofe, C. Williamson, and R. A. Grünewald, "Gluten ataxia," *The Cerebellum*, vol. 7, no. 3, pp. 494–498, 2008.

[37] C.-S. Liu, B.-W. Soong, Y.-C. Lee et al., "Gluten sensitivity: associated sporadic cerebellar ataxia in Taiwan," *Acta Neurologica Taiwanica*, vol. 19, no. 4, pp. 263–269, 2010.

[38] M. Hadjivassiliou, P. Aeschlimann, D. S. Sanders et al., "Transglutaminase 6 antibodies in the diagnosis of gluten ataxia," *Neurology*, vol. 80, no. 19, pp. 1740–1745, 2013.

[39] P. Collin, T. Pirttilä, T. Nurmikko, H. Somer, T. Erilä, and O. Keyriläinen, "Celiac disease, brain atrophy, and dementia," *Neurology*, vol. 41, no. 3, pp. 372–375, 1991.

[40] A. J. Wills, "The neurology and neuropathology of coeliac disease," *Neuropathology and Applied Neurobiology*, vol. 26, no. 6, pp. 493–496, 2000.

[41] H. J. Freeman, "Neurological disorders in adult celiac disease," *The Canadian Journal of Gastroenterology*, vol. 22, no. 11, pp. 909–911, 2008.

[42] W. T. Hu, J. A. Murray, M. C. Greenaway, J. E. Parisi, and K. A. Josephs, "Cognitive impairment and celiac disease," *Archives of Neurology*, vol. 63, no. 10, pp. 1440–1446, 2006.

[43] M. Hadjivassiliou, A. Gibson, G. A. B. Davies-Jones, A. J. Lobo, T. J. Stephenson, and A. Milford-Ward, "Does cryptic gluten sensitivity play a part in neurological illness?" *The Lancet*, vol. 347, no. 8998, pp. 369–371, 1996.

[44] P. M. Kris-Etherton, W. S. Harris, and L. J. Appel, "Fish consumption, fish oil, omega-3 fatty acids, and cardiovascular disease," *Circulation*, vol. 106, no. 21, pp. 2747–2757, 2002.

[45] S. Liang, L. M. Steffen, B. T. Steffen et al., "APOE genotype modifies the association between plasma omega-3 fatty acids and plasma lipids in the Multi-Ethnic Study of Atherosclerosis (MESA)," *Atherosclerosis*, vol. 9150, no. 13, pp. 00114–00017, 2013.

[46] E. Olano-Martin, E. Anil, M. J. Caslake et al., "Contribution of apolipoprotein E genotype and docosahexaenoic acid to the LDL-cholesterol response to fish oil," *Atherosclerosis*, vol. 209, no. 1, pp. 104–110, 2010.

[47] H. Sanada, J. E. Jones, and P. A. Jose, "Genetics of salt-sensitive hypertension," *Current Hypertension Reports*, vol. 13, no. 1, pp. 55–66, 2011.

[48] D. Gu, Q. Zhao, T. N. Kelly et al., "The role of the kallikrein-kinin system genes in the salt sensitivity of blood pressure: the GenSalt Study," *The American Journal of Epidemiology*, vol. 176, supplement 7, pp. S72–S80, 2012.

[49] C. M. Rebholz, D. Gu, J. Chen et al., "Physical activity reduces salt sensitivity of blood pressure: the Genetic Epidemiology Network of Salt Sensitivity Study," *The American Journal of Epidemiology*, vol. 176, supplement 7, pp. S106–S113, 2012.

[50] M. L. Fernandez, "Rethinking dietary cholesterol," *Current Opinion in Clinical Nutrition & Metabolic Care*, vol. 15, no. 2, pp. 117–121, 2012.

[51] M. Kratz, "Dietary cholesterol, atherosclerosis and coronary heart disease," *Handbook of Experimental Pharmacology*, no. 170, pp. 195–213, 2005.

[52] Y. Rong, L. Chen, T. Zhu et al., "Egg consumption and risk of coronary heart disease and stroke: dose-response meta-analysis of prospective cohort studies," *The British Medical Journal*, vol. 346, article e8539, 2013.

[53] T. W. Buford, M. D. Roberts, and T. S. Church, "Toward exercise as personalized medicine," *Sports Medicine*, vol. 43, no. 3, pp. 157–165, 2013.

[54] L. Pérusse, T. Rankinen, J. M. Hagberg et al., "Advances in exercise, fitness, and performance genomics in 2012," *Medicine and Science in Sports and Exercise*, vol. 45, no. 5, pp. 824–831, 2013.

[55] P. T. Williams and P. D. Thompson, "Walking versus running for hypertension, cholesterol, and diabetes mellitus risk reduction," *Arteriosclerosis, Thrombosis and Vascular Biology*, 2013.

[56] T. Rankinen, Y. J. Sung, M. A. Sarzynski, T. K. Rice, D. C. Rao, and C. Bouchard, "Heritability of submaximal exercise heart rate response to exercise training is accounted for by nine SNPs," *Journal of Applied Physiology*, vol. 112, no. 5, pp. 892–897, 2012.

[57] I. I. Ahmetov, A. G. Williams, D. V. Popov et al., "The combined impact of metabolic gene polymorphisms on elite endurance athlete status and related phenotypes," *Human Genetics*, vol. 126, no. 6, pp. 751–761, 2009.

[58] J. M. Hagberg, T. Rankinen, R. J. Loos et al., "Advances in exercise, fitness, and performance genomics in 2010," *Medicine and Science in Sports and Exercise*, vol. 43, no. 5, pp. 743–752, 2011.

[59] N. Chainani-Wu, G. Weidner, D. M. Purnell et al., "Changes in emerging cardiac biomarkers after an intensive lifestyle intervention," *The American Journal of Cardiology*, vol. 108, no. 4, pp. 498–507, 2011.

[60] J. A. Dusek, H. H. Otu, A. L. Wohlhueter et al., "Genomic counter-stress changes induced by the relaxation response," *Plos One*, vol. 3, no. 7, Article ID e2576, 2008.

[61] D. S. Black, S. W. Cole, M. R. Irwin et al., "Yogic meditation reverses NF-κB and IRF-related transcriptome dynamics in leukocytes of family dementia caregivers in a randomized controlled trial," *Psychoneuroendocrinology*, vol. 38, no. 3, pp. 348–355, 2013.

[62] T. Y. Zhang, B. Labonté, X. L. Wen, G. Turecki, and M. J. Meaney, "Epigenetic mechanisms for the early environmental regulation of hippocampal glucocorticoid receptor gene expression in rodents and humans," *Neuropsychopharmacology*, vol. 38, no. 1, pp. 111–123, 2013.

[63] I. N. Karatoreos and B. S. McEwen, "Annual research review: the neurobiology and physiology of resilience and adaptation across the life course," *Journal of Child Psychology and Psychiatry*, vol. 54, no. 4, pp. 337–347, 2013.

[64] G. Bagdy, G. Juhasz, and X. Gonda, "A new clinical evidence-based gene-environment interaction model of depression," *Neuropsychopharmacologia Hungarica*, vol. 14, no. 4, pp. 213–220, 2012.

[65] S. D. Norrholm, T. Jovanovic, A. K. Smith et al., "Differential genetic and epigenetic regulation of catechol-O-methyltransferase is associated with impaired fear inhibition in posttraumatic stress disorder," *Frontiers in Behavioral Neuroscience*, vol. 7, article 30, 2013.

[66] I. T. Petersen, J. E. Bates, J. A. Goodnight et al., "Interaction between serotonin transporter polymorphism (5-HTTLPR) and stressful life events in adolescents' trajectories of anxious/depressed symptoms," *Developmental Psychology*, vol. 48, no. 5, pp. 1463–1475, 2012.

[67] S. de Mel, K. Nordlind, M. Holst, M. Frohm-Nilsson, and S. B. Lonne-Rahm, "Polymorphisms in the serotonin transporter gene of patients with atopic dermatitis-association with personality traits related to high level of anxiety," *Immunopharmacology and Immunotoxicology*, vol. 34, no. 3, pp. 534–538, 2012.

[68] S. M. Rappaport, "Implications of the exposome for exposure science," *Journal of Exposure Science and Environmental Epidemiology*, vol. 21, no. 1, pp. 5–9, 2011.

[69] C. P. Wild, "Complementing the genome with an "exposome": the outstanding challenge of environmental exposure measurement in molecular epidemiology," *Cancer Epidemiology Biomarkers and Prevention*, vol. 14, no. 8, pp. 1847–1850, 2005.

[70] J. D. Pleil, "Categorizing biomarkers of the human exposome and developing metrics for assessing environmental sustainability," *Journal of Toxicology and Environmental Health B*, vol. 15, no. 4, pp. 264–280, 2012.

[71] K. W. Gong, W. Zhao, N. Li et al., "Air-pollutant chemicals and oxidized lipids exhibit genome-wide synergistic effects on endothelial cells," *Genome Biology*, vol. 8, no. 7, article R149, 2007.

[72] T. L. M. Hectors, C. Vanparys, K. van der Ven et al., "Environmental pollutants and type 2 diabetes: a review of mechanisms that can disrupt beta cell function," *Diabetologia*, vol. 54, no. 6, pp. 1273–1290, 2011.

[73] C. J. Everett, I. Frithsen, and M. Player, "Relationship of polychlorinated biphenyls with type 2 diabetes and hypertension," *Journal of Environmental Monitoring*, vol. 13, no. 2, pp. 241–251, 2011.

[74] S. Lim, Y. M. Cho, K. S. Park, and H. K. Lee, "Persistent organic pollutants, mitochondrial dysfunction, and metabolic syndrome," *Annals of the New York Academy of Sciences*, vol. 1201, pp. 166–176, 2010.

[75] H. Wu, K. A. Bertrand, A. L. Choi et al., "Persistent organic pollutants and type 2 diabetes: a prospective analysis in the nurses' health study and meta-analysis," *Environmental Health Perspectives*, vol. 121, no. 2, pp. 153–161, 2013.

[76] K. A. Thayer, J. J. Heindel, J. R. Bucher, and M. A. Gallo, "Role of environmental chemicals in diabetes and obesity: a National Toxicology Program workshop review," *Environmental Health Perspectives*, vol. 120, no. 6, pp. 779–789, 2012.

[77] M. Porta, J. Pumarega, and M. Gasull, "Number of persistent organic pollutants detected at high concentrations in a general population," *Environment International*, vol. 44, no. 1, pp. 106–111, 2012.

[78] J. McGraw and D. Waller, "Cytochrome P450 variations in different ethnic populations," *Expert Opinion on Drug Metabolism & Toxicology*, vol. 8, no. 3, pp. 371–382, 2012.

[79] J. Sirivarasai, W. Wananukul, S. Kaojarern et al., "Association between inflammatory marker, environmental lead exposure, and glutathione S-transferase gene," *BioMed Research International*, vol. 2013, Article ID 474963, 6 pages, 2013.

[80] U. Görman, J. C. Mathers, K. A. Grimaldi, J. Ahlgren, and K. Nordström, "Do we know enough? A scientific and ethical analysis of the basis for genetic-based personalized nutrition," *Genes and Nutrition*. In press.

[81] D. E. Nielsen and A. El-Sohemy, "A randomized trial of genetic information for personalized nutrition," *Genes and Nutrition*, vol. 7, no. 4, pp. 559–566, 2012.

[82] T. Shah, D. Zabaneh, T. Gaunt et al., "Gene-centric analysis identifies variants associated with interleukin-6 levels and shared pathways with other inflammation markers," *Circulation Cardiovascular Genetics*, vol. 6, no. 2, pp. 163–170, 2013.

2

Intervention Based Exclusively on Stage-Matched Printed Educational Materials Regarding Healthy Eating Does Not Result in Changes to Adolescents' Dietary Behavior

Natacha Toral[1] and Betzabeth Slater[2]

[1] *Nutrition Department, Health Sciences School, University of Brasília, Campus Universitário Darcy Ribeiro, Asa Norte, 70910-900 Brasília, DF, Brazil*
[2] *Nutrition Department, Public Health School, University of Sao Paulo, Avenida Dr. Arnaldo, 715, 2 No. andar, 01246-904 São Paulo, SP, Brazil*

Correspondence should be addressed to Natacha Toral, natachatoral@hotmail.com

Academic Editors: L. Kuller and I. Zakeri

Purpose. To assess the impact of a six-month stage-based intervention on fruit and vegetable intake, regarding perceived benefits and barriers, and self-efficacy among adolescents. *Design.* Randomized treatment-control, pre-post design. *Subjects/Setting.* Schools were randomized between control and experimental groups. 860 adolescents from ten public schools in Brasília, Federal District, Brazil were evaluated at baseline; 771 (81%) completed the study. *Intervention.* Experimental group received monthly magazines and newsletters aimed at promotion of healthy eating. *Measures.* Self-reported fruit and vegetable intake, stages of change, self-efficacy and decisional balance scores were evaluated at baseline and post-intervention in both groups. *Analysis.* The effectiveness of the intervention was evaluated using the analysis of covariance model (ANCOVA) and repeated measurement analysis by means of weighted least squares. Comparison between the proportions of adolescents who advanced through the stages during the intervention was performed using the Mantel-Haenszel chi-square test. *Results.* After adjusting for sex and age, study variables showed no modifications through the proposed intervention. There was no statistical difference in participant mobility in the intervention and control groups between the stages of change, throughout the study. *Conclusion.* A nutritional intervention based exclusively on distribution of stage-matched printed educational materials was insufficient to change adolescents' dietary behavior.

1. Introduction

The most common description of the dietary practices currently adopted during adolescence consists of fat, sugar, and sodium-rich diets, with little addition of fruits and vegetables [1, 2]. This picture correlates with increasingly early appearance of chronic diseases among adolescents, such as obesity and diabetes, which have a great public health impact [3]. According to the National Survey on Students' Health, conducted in Brazil in 2009, about one third of adolescents reported eating fruits and vegetables on at least five days of the week [4]. This intake level is much lower than the consumption of about 400 g of these foods a day that is recommended in order to prevent chronic diseases [3]. Therefore, there is an urgent need to implement strategies that can promote healthy dietary habits among adolescents.

In this regard, one possibility would be to adopt interventions based on behavioral theories, such as the transtheoretical model. This model makes it possible to determine *stages of change*, which represent *when* the behavioral change occurs and what the individual's degree of motivation toward accomplishing it is. In applying the theory to dietary behavior, individuals can be classified in one of five stages of change [5], namely: *precontemplation,* when they do not intend to change their dietary habits in the near future; *contemplation*, when they acknowledge that their dietary habits are inadequate, but still see difficulty in changing their habits; *preparation,* when they have decided to change their dietary habits within the next thirty days; *action*, when they have already changed some dietary habits over the last few months; *maintenance*, when they have kept to the changes for over six months.

In addition to the stages of change, the model encompasses three other constructs: the *decisional balance*, which deals with the balance that individuals make between the benefits and barriers relating to having a healthy diet; *self-efficacy*, which refers to individuals' self-confidence regarding their real ability to change their dietary behavior; the *processes of change*, which are individuals' experiences and feelings relating to advancing through the stages of change [5].

Since the basis for understanding the processes of change at different times was established, several studies among young people have shown positive results from nutritional interventions directed toward the stages of change. In addition to advancing through the stages with tailored interventions, individuals perceive more benefits and fewer barriers, present greater self-efficacy, and start to have a healthier diet, including greater fruit and vegetable intake [6–9].

2. Purpose

The objective of this study was to assess the impact of a stage-based intervention using printed educational materials, directed toward greater fruit and vegetable intake, along with the decisional balance relating to the benefits and barriers perceived and the self-efficacy, among adolescents in public schools in Brasília, Federal District, Brazil.

3. Methods

3.1. Design. This was a randomized trial in which a six-month nutritional intervention was developed during the 2009 school year. Two groups were assessed (intervention and control) in order to identify the effects of an intervention based on printed educational materials for promoting healthy dietary habits, which were distributed to the adolescents every month, both in classrooms and by mail. The materials were directed toward the participants' stages of change. This study was approved by the Research Ethics Committee of the School of Public Health, University of São Paulo.

3.2. Sample. The sampling process aimed toward obtaining a representative sample of adolescents in the 7th and 8th school years in Brasília. In order to calculate this, the 2006 School Census was used: at that time, there were 15 public schools in Brasília with 7th and 8th year students, with a total of 5,785 students enrolled [10]. In addition, the following statistical factors were used: a significance level of 5%, test power of 80%, correlation coefficient of 0.55 between observations at the two times and effect size of 0.10 between the null hypothesis of equal means in the two groups, and the alternative hypothesis of different means in the two groups. Thus, the minimum number of participants was estimated to be 706, with 353 in each group (control and intervention). Schools (not students) were randomized to avoid the possibility of exchanging experiences within the same social group. Four schools were randomly selected for the intervention group and six schools for the control group in order to achieve the minimum number calculated. All 7th and 8th year students in the ten schools were invited to participate in the study.

3.3. Measures. In addition to age (in years), the variables of sex, nutritional status, and family income (as multiples of the Brazilian minimum monthly salary) were evaluated. Nutritional status was assessed from weight and height measurements, which were taken in duplicate to investigate the body mass index according to age [11].

3.3.1. Self-Reported Fruit and Vegetables Consumption. Initially, each adolescent was introduced to the concept of servings of fruits and vegetables by means of an illustrated leaflet. This showed that one serving of vegetables was equivalent to a dessert plate (or cup) of raw vegetables or half a dessert plate (or half a cup) of cooked vegetables, excluding potatoes and other starchy vegetables. In the case of fruits, for instance, one serving was equivalent to a medium-sized banana or orange, a small-sized apple, a medium-sized slice of pineapple or watermelon, a small-sized slice of papaya, or a small bunch of grapes. Next, the participants were asked about their habitual intake of such foods, in servings. Their answers were recorded in categories ranging from less than one serving a day to five or more servings a day.

In order to assess the adequacy of the fruit and vegetable intake, the recommended daily intake of these foods (400 g) [3], corresponding to about five servings a day, was taken into consideration. Thus, only the last option of self-reported consumption (five or more servings a day) was considered to be a healthy practice.

3.3.2. Stages of Change. In order to classify the adolescents in the five stages of change regarding their fruit and vegetable consumption, an algorithm was used. This consisted of a questionnaire with a limited number of questions for which the answers are mutually exclusive, with a format that is similar to what has been described by several authors [8, 9, 12].

If the self-reported habitual fruit and vegetable consumption was inadequate, that is, less than five servings a day, the adolescents were asked about their intentions with regard to increasing their consumption of these foods in the near future. If they said that they had no intention of changing their dietary habits, they were classified as at the *precontemplation* stage. If they said that they did have some intention, they were classified as at the *contemplation* stage if they intended to increase their consumption of fruits and vegetables within the next six months or at the *preparation* stage if they showed an intention to increase their consumption within the next 30 days.

If the participants' habitual consumption of fruits and vegetables was adequate, that is, five or more servings a day, they were asked how long they had had this habit. If this was a recent habit, of less than six months, they were classified in the *action* stage; if they reported having this habit for six months or more, they were classified in the *maintenance* stage.

3.3.3. Decisional Balance. A seven-item scale relating to the barriers faced by individuals when trying to eat in a healthy manner was included, along with a seven-item scale relating to the benefits identified by these individuals when following an adequate diet. Each item consisted of a sentence in which the participants expressed their agreement or disagreement with its contents, by means of a five-point Likert scale, ranging from 1—"I do not agree at all" to 5—"I strongly agree." The items were selected from previous studies, which had shown relatively moderate-to-high internal consistency coefficients (Cronbach's α) [12–15], as well as a qualitative study on Brazilian adolescents who had spoken of their main difficulties in eating in a healthy manner [16].

3.3.4. Self-Efficacy. This variable was assessed using a set of eight items. The participants expressed their agreement or disagreement with the content of these items on five-point Likert scales, ranging from 1—"I'm sure I cannot do this" to 5—"I'm sure I can do it." The items were selected using the same criteria as presented regarding preparation of the scale for decisional balance [12, 14, 15].

3.3.5. Previous Nutritional Guidance. In the initial assessment, all participants in the intervention group were asked whether they had received any nutritional guidance over the past year from a nutritionist or other healthcare professional.

3.4. Intervention. All adolescents in both the control and the intervention group were evaluated according to the variables presented above. After the six-month intervention, all the participants were assessed again. At the end of the first and second interviews, the participants in both groups received a folder presenting the 10 steps toward healthy eating during adolescence, as described by the Brazilian Ministry of Health [17], along with a record of their anthropometric measurements and their nutritional status at that time.

Every month, the intervention group received colorful printed magazines that promoted healthy eating and information newsletters directed toward the participants' stages of change that had been identified at the beginning of the study, with the aim of promoting fruit and vegetable consumption. The magazines were handed out at the schools and the newsletters were mailed.

The topics presented in the six magazines developed for the study were the means for overcoming the difficulties in eating healthily; the importance of breakfast and the right distribution of meals during the day; the relationship between nutritional status and adolescents' physical activity; the role of nutrients in adolescents' diets, the concepts of the terms *diet* and *light* and the importance of nutrition labeling; diet-related health problems such as diabetes, obesity, and eating disorders.

The basis for developing the magazines was the discourse of participants in a qualitative study conducted among focus groups that preceded this study [16]. The participants' testimonies were analyzed with a view to characterizing the educational materials for promoting healthy eating, particularly regarding their visual presentation and content, so that the material would be well accepted and understood by the adolescents.

Since previous studies found that high percentages of the adolescents were classified in the stages of change prior to action, that is, precontemplation and contemplation [2, 18], the magazines focused on the early stages. In this sense, the main objectives of the magazines were to increase knowledge about healthy eating through playful means, such as comics and games; to present ways to overcome barriers that hinder adoption of an appropriate diet and emphasize the benefits from following it, taking into account young people's lifestyles; to present curiosities about foods and healthy and practical recipes, along with tips on different cultural aspects of food, in such a way as to raise awareness about and reflect on diet and to increase interest in the subject.

The basis for developing the newsletters was stage-based materials for promoting regular consumption of fruits and vegetables that have been used in several studies, with satisfactory results among young adults [8, 9, 19, 20]. The newsletters took into account the *processes of change* needed to determine the progress from one stage to another [5].

The newsletters for the adolescents at the precontemplation stage covered the processes of change relating to *raising awareness, dramatic relief,* and *reevaluation of the environment*, so as to raise their awareness about the inadequacy of their intake of certain foods and promote acceptance that a dietary change was needed [21].

The materials for the adolescents classified in the contemplation and preparation stages included activities relating to the processes of change consisting of *self-reevaluation* and *self-liberation,* with strategies to increase their confidence in their own ability to improve their dietary habits, resolve their ambivalence about the commitment to change, and facilitate development of a specific plan for modifying their dietary behavior [21].

In the newsletters targeted toward individuals at the action and maintenance stages, the strategies emphasized consisted of maintaining an adequate intake of fruits and vegetables and preventing relapse (process of change: *stimulus control*), along with offering reward and reinforcement for keeping to the appropriate behavior (process of change: *contingency management*).

3.5. Analysis. Comparison of the variables between the control and intervention groups at the baseline was performed using the chisquare test for categorical data and Student's t test for independent samples for continuous variables.

The effect of the intervention was assessed by analyzing the changes in the components of the transtheoretical model (stages of change, decisional balance, and self-efficacy) and the changes in fruit and vegetable intake. Analysis of covariance (ANCOVA) models with adjustments for sex, age, and baseline values were used for each continuous outcome, that is, decisional balance between benefits and barriers and self-efficacy. A model for repeated measurement analysis with weighted minimum squares was used for categorized outcomes, that is, stages of change and fruit and vegetable intake. The same analyses were also performed with selection of only the group of adolescents that had not received nutritional guidance prior to the intervention.

The proportions of the adolescents who progressed through each stage of change over the course of the intervention were also assessed by means of Mantel-Haenszel chisquare analyses.

A 5% significance level was used. The analyses were conducted using the Statistical Analysis Software (SAS version 9.2; SAS Institute Inc., Cary, NC, USA) and the Statistical Package for the Social Sciences (SPSS for Windows, version 13.0; SPSS Inc., Chicago, Ill, USA).

The adolescents who participated in the survey had handed over a free and informed consent statement signed by their parents or guardians. This study was approved by the Research Ethics Committee of the School of Public Health, University of São Paulo.

4. Results

This study included initial participation by 860 students: 373 in the control group and 487 in the intervention group. In total, 771 participants completed the study, representing 81% followup. The losses were due to transfers of students to other schools ($n = 54$) and absence of participants on the days when interviews were conducted ($n = 35$).

More than half of the participants were aged between 11 and 13 years, and 59.5% were female (Table 1). It was found that over a third of the adolescents came from low-income families (less than two Brazilian minimum monthly salaries, that is, around US$ 460.00). It was observed that 18.1% were overweight to some extent and that only 10.9% reported consuming an adequate amount of fruits and vegetables (minimum of 5 servings a day).

At the baseline, there were no significant differences between the control and intervention groups regarding the category variables, with the exception of gender distribution, given that there was a higher percentage of girls in the control group (Table 1). There were also no significant differences between the groups regarding the decisional balance scores for barriers ($P = 0.883$) and benefits ($P = 0.136$), or regarding the self-efficacy scores ($P = 0.196$). Among the participants in the intervention group, it was found that 84.0% ($n = 409$) had not received any nutritional guidance before the start of the intervention.

The model for repeated measurements analysis using weighted minimum squares for categorized outcomes showed that the proposed intervention did not produce any significant changes to fruit and vegetable intake ($P = 0.626$) or to the stages of change ($P = 0.905$) (Table 2). Similarly, following the covariance analysis model applied to continuous variables, it was observed that the intervention did not result in any significant effects on the different variables of the transtheoretical model (Table 3). After adjusting for sex and age, no differences were observed between the control and intervention groups concerning the decisional balance for benefits ($P = 0.288$) or barriers ($P = 0.415$), or regarding participants' self-efficacy ($P = 0.775$).

The same analyses for assessing the impact of the intervention that were conducted on the full sample were also conducted by selecting only the participants who had not received prior nutritional guidance. This analysis showed that the absence of significant effects was maintained.

Comparing the control and intervention groups, there were no differences between the proportions of adolescents who progressed from precontemplation ($P = 0.5613$), contemplation ($P = 0.2844$) and preparation ($P = 0.5779$) to other stages, or between the proportions of the adolescents who remained in the action and maintenance stages ($P = 0.4057$). Thus, there were no statistical differences between the changes in either group regarding participants' mobility among the stages of change resulting from the proposed intervention.

5. Discussion

In the present study, high prevalence of inadequate fruit and vegetable intake among school children was observed, as also shown in several national studies conducted among Brazilian adolescents from different regions. [18, 22, 23] Likewise, studies conducted in many countries with different socioeconomic and cultural contexts, such as Sweden [1], Costa Rica [24], Australia [25], and USA [26], have also shown that dietary habits at this stage of life are frequently imbalanced.

This, together with the high percentage of overweight adolescents found in the present study, highlights the urgent need for impactful nutritional interventions in order to promote healthy dietary practices and motivate young people to adopt the nutritional recommendations. It should be emphasized that adolescence is an important period for establishing the dietary behavior that will be maintained in adulthood, and it is a stage in which there is greater independence in relation to choosing food, compared with childhood [27]. Overall, assessments of adolescent health have shown alarming results. Several Brazilian studies conducted among schoolchildren have shown high prevalence of cardiovascular risk factors at this early stage of life, reinforcing the importance of actions to promote health within the school environment [28–30].

It should be noted that the low fruit and vegetable intake among the participants in the present study may have been associated not only with the individuals' ages, but also with their families' socioeconomic conditions. Family income and schooling level have been seen to be determinants of the low intake of these foods in Brazil [31, 32]. According to Claro et al. [33], reducing the price of fruits and vegetables, which could be made possible through public policies and increases

Table 1: Comparability between the intervention and control groups, regarding baseline characteristics.

Variables	Total		Control Group		Intervention Group		*P* value
	n	%	*n*	%	*n*	%	
Age							
11–13 yrs	489	56.9%	207	55.5%	282	57.9%	
14–16 yrs	365	42.4%	163	43.7%	202	41.5%	0.459
17–19 yrs	6	0.7%	3	0.8%	3	0.6%	
Gender							
Male	348	40.5%	135	36.2%	213	43.7%	0.030
Female	512	59.5%	238	63.8%	274	56.3%	
Family income							
<2 BMMS*	294	34.2%	120	32.2%	174	35.7%	
2–4.9 BMMS*	286	33.2%	118	31.6%	168	34.5%	0.130
≥5 BMMS*	200	23.3%	100	26.8%	100	20.5%	
Didn't know/no answer	80	9.3%	35	9.4%	45	9.3%	
Nutritional status							
Thinness	23	2.6%	8	2.2%	15	3.1%	
Adequate	682	79.3%	304	81.5%	378	77.6%	0.544
Overweight	126	14.7%	50	13.4%	76	15.6%	
Obesity	29	3.4%	11	2.9%	18	3.7%	
Fruit/vegetable intake							
Adequate	94	10.9%	43	11.5%	51	10.5%	0.660
Inadequate	766	89.1%	330	88.5%	436	89.5%	
Stages of change							
Precontemplation	376	43.7%	159	42.6%	217	44.6%	
Contemplation	117	13.6%	46	12.3%	71	14.6%	
Preparation	273	31.7%	125	33.5%	148	30.4%	0.377
Action	16	1.9%	8	2.1%	8	1.6%	
Maintenance	78	9.1%	35	9.4%	43	8.8%	
Total	**860**	**100%**	**373**	**100%**	**487**	**100%**	

* BMMS: Brazilian minimum monthly salary.

in family income, is one way to increase the participation of these foods in the Brazilian diet.

Unlike what was expected, the intervention proposed was ineffective in changing these adolescents' dietary behavior regarding their consumption of fruits and vegetables. Other studies with similar methodology have been conducted among young people, aimed at promoting the consumption of these foods, and have shown positive results after nutritional interventions targeted at stages of change. However, it should be noted that the major difference between the present study and other studies in the literature was that they included other nutritional intervention strategies in addition to distribution of educational materials to participants in order to promote fruit and vegetable consumption and change their dietary behavior [6, 8, 9].

According to Brinley et al. [6], an intervention with educational materials, lectures, and food tasting for six weeks resulted in advances through the stages of change for about 27% of the schoolchildren. In the study conducted by Richards et al. [8], the intervention among young students included sending personal newsletters directed toward the stages of change, along with motivational interviews and emails, over a four-month period. These authors found that the fruit and vegetable intake was significantly higher among the participants in the intervention group at the end of the study. Another nutritional intervention that lasted for six months included mailed printed materials targeted at the stages of change and two educational telephone calls to motivate change [9]. As a result, greater fruit and vegetable intake and more notable progression to the action and maintenance stages were observed in the intervention group.

As mentioned earlier, the printed materials used in studies by Richards et al. [8] and Nitzke et al. [9] were adopted as the basis for developing the materials of the present study. The original documents were accessed in full, prior to conducting the present study, with permission from the authors. The present study maintained a similar approach in the strategies used in the materials to promote consumption of fruits and vegetables, with adaptation of the language, content, and visual presentation for the Brazilian adolescent

Table 2: Comparability between the intervention and control groups regarding fruit and vegetable intake and stages of change after the proposed intervention (analysis of the repeated measurements model using weighted minimum squares).

Variables	Control Group		Intervention Group		*P* value
	n	%	*n*	%	
Fruit/vegetable intake					
Adequate	27	8.4%	42	9.4%	0.626
Inadequate	296	91.6%	406	90.6%	
Stages of change					
Precontemplation	134	41.5%	195	43.5%	
Contemplation	67	20.7%	89	19.9%	
Preparation	95	29.4%	122	27.2%	0.905
Action	5	1.6%	9	2.0%	
Maintenance	22	6.8%	33	7.4%	
Total	**323**	**100%**	**448**	**100%**	

Table 3: Comparability between the intervention and control groups regarding decisional balance for benefits ("pros" scores) and barriers ("cons" scores) and self-efficacy, adjusted for sex and age, after the proposed intervention (analysis of covariance, ANCOVA).

Variables	Control Group		Intervention Group		*P* value
	Mean	Standard Error	Mean	Standard Error	
Pros scores	28.73	0.17	28.97	0.14	0.2885
Cons scores	13.50	0.16	13.33	0.13	0.4153
Self-efficacy scores	31.62	0.20	31.69	0.17	0.7749

audience, given that the previous studies were directed towards young Americans aged 18 to 24 years.

It can, therefore, be said that additional motivation strategies should be included in parallel with intervention studies based on the distribution of printed materials tailored to the stages of change. Such strategies appear to be of fundamental importance for achieving a positive impact. On the other hand, recent criticism of the use of the transtheoretical model has suggested that interventions based on this theory are, in general, more intense and personalized than are the conditions presented to the control group. In other words, such interventions promote greater proximity and involvement between the researchers and the participants in the intervention group and contacts of greater frequency and of a more personal nature than in the control group. Consequently, the positive impact observed in intervention studies in this format could be a result from their intensity and not from the fact that they were based on the transtheoretical model [34].

Other important matters may explain the lack of impact from the proposed intervention in this study, such as the lack of family and teacher involvement in motivating behavioral changes. The family represents a fundamental social context in which behavior, actions, and habits of life are affected [35], including dietary practices. Families provide an important support network in the process of nutritional education for young people, especially in programs for prevention and treatment of obesity [36].

In addition, family participation in nutritional interventions is relevant given that often it is not the adolescent who makes decisions about the food available at home. The lack of autonomy in selecting foods that are consumed at home was shown in the study by Silva et al. [23], in which the mothers were responsible for the preparation of 44.7% of the food eaten by the students while the students were only responsible for 12.6% of the preparations.

Direct involvement by teachers in interventions is a debatable point, considering that Sichieri and Souza [37] showed that obesity prevention programs among children and adolescents are most effective when conducted by people devoted exclusively to this purpose than when conducted by teachers. This is because teachers are often involved in other school activities or are poorly motivated and do not receive specialized training and proper supervision for administering the intervention as proposed.

Likewise, the present study may not have had sufficient duration to promote changes in dietary behavior. The six-month duration was determined based on two points: the possibility of completing the study during the school year, from its submission to and approval by the school directors, until the final assessment of the students in both groups, and the fact that changing the stage from *action* to *maintenance* takes six months, which would make it possible to see any advance between the final stages.

Although the duration of previous interventions was less than or equal to six months, the literature has shown that studies of longer duration allow greater exposure of individuals to the information transmitted and favor behavioral changes [37]. However, it should be noted that long-term interventions imply higher costs and, when conducted in school environments, they compete with activities conducted in the classroom.

Another limitation of the present study relates to the assessment of food intake measurements through the categorized options. Small increases in the weekly consumption of fruits and vegetables that remained less than one serving (e.g., from two to four times a week) could not be identified through the evaluation adopted, since the first option corresponded to consumption of these foods "less than once a day." Other forms of assessment of fruit and vegetable intake with greater sensitivity to small changes need to be incorporated, especially among groups in which there are significant percentages of individuals with inadequate dietary practices.

6. Conclusion

This study showed that a nutritional intervention exclusively based on distribution of printed educational materials targeted at individuals' stages of change was not enough to change the dietary habits of adolescents. No significant changes to the participants' fruit and vegetable intake, benefits, and barriers or perceived self-efficacy were identified. This indicates the complexity of the issues involved in adolescents' dietary behavior and emphasizes the major difficulties that need to be overcome in promoting healthy dietary practices in this group.

Interventions aimed at adolescents should be adapted so that, in addition to incorporating stage-matched printed educational materials, they also include other strategies for motivating them to adopt a healthy diet. It is also important to involve the social network that surrounds adolescents, in order to provide support for behavioral changes, and consider the duration of the nutritional intervention and the assessment measurements that can identify small changes in dietary habits.

Acknowledgments

This research was supported by an award provided by the International Life Sciences Institute (ILSI), Brazil, a nongovernmental and nonprofit organization. The language translation was supported by a grant from the Deanship for Research and Post-graduation of the University of Brasília.

References

[1] G. Samuelson, "Dietary habits and nutritional status in adolescents over Europe. An Overview of current studies in the Nordic countries," *European Journal of Clinical Nutrition*, vol. 54, supplement 1, pp. S21–S28, 2000.

[2] N. Toral, B. Slater, I. D. P. Cintra, and M. Fisberg, "Adolescent eating behavior regarding fruit and vegetable intakes," *Revista de Nutricao*, vol. 19, no. 3, pp. 331–340, 2006.

[3] World Health Organization, "Diet, nutrition and the prevention of chronic diseases," Tech. Rep. Series 916, Geneva, Switzerland, 2003.

[4] Instituto Brasileiro de Geografia e Estatística, Pesquisa Nacional de Saúde do Escolar, 2010, http://www.ibge.gov.br/home/estatistica/populacao/pense/pense.pdf.

[5] J. O. Prochaska and W. F. Velicer, "The transtheoretical model of health behavior change," *American Journal of Health Promotion*, vol. 12, no. 1, pp. 38–48, 1997.

[6] C. Brinley, C. Barrar, and N. Cotugna, "Stages of change tools to increase fruit and vegetable consumption in high school students," *Journal of Nutrition Education and Behavior*, vol. 33, no. 1, pp. 57–58, 2001.

[7] M. Frenn, S. Malin, and N. K. Bansal, "Stage-based interventions for low-fat diet with middle school students," *Journal of Pediatric Nursing*, vol. 18, no. 1, pp. 36–45, 2003.

[8] A. Richards, K. K. Kattelmann, and C. Ren, "Motivating 18- to 24-year-olds to increase their fruit and vegetable consumption," *Journal of the American Dietetic Association*, vol. 106, no. 9, pp. 1405–1411, 2006.

[9] S. Nitzke, K. Kritsch, L. Boeckner et al., "A stage-tailored multi-modal intervention increases fruit and vegetable intakes of low-income young adults," *American Journal of Health Promotion*, vol. 22, no. 1, pp. 6–14, 2007.

[10] Brazil, Ministry of Education, National Institute of Eduational Studies and Researches Anísio Teixeira, *Results of the School Census 2006*, Ministry of Education, Brasília, Brazil, 2006.

[11] M. De Onis, A. W. Onyango, E. Borghi, A. Siyam, C. Nishida, and J. Siekmann, "Development of a WHO growth reference for school-aged children and adolescents," *Bulletin of the World Health Organization*, vol. 85, no. 9, pp. 660–667, 2007.

[12] J. Ma, N. M. Betts, T. Horacek, C. Georgiou, A. White, and S. Nitzke, "The importance of decisional balance and self-efficacy in relation to stages of change for fruit and vegetable intakes by young adults," *American Journal of Health Promotion*, vol. 16, no. 3, pp. 157–166, 2002.

[13] A. M. C. Ling and C. Horwath, "Perceived benefits and barriers of increased fruit and vegetable consumption: validation of a decisional balance scale," *Journal of Nutrition Education and Behavior*, vol. 33, no. 5, pp. 257–265, 2001.

[14] E. De Vet, J. De Nooijer, N. K. De Vries, and J. Brug, "Determinants of forward stage transition from precontemplation and contemplation for fruit consumption," *American Journal of Health Promotion*, vol. 19, no. 4, pp. 278–285, 2005.

[15] M. F. Zabinski, T. Daly, G. J. Norman et al., "Psychosocial correlates of fruit, vegetable, and dietary fat intake among adolescent boys and girls," *Journal of the American Dietetic Association*, vol. 106, no. 6, pp. 814–821, 2006.

[16] N. Toral, M. A. Conti, and B. Slater, "Healthy eating according to teenagers: perceptions, barriers, and expected characteristics of teaching materials," *Cadernos de Saude Publica*, vol. 25, no. 11, pp. 2386–2394, 2009.

[17] Brazil, Ministry of Health, General Food and Nutrition Policy Coordination, "Healthy Eating to Adolescents: Follow the 10 Steps," Ministry of Health, Brasília, Brazil, 2010, http://189.28.128.100/nutricao/docs/geral/10passosAdolescentes.pdf.

[18] N. Toral and B. Slater, "Perception of eating practices and stages of change among Brazilian adolescents," *Preventive Medicine*, vol. 48, no. 3, pp. 279–283, 2009.

[19] J. S. Ruud, N. Betts, K. Kritch, S. Nitzke, B. Lohse, and L. Boeckner, "Acceptability of stage-tailored newsletters about fruits and vegetables by young adults," *Journal of the American Dietetic Association*, vol. 105, no. 11, pp. 1774–1778, 2005.

[20] A. Park, S. Nitzke, K. Kritsch et al., "Internet-based interventions have potential to affect short-term mediators and indicators of dietary behavior of young adults," *Journal of Nutrition Education and Behavior*, vol. 40, no. 5, pp. 288–297, 2008.

[21] J. Di Noia, I. R. Contento, and J. O. Prochaska, "Computer-mediated intervention tailored on transtheoretical model stages and processes of change increases fruit and vegetable consumption among urban African-American adolescents," *American Journal of Health Promotion*, vol. 22, no. 5, pp. 336–341, 2008.

[22] M. V. Nahas, M. V. G. de Barros, B. D. Goldfine et al., "Physical activity and eating habits in public high schools from different regions in Brazil: the Saude na Boa project," *Revista Brasileira de Epidemiologia*, vol. 12, no. 2, pp. 270–277, 2009.

[23] A. R. da Silva, M. M. Damasceno, N. B. Marinho et al., "The feeding habits of adolescents from public schools in Fortaleza, CE, Brazil," *Revista Brasileira de Enfermagem*, vol. 62, no. 1, pp. 18–24, 2009.

[24] R. M. Rojas, "Fruits and vegetables consumption among Costa Rican adolescents," *Archivos Latinoamericanos de Nutricion*, vol. 51, no. 1, pp. 81–85, 2001.

[25] A. C. Bell and B. A. Swinburn, "What are the key food groups to target for preventing obesity and improving nutrition in schools?" *European Journal of Clinical Nutrition*, vol. 58, no. 2, pp. 258–263, 2004.

[26] P. M. Guenther, K. W. Dodd, J. Reedy, and S. M. Krebs-Smith, "Most Americans eat much less than recommended amounts of fruits and vegetables," *Journal of the American Dietetic Association*, vol. 106, no. 9, pp. 1371–1379, 2006.

[27] D. C. Cusatis and B. M. Shannon, "Influences on adolescent eating behavior," *Journal of Adolescent Health*, vol. 18, no. 1, pp. 27–34, 1996.
[28] M. R. Cuce Nobre, R. Z. De Lima Domingues, A. R. Da Silva, F. A. Basile Colugnati, and J. A. D. A. Carrazedo Taddei, "Prevalence of overweight, obesity and lyfe style associated with cardiovascular risk among middle school students," *Revista da Associacao Medica Brasileira*, vol. 52, no. 2, pp. 118–124, 2006.
[29] R. Q. C. Ribeiro, P. A. Lotufo, J. A. Lamounier, R. G. Oliveira, J. F. Soares, and D. A. Botter, "Additional cardiovascular risk factors associated with excess weigth in children and adolescents. The Belo Horizonte heart study," *Arquivos Brasileiros de Cardiologia*, vol. 86, no. 6, pp. 408–418, 2006.
[30] M. Romanzini, F. F. Reichert, A. D. S. Lopes, E. L. Petroski, and J. C. De Farias, "Prevalence of cardiovascular risk factors in adolescents," *Cadernos de Saude Publica*, vol. 24, no. 11, pp. 2573–2581, 2008.
[31] P. C. Jaime, I. C. R. Figueiredo, E. C. de Moura, and D. C. Malta, "Factors associated with fruit and vegetable consumption in Brazil, 2006," *Revista de Saude Publica*, vol. 43, no. 2, pp. 57–64, 2009.
[32] M. B. Neutzling, A. J. Rombaldi, M. R. Azevedo, and P. C. Hallal, "Factors associated with fruit and vegetable intake among adults in a southern Brazilian city," *Cadernos de Saude Publica*, vol. 25, no. 11, pp. 2365–2374, 2009.
[33] R. M. Claro, H. C. Esvael do Carmo, F. M. Sarti Machado, and C. A. Monteiro, "Income, food prices, and participation of fruit and vegetables in the diet," *Revista de Saude Publica*, vol. 41, no. 4, pp. 557–564, 2007.
[34] C. Bridle, R. P. Riemsma, J. Pattenden et al., "Systematic review of the effectiveness of health behavior interventions based on the transtheoretical model," *Psychology and Health*, vol. 20, no. 3, pp. 283–301, 2005.
[35] M. L. Zanetti, M. V. Biagg, M. A. dos Santos, D. S. Péres, and C. R. Teixeira, "The care for the diabetic patient and family repercussion," *Revista Brasileira de Enfermagem*, vol. 61, no. 2, pp. 186–192, 2008.
[36] K. M. Young, J. J. Northern, K. M. Lister, J. A. Drummond, and W. H. O'Brien, "A meta-analysis of family-behavioral weight-loss treatments for children," *Clinical Psychology Review*, vol. 27, no. 2, pp. 240–249, 2007.
[37] R. Sichieri and R. A. De Souza, "Strategies for obesity prevention in children and adolescents," *Cadernos de Saude Publica*, vol. 24, supplement 2, pp. S209–S223, 2008.

3

Fetal and Neonatal Levels of Omega-3: Effects on Neurodevelopment, Nutrition, and Growth

Juliana Rombaldi Bernardi, Renata de Souza Escobar, Charles Francisco Ferreira, and Patrícia Pelufo Silveira

Núcleo de Estudos da Saúde da Criança e do Adolescente, Hospital de Clínicas de Porto Alegre (HCPA), Universidade Federal do Rio Grande do Sul, Rua Ramiro Barcelos 2350, 90035-903, Porto Alegre, RS, Brazil

Correspondence should be addressed to Patrícia Pelufo Silveira, 00032386@ufrgs.br

Academic Editors: C. Capurso, P. Pérez-Martínez, and Y. Vandenplas

Nutrition in pregnancy, during lactation, childhood, and later stages has a fundamental influence on overall development. There is a growing research interest on the role of key dietary nutrients in fetal health. Omega-3 polyunsaturated fatty acids (n-3 LCPUFAs) play an important role in brain development and function. Evidence from animal models of dietary n-3 LCPUFAs deficiency suggests that these fatty acids promote early brain development and regulate behavioral and neurochemical aspects related to mood disorders (stress responses, depression, and aggression and growth, memory, and cognitive functions). Preclinical and clinical studies suggest the role of n-3 LCPUFAs on neurodevelopment and growth. n-3 LCPUFAs may be an effective adjunctive factor for neural development, growth, and cognitive development, but further large-scale, well-controlled trials and preclinical studies are needed to examine its clinical mechanisms and possible benefits. The present paper discusses the use of n-3 LCPUFAs during different developmental stages and the investigation of different sources of consumption. The paper summarizes the role of n-3 LCPUFAs levels during critical periods and their effects on the children's neurodevelopment, nutrition, and growth.

1. Introduction

Arachidonic acid (AA; 20:4n-6) and Docosahexaenoic acid (DHA; 22:5n-3) are essential for brain growth and cognitive development; they also accumulate rapidly in the brain and retina during the later stages of gestation and early postnatal life [1–3].

During pregnancy, AA and DHA are transported across the placenta into fetal venous blood [4, 5]. Nutrition in pregnancy has a significant influence on fetal development. In this sense, there is an increasing interest on the role of key dietary nutrients in subsequent health status or diseases [6]. The major effects of higher levels of omega-3 polyunsaturated fatty acids (n-3 LCPUFAs) during pregnancy are associated with the development of brain and nerve tissues during the period of maximum intrauterine accretion [7].

After birth, breast milk is the source of AA and DHA to the neonate; the content of essential polyunsaturated fatty acids (PUFAs) in breast milk is dependent on the maternal intake of these fatty acids [8, 9]. The content of essential PUFAs may be low in populations eating primarily plant-based diets with no or limited fish intake [10]. The consumption of PUFAs is essential for the development of the brain and nervous system of children and teenagers [11].

The contribution of DHA for better neurodevelopment has been documented in breastfed infants. However, the effects of different levels of DHA in human milk and maternal DHA supplementation limited to the lactation period are still under investigation [7]. In foods, the most important source of DHA is fish and fish oil [12]. Sea fish are generally a better source of DHA than freshwater fish [10]. Hence, in many studies the consumption of marine foods is evaluated separately.

Researchers and mothers have turned to fish oil supplements, which are generally low in contaminants (methylmercury) and can provide substantially higher doses of n-3 LCPUFAs than most adults are able to consume in their diets [13]. In a recent review of studies in 13 countries within the lower and middle worldwide brackets of gross domestic product (GDP), there was a strong positive association between the economic status of the country (GDP) and the supply of total fat and n-3 LCPUFAs. In families living on a primarily plant-based diet, most of the fat and PUFAs intake come from vegetable oils and cereals [10].

It is evident that several worldwide health agencies recognize the importance of increasing dietary intake of n-3 LCPUFAs. The daily DHA recommendation during pregnancy from the Expert Committee ranges from 200–300 mg/daily (modified from [14]). For the first 6 months of life of preterm and term infants, dietary intakes of n-3 LCPUFAs should correspond to 0.45–1.5 energy% of total of fatty acids, and with an n-6 LCPUFAs to n-3 LCPUFAs ratio of 4–10 (modified from [15]). The Institute of Medicine (IOM) recommends a range of 0.6–1.2 energy% in n-3 LCPUFAs and a range of 5–10 energy% in n-6 PUFAs in children and adults [16].

In the present paper, we review the scientific evidence that relates n-3 LCPUFAs levels during these critical periods to children's neurodevelopment, nutrition, and growth. PubMed database was used to identify relevant studies, and reference lists from retrieved studies were reviewed. Study selections were limited to English and Portuguese studies involving humans and experimental studies, from 1980 to 2012.

2. Dietary Intake and Total Fat Status

In Iran, authors found a significant difference in the total n-3 LCPUFAs and DHA in breast milk in women in coastal cities compared with those in inland cities. Coastal mothers showed a significantly higher intake of fish or seafood compared with inland mothers ($P < 0.001$). The dietary intake of fish and seafood was assessed using a structured interview, called food frequency questionnaire (FFQ). Breast milk was collected from the mother's breasts by hand, pumping eight to 72 h after delivery. The study showed that dietary fish and seafood intake by the mother influenced the DHA content of breast milk.

A randomized controlled trial investigated direct supplementation of high dose fish oil to term infants in the early postnatal period (with regard to feeding practices). Infants were supplemented daily, from birth to six months, with fish oil supplement or placebo. The results indicate that direct fish oil supplementation can significantly elevate DHA levels in infancy. The study showed a successful strategy for raising infant DHA status [18]. In breastfed infants, DHA levels in breast milk were determinant for their DHA status [18].

3. Impact of Fatty Acids Status on Neurobehavioral Development

Long-chain polyunsaturated fatty acids (LCPUFAs) play an important role in the central nervous system (CNS) and are essential for early brain development. LCPUFAs comprise approximately 15 to 30% of the brain's dry weight [19]. LCPUFAs are involved in the functioning and architecture of the central nervous system; the function of LCPUFA is demonstrated, in part, through the dependence on LCPUFA through different stages in life. The brain's structure is lipid and consists mainly of phosphoglycerides and cholesterol rich in AA and DHA [20]. Studies show that DHA affects blood-brain barrier functions and neuronal membrane fluidity; it also regulates neurotransmission systems such as serotonergic, dopaminergic, norepinephrinergic, and acetylcholinergic systems [21, 22]. DHA has a significant effect on neuronal membrane dynamics and therefore on transporter, receptor, and neurotransmitter functions [19].

The fastest stage of neural development is during fetal growth. However, there is also significant development during the first five years of postnatal life. At this time, environmental factors, including nutrient intake, play a critical role in the development of the brain's cytoarchitecture [23]. n-3 and n-6 LCPUFA are required for proper brain function and for the development of a mature brain. n-3 and n-6 LCPUFA are important due to their effects on electrophysiology and cell membrane structures [24]. Human milk fatty acid composition depends on short-term and long-term maternal diet [25]. The early diet can provide the proper amount of DHA and n-6 LCPUFA to the infant's brain [26]. The psychophysiology of n-3 LCPUFAs indicates the potential effects of n-3 LCPUFAs in relation to direct changes in the brain; the potential effects include changes in cognitive measures [27].

During the third trimester of pregnancy, fetuses require approximately 40 to 60 mg of n-3 LCPUFAs per kilogram of body weight per day [28]. During the last gestational trimester and first postnatal months, there is significant growth of the human brain and a large increase in cerebral volume of DHA and AA [29]. During prenatal and perinatal growth, significant amounts of AA and DHA accumulate in the brain and hence the physiological demand for these nutrients [28].

Studies have shown evidence for the neurodevelopmental benefits of dietary PUFA during pregnancy and infancy [27, 29, 30]. In addition to the neural tissue, the retinal tissue also accumulates LCPUFA DHA during gestation. In retina rod cells, DHA accounts for 50 to 60% of the fatty acids used in the polar phosphoglycerides of the plates [20, 22]. Preterm infants are denied the full intrauterine supply of DHA available to term infants [31]; therefore, preterm infants depend on a diet that supplies all the DHA needed for growth and development.

Several studies have shown the cognitive benefits of high levels of consumption of n-3 LCPUFA in elderly populations [32–34]. There is a link between EPA and the central nervous system, which has been shown in studies that indicate that n-3 LCPUFA levels are associated with protection against certain diseases including Alzheimer's and multiple sclerosis. In animal study, author showed that EPA stimulates the expression of myelin-related proteins in rat brains. Better myelination may be associated with improved segregation of electrochemical signals transmitted to the axons; this may lead to faster speed of information processing and improved cognition among people with high levels of n-3 LCPUFAs consumption [36].

3.1. Dietary Consumption: n-3 LCPUFAs. Reference [37] showed a positive association between DHA concentrations in breast milk and infant scores on the NBAS (Brazelton Neonatal Behavioral Assessment Scale) Range of State cluster score. The results suggest that DHA is related to infant's superior ability to maintain optimal arousal.

Maternal intake of n-3 LCPUFA and breastfeeding predicted oppositional defiant and conduct disorder and comorbid externalizing disorder, before adjustment for confounding factors. However, there was no association between intake of n-3 LCPUFA by the mother or child with any type of externalizing disorder once sociodemographic factors were taken into account [38]. Studies show inconsistent results about the effects of n-3 LCPUFA on externalizing disorders: some studies report positive effects of n-3 LCPUFA [39, 40], but others have shown less conclusive results [41].

Confounding factors associated with inherited factors such as maternal IQ [42] and maternal nutrition present serious challenges in these studies. Prenatal exposure may persist into the postnatal environment; therefore, the identification of the precise timing of factors poses a scientific challenge. Nutrition, of course, has an essential role in mental development during different life stages. Reference [43] showed that breastfeeding is associated with positive effects on cognitive development. However, the evidence about the parallel effects of breastfeeding on emotional development is inconsistent [38, 44, 45]. There are also nonnutritional reasons why breastfeeding may influence mental health, including closeness and reciprocity [46].

Reference [47], in a double-blind randomized controlled trial, investigated the effects of raising intakes of EPA and DHA on depressed mood in mild to moderately depressed individuals who were not receiving conventional treatments for depression. The results did not show a significant effect of n-3 LCPUFA supplementation on depressed moods. Participants in the intervention group received three daily doses of 630 mg EPA, 850 mg DHA, 870 mg olive oil, 7,5 mg mixed tocopherols, and 12 mg orange oil (which was included to improve palatability and blinding) for 12 weeks. The measures of depressed mood for the experimental group were not better than those for the placebo group.

A review of studies that investigated the effects of n-3 LCPUFAs and mental illness found consistent evidence about the beneficial effects of n-3 LCPUFAs in relation to mood disorders. The results of studies that investigated an association between n-3 LCPUFAs and schizophrenia, borderline personality, attention deficit hyperactivity, and symptoms of anxiety are inconclusive. The results do not support indication of monotherapy or adjunctive treatment for mental illnesses [48].

However, there is evidence of n-3 LCPUFAs deficiency identified in women who develop postpartum depression. Postpartum depression is a serious mood disorder with the same symptoms as major depressive disorders (depressed mood, loss of interest in pleasurable activities, changes in sleep patterns and weight, and reduced cognitive abilities and concentration) [49, 50].

Observational studies show that prevalence of postpartum depression may be associated with n-3 LCPUFAs (FAs) intake and status. However, there are few controlled trials that have evaluated the effects of increasing the intakes of FAs on depression symptoms in postpartum women. Most interventions studies investigated a reduced number of patients and typically provided fish oil-based supplements that contained high doses of EPA and DHA [51]. Prenatal fish consumption was not predictive of postnatal depression (PND); also, postnatal n-3 status was not associated with postnatal depression. However, prenatal fish consumption predicted n-3 status in mothers after birth. Based on these findings, it is difficult to assess the efficacy of n-3 LCPUFAs for the treatment of PND [52].

3.2. Supplementation: n-3 LCPUFAs. A recent review showed unclear effects of maternal prenatal and postnatal LC-PUFAs supplementation on global neurobehavioral outcomes for children born to term. However, n-3 LCPUFAs supplementation for breastfeeding women of preterm infants improved performance on tests of global neurodevelopment [53].

Fish oil supplementation (4 g of fish oil with 1.1 g EPA and 2.2 DHA/daily) starting at 20 weeks of pregnancy until birth significantly increased the fatty acid composition of maternal and neonatal erythrocytes in comparison with olive oil supplementation. The effects were partially sustained until at least 6 weeks postpartum. Similarly, administration of n-6 polyunsaturated fatty acids AA was associated with significantly lower erythrocytes in neonates in the fish oil group in comparison with controls [54].

A DOMInO (DHA to Optimize Mother Infant Outcome) study with 2,399 women investigated whether DHA supplementation during the second half of gestation reduced the risk for depressed maternal mood (Edinburgh Postnatal Depression Scale) during the postpartum period. Women in the DHA group consumed 3 daily capsules of fish oil that contained a total of 800 mg DHA and 100 mg EPA (eicosapentaenoic acid); women in the control group consumed similar supplement levels of vegetable oil. The group given DHA did not show significant reduction in the rates of PND [55].

In the same study, researchers investigated early cognitive development in the offspring at 18 months of age. The results did not show an overall effect of DHA on development (assessed using the Bayley Scales of Infant and Toddler Development including cognitive scores and language scores [55]). With the objective of determining whether DHA deficiency occurs in pregnant women and contributes to poor infant development, 200 mg/g of DHA was administered to women from 16 weeks of gestation until delivery. The results showed a visual acuity below average among infants in the placebo than in the DHA intervention group [56].

Daily maternal supplementation with 1.6 g EPA or 1.1 g DHA from the 25th gestational week to an average 3-4 months in early breastfeeding decreased the risk for food allergies and IgE-associated eczema during the first year of life. The effects were shown in infants with a family history of allergic disease compared with a placebo group [57].

Supplementation with a relatively high dose of fish oil (1.1 g EPA and 2.2 g DHA/daily) during the last 20 weeks of pregnancy is not only safe but also has potential beneficial effects, but the effects need to be further investigated. At age 2.5 years, children in the fish oil-supplemented group showed a significantly higher score for hand-eye coordination than children in the placebo group. There was a correlation between hand-eye coordination scores with n-3 LCPUFAs levels in cord blood erythrocytes, and a negative correlation with n-6 PUFA [58].

Reference [29] found that giving pregnant and lactating women n-3 very long-chain PUFAs supplementation was associated with higher IQ scores at 4 years of age in comparison with maternal supplementation with n-6 long-chain PUFAs. There were no significant differences on the Kaufman Assessment Battery for Children test at 7 years of age between children whose mothers had taken cod liver oil (n-3 LCPUFAs rich) or corn oil (n-6 PUFA rich) [59].

A multicenter, randomized controlled trial from DINO (Docosahexaenoic Acid for the Improvement of Neurodevelopmental Outcome in Preterm Infants) with 657 lactating administered six 500 mg DHA-rich tuna oil capsules per day (for breast milk DHA concentration). The study showed that a DHA dose of approximately 1% total fatty acids in early life did not increase Bayley Mental Developmental (MDI) scores of preterm infants with less than 33 weeks of gestation. However, the dosage improved the MDI scores of girls [60].

In another study, breast-feeding women received identical capsules containing either DHA algal oil (200 mg/d of DHA) or a vegetable oil (no DHA) from delivery until 4 months postpartum. The results showed that at 5 years, there were no differences in visual function (Bailey-Lovie acuity chart), transient visual evoked potential, or sweep visual evoked potential testing between children whose mothers received DHA versus placebo. However, children whose mothers received DHA versus placebo performed significantly better on the Sustained Attention Subscale of the Leiter International Performance Scale. There were no statistically significant differences between groups on other neuropsychological domains [61].

Yet another study was carried out with the objective of determining the effect of DHA supplementation on neurodevelopment status and visual function. Breastfeeding mothers were administered capsules containing either high-DHA concentration algal oil (200 mg DHA/day) or a vegetable oil (no DHA) to breastfeeding women for 4 months after delivery. The intervention group showed 50% greater content of maternal plasma phospholipids DHA, 75% greater content of DHA in milk lipids, and 35% greater content of DHA in infant plasma phospholipids. However, higher infant plasma phospholipids DHA content did not show effects on visual acuity at either 4 or 8 months of age [62].

The DINO Trial DHA found that supplementation for infants <33 weeks gestation with tuna oil capsules reduced the incidence of bronchopulmonary dysplasia in boys and in all infants with a birth weight <1250 g; it also reduced the incidence of reported hay fever in boys at either 12 or 18 months [63].

Reference [64] compared the content of DHA in breast milk in three groups: mothers with habitual high fish intake, with fish oil supplementation and with olive oil supplementation. The authors described a small effect of DHA levels in breast milk on early language development (word production) of breast-fed infants. No beneficial effect was reported for problem solving, though the data suggest there may be an effect in girls.

Reference [65], in a follow-up study, evaluated IQ, receptive and expressive vocabulary, visual-motor function, and visual acuity in formula-fed and breast-fed infants. Healthy term infants ($n = 197$) less than a week old were randomized to be fed formulas for one year, one containing DHA or another containing both AA and DHA; there was also a group of infants who were exclusively breastfed for at least 3 months. At 39 months, IQ, receptive and expressive language, visual-motor function, and visual acuity were not different between the randomized formula groups or between the breastfed and formula groups. Growth achievement, red blood cell fatty acid levels, and morbidity did not differ between the groups [66].

3.3. Use of Food Supplements with n-3 LCPUFAs. In an observational study of subjects born in 1936 whose mental ability was tested in 1947 and who were followed up in 2000-2001, the childhood IQ did not differ significantly by category of food supplement use. However, at the age of 64 years, cognitive function was higher in food supplement users than in nonusers, before adjustment for childhood IQ [67]. In a nested case-control study, erythrocyte membrane n-3 content was higher in fish oil supplement users than in nonusers, but cognitive function did not differ significantly between the groups [67].

4. Impact of Fatty Acids Status on Nutrition and Growth

A recent review limited to human studies published in English from 2000 until 2010 on n-3 and growth suggests that n-3 (DHA in particular) during pregnancy, lactation and early life may be associated with significant benefits for infant growth and development in developing countries. Studies in developing countries show that a higher n-3 intake or supplementation during pregnancy may result in improvements in birth weight, length, and gestational age. Limited data from developing countries suggest that ALA or DHA supplementation during lactation and in infants may be beneficial for growth and development of young children; these benefits are more pronounced in undernourished children. However, there is no evidence of improvements in growth following n-3 supplementation in children >2 years of age [68].

4.1. Dietary Consumption of n-3 Fatty Acid. Reference [69] compared the levels of the main long-chain PUFA between birth and the first year of age. The results showed a significant decrease with age in the proportion of these fatty acids in the plasma of children. At one year of age, the percentage of DHA in the extended breastfeeding group (more than 6 months) differed significantly from the other groups, that is, medium term breastfeeding (more than 3 and less than 5 months) and exclusive formula feeding.

An interventional study carried out in Brazil showed that postnatal sardine consumption (100 g of sardines two or three times a week) contributed to an increase omega-3 series fatty acids (DHA and DPA) on the composition of breast milk of mothers at 15 and 30 days into the study [70].

In a prospective, observational cohort study with 2109 subjects who were enrolled in the Project Viva, in the USA, the authors investigated if maternal marine n-3 LCPUFAs and seafood intake were associated with birth weight, birthweight for gestational-age z value (fetal growth), length of gestation, low birth weight, preterm delivery, and babies small for gestational age. The study showed that increased consumption of the n-3 LCPUFAs DHA and EPA was associated with a modest decrease in fetal growth. The study did not show any association between higher seafood or n-3 LCPUFAs intake and length of gestation [71].

A prospective study with 62099 women in Norway (Norwegian Mother and Child Cohort Study-MoBa) investigated the influence of maternal intakes of seafood and supplementary n-3 LCPUFAs in infant birth weight, length, and head circumference. The researchers found that maternal seafood consumption was positively associated with birth size, driven by lean fish intake, while supplementary n-3 intake was negatively associated with infant head circumference [72].

4.2. Supplementation with n-3 LCPUFAs

4.2.1. Experimental Studies. A study was conducted with 22 Lister Hooded rats that are divided into two groups: the control group (CG) which received a casein-based diet, and the flaxseed group (FG) which received 25% flaxseed diet supplement, and 14% casein showed that, during gestation and lactation, the FG was similar to the CG group in relation to food intake and litter size. The same result was observed for milk fat content and total energy value. At weaning, the FG group was similar to the CG group in both in offspring body weight and in weight gain of pups during lactation [73]. However, a study using only female Wistar rats ($n = 16$) and the same group division (FG and CG) showed that mothers on the flaxseed diet gained less weight during lactation and their offspring had lower body weight only after weaning. At 170 days, lower hemoglobin levels were observed in the FG group, but there was no statistically significant difference in visceral fat mass between groups [74].

A study with female Wistar rats ($n = 18$) administered three types of diet: control group (CG) with 7% soy oil; flaxseed group (FG) with 10% flaxseed diet (25 g), both fed ad libitum diets and a modified control group (MCG) with 10% soy oil, pair-fed with the FG. The diets were given to dams during preconception, pregnancy, and lactation and to their pups after weaning. The offspring of FG dams showed lower body mass than those of CG dams. The content of DHA in the hippocampus was higher in the FG, followed by the MCG compared with the CG. Hippocampal DHA content correlated with better spatial memory performance in the FG, whereas AA content correlated with longer time in solving tasks [75].

4.2.2. Clinical Studies. A recent review shows that LC-PUFAs supplementation during pregnancy is associated with modest increases in birth size in both low-income and high-income populations. However, postnatal supplementation with LC-PUFAs did not influence infant growth [53].

Babies born of primiparous Mexican women who received 400 mg/d of algal DHA during the second half of the pregnancy term were heavier and had larger head circumferences at birth than children whose mothers received placebo (olive oil). However, no effect was observed in multiparous mothers. Children of primiparous women who were given DHA were taller at 18 months than those of primiparous women given placebo. The authors suggest that since primiparous women were, on average, younger than the multiparous women, their own body stores of DHA are not well established and available to the fetus and infant [76].

Reference [62] found that there were no statistically significant differences in weight, length, or head circumference between the 2 groups of infants at any time (high-DHA algal oil or a vegetable oil without DHA for 4 months after delivery). At all ages, these measures were within the normal range for age in both groups.

Supplementation with fish oil (1.1 g EPA and 2.2 DHA/daily) or olive oil starting at 18–20 weeks of pregnancy and continued until delivery showed similar growth measurements in the two groups at age $2^{1/2}$ years [58].

A randomized, double-blind trial gave lactating mothers fish oil or olive oil supplements for 4 months; the study followed infant development for 2.5 years and showed that children from the fish oil group had larger head circumference and higher BMI than those in the olive oil group after adjustment for relevant confounds. Both body composition and head circumference at 2.5 years of age positively correlated with the DHA content of maternal red blood cells at the end of the intervention [77].

5. Conclusions

Experimental, biochemical, and epidemiological evidence support the hypothesis that low n-3 polyunsaturated fatty acids (n-3 LCPUFA) levels are associated with dysfunctional brain development and impaired growth; the evidence also shows that n-3 supplementation is useful for improvement of specific parameters, especially those related to memory and cognition. However, the precise definition of the method of use and dosages is still unclear. Large-scale, well-controlled trials should be carried out to confirm the efficacy of the acids and establish the minimum dose and length of supplementation to significantly improve clinical outcomes. It is also important to determine the use of the acids on different stages of development. n-3 LCPUFAs represent an attractive supplementary alternative, because they are perceived as a natural substance rather than an artificial supplement. In sum, the dietary consumption and supplementation of n-3 LCPUFAs could provide physical and mental health benefits for development.

Acknowledgments

The authors would like to acknowledge the contribution of Carla Dalmaz (Biochemistry Department, UFRGS, Brazil) in the discussion and preparation of the early draft of this paper. There is no conflict of interests, either financial or of any other nature in relation to the present work. Financial support was received from ARD/FAPERGS 2010 (Silveira PP, 10/0474-2); Universal National Counsel of Technological and Scientific Development (CNPq)—Brazil 2010 (Silveira PP, 478820/2010-0); FIPE/HCPA (GPPG 09-410); Foundation for the Coordination of Higher Education and Graduate Training (CAPES); INCT Translational Medicine (CNPq) 573671/2008-7.

References

[1] M. T. Clandinin, J. E. Chappell, and S. Leong, "Extrauterine fatty acid accretion in infant brain: implications for fatty acid requirements," *Early Human Development*, vol. 4, no. 2, pp. 131–138, 1980.

[2] M. T. Clandinin, J. E. Chappell, and S. Leong, "Intrauterine fatty acid accretion rates in human brain: implications for fatty acid requirements," *Early Human Development*, vol. 4, no. 2, pp. 121–129, 1980.

[3] M. Martinez, "Tissue levels of polyunsaturated fatty acids during early human development," *Journal of Pediatrics*, vol. 120, no. 4, part 2, pp. 129–138, 1992.

[4] F. M. Campbell, A. M. Clohessy, M. J. Gordon, K. R. Page, and A. K. Dutta-Roy, "Uptake of long chain fatty acids by human placental choriocarcinoma (BeWo) cells: role of plasma membrane fatty acid-binding protein," *Journal of Lipid Research*, vol. 38, no. 12, pp. 2558–2568, 1997.

[5] A. K. Dutta-Roy, "Transport mechanisms for long-chain polyunsaturated fatty acids in the human placenta," *American Journal of Clinical Nutrition*, vol. 71, no. 1, supplement, pp. 315S–22S, 2000.

[6] S. L. Prescott and J. A. Dunstan, "Prenatal fatty acid status and immune development: the pathways and the evidence," *Lipids*, vol. 42, no. 9, pp. 801–810, 2007.

[7] C. Agostoni, "Docosahexaenoic acid (DHA): from the maternal-foetal dyad to the complementary feeding period," *Early Human Development*, vol. 86, supplement 1, pp. 3–6, 2010.

[8] W. S. Harris, W. E. Connor, and S. Lindsey, "Will dietary ω-3 fatty acids change the composition of human milk?" *American Journal of Clinical Nutrition*, vol. 40, no. 4, pp. 780–785, 1984.

[9] I. B. Helland, K. Saarem, O. D. Saugstad, and C. A. Drevon, "Fatty acid composition in maternal milk and plasma during supplementation with cod liver oil," *European Journal of Clinical Nutrition*, vol. 52, no. 11, pp. 839–845, 1998.

[10] K. F. Michaelsen, K. G. Dewey, A. B. Perez-Exposito, M. Nurhasan, L. Lauritzen, and N. Roos, "Food sources and intake of n-6 and n-3 fatty acids in low-income countries with emphasis on infants, young children (6–24 months), and pregnant and lactating women," *Maternal and Child Nutrition*, vol. 7, no. 2, pp. 124–140, 2011.

[11] J. P. Schuchardt, M. Huss, M. Stauss-Grabo, and A. Hahn, "Significance of long-chain polyunsaturated fatty acids (PUFAs) for the development and behaviour of children," *European Journal of Pediatrics*, vol. 169, no. 2, pp. 149–164, 2010.

[12] M. Gil-Campos and J. Dalmau Serra, "Importance of docosahexaenoic acid (DHA): functions and recommendations for its ingestion in infants," *Anales de Pediatria*, vol. 73, no. 3, pp. 142.e1–148.e1, 2010.

[13] E. Oken and M. B. Belfort, "Fish, fish oil, and pregnancy," *Journal of the American Medical Association*, vol. 304, no. 15, pp. 1717–1718, 2010.

[14] R. G. Jordan, "Prenatal omega-3 fatty acids: review and recommendations," *Journal of Midwifery and Women's Health*, vol. 55, no. 6, pp. 520–528, 2010.

[15] P. Guesnet and J. M. Alessandri, "Docosahexaenoic acid (DHA) and the developing central nervous system (CNS)—implications for dietary recommendations," *Biochimie*, vol. 93, no. 1, pp. 7–12, 2011.

[16] P. Trumbo, S. Schlicker, A. A. Yates, and M. Poos, "Dietary reference intakes for energy, carbohydrate, fiber, fat, fatty acids, cholesterol, protein and amino acids," *Journal of the American Dietetic Association*, vol. 102, no. 11, pp. 1621–1630, 2002.

[17] B. Olang, M. Hajifaraji, M. A. Ali et al., "Docosahexaenoic acid in breast milk reflects maternal fish intake in Iranian mothers," *Food and Nutrition Sciences*, vol. 3, pp. 441–446, 2012.

[18] S. J. Meldrum, N. D'Vaz, Y. Casadio et al., "Determinants of DHA levels in early infancy: differential effects of breast milk and direct fish oil supplementation," *Prostaglandins Leukot Essent Fatty Acids*, vol. 86, no. 6, pp. 233–239, 2012.

[19] B. Hallahan and M. R. Garland, "Essential fatty acids and mental health," *British Journal of Psychiatry*, vol. 186, pp. 275–277, 2005.

[20] M. A. Crawford, "The role of dietary fatty acids in biology: their place in the evolution of the human brain," *Nutrition Reviews*, vol. 50, no. 4, part 2, pp. 3–11, 1992.

[21] G. Fontani, F. Corradeschi, A. Felici, F. Alfatti, S. Migliorini, and L. Lodi, "Cognitive and physiological effects of Omega-3 polyunsaturated fatty acid supplementation in healthy subjects," *European Journal of Clinical Investigation*, vol. 35, no. 11, pp. 691–699, 2005.

[22] P. M. Kidd, "Omega-3 DHA and EPA for cognition, behavior, and mood: clinical findings and structural-functional synergies with cell membrane phospholipids," *Alternative Medicine Review*, vol. 12, no. 3, pp. 207–227, 2007.

[23] P. Levitt, "Structural and functional maturation of the developing primate brain," *Journal of Pediatrics*, vol. 143, no. 4, supplement, pp. S35–S45, 2003.

[24] K. Kitajka, A. J. Sinclair, R. S. Weisinger et al., "Effects of dietary omega-3 polyunsaturated fatty acids on brain gene expression," *Proceedings of the National Academy of Sciences of the United States of America*, vol. 101, no. 30, pp. 10931–10936, 2004.

[25] M. H. Jørgensen, O. Hernell, E. L. Hughes, and K. F. Michaelsen, "Is there a relation between Docosahexaenoic acid concentration in mothers' milk and visual development in term infants?" *Journal of Pediatric Gastroenterology and Nutrition*, vol. 32, no. 3, pp. 293–296, 2001.

[26] E. M. Novak, R. A. Dyer, and S. M. Innis, "High dietary ω-6 fatty acids contribute to reduced docosahexaenoic acid in the developing brain and inhibit secondary neurite growth," *Brain Research*, vol. 1237, pp. 136–145, 2008.

[27] J. L. Daniels, M. P. Longnecker, A. S. Rowland, and J. Golding, "Fish intake during pregnancy and early cognitive development of offspring," *Epidemiology*, vol. 15, no. 4, pp. 394–402, 2004.

[28] M. T. Clandinin, J. E. Chappell, and J. E. E. Van Aerde, "Requirements of newborn infants for long chain polyunsaturated fatty acids," *Acta Paediatrica Scandinavica, Supplement*, vol. 78, no. 351, pp. 63–71, 1989.

[29] I. B. Helland, L. Smith, K. Saarem, O. D. Saugstad, and C. A. Drevon, "Maternal supplementation with very-long-chain n-3 fatty acids during pregnancy and lactation augments children's IQ at 4 years of age," *Pediatrics*, vol. 111, no. 1, pp. e39–e44, 2003.

[30] E. Larque, H. Demmelmair, and B. Koletzko, "Perinatal supply and metabolism of long-chain polyunsaturated fatty acids: importance for the early development of the nervous system," *Annals of the New York Academy of Sciences*, vol. 967, pp. 299–310, 2002.

[31] M. T. Clandinin, J. E. Chappell, and T. Heim, "Fatty acid utilization in perinatal de novo synthesis of tissues," *Early Human Development*, vol. 5, no. 4, pp. 355–366, 1981.

[32] M. C. Morris, D. A. Evans, J. L. Bienias et al., "Consumption of fish and n-3 fatty acids and risk of incident Alzheimer disease," *Archives of Neurology*, vol. 60, no. 7, pp. 940–946, 2003.

[33] M. H. Eskelinen, T. Ngandu, E. L. Helkala et al., "Fat intake at midlife and cognitive impairment later in life: a population-based CAIDE study," *International Journal of Geriatric Psychiatry*, vol. 23, no. 7, pp. 741–747, 2008.

[34] V. Solfrizzi, A. M. Colacicco, A. D'Introno et al., "Dietary fatty acids intakes and rate of mild cognitive impairment. The Italian Longitudinal Study on Aging," *Experimental Gerontology*, vol. 41, no. 6, pp. 619–627, 2006.

[35] S. Salvati, F. Natali, L. Attorri et al., "Eicosapentaenoic acid stimulates the expression of myelin proteins in rat brain," *Journal of Neuroscience Research*, vol. 86, no. 4, pp. 776–784, 2008.

[36] M. K. Georgieff, "Nutrition and the developing brain: nutrient priorities and measurement," *American Journal of Clinical Nutrition*, vol. 85, no. 2, pp. 614S–620S, 2007.

[37] S. L. Hart, L. M. Boylan, S. R. Carroll et al., "Brief report: newborn behavior differs with decosahexaenoic acid levels in breast milk," *Journal of Pediatric Psychology*, vol. 31, no. 2, pp. 221–226, 2006.

[38] A. Waylen, T. Ford, R. Goodman, M. Samara, and D. Wolke, "Can early intake of dietary omega-3 predict childhood externalizing behaviour?" *Acta Paediatrica, International Journal of Paediatrics*, vol. 98, no. 11, pp. 1805–1808, 2009.

[39] N. Sinn and J. Bryan, "Effect of supplementation with polyunsaturated fatty acids and micronutrients on learning and behavior problems associated with child ADHD," *Journal of Developmental and Behavioral Pediatrics*, vol. 28, no. 2, pp. 82–91, 2007.

[40] A. J. Richardson and P. Montgomery, "The Oxford-Durham study: a randomized, controlled trial of dietary supplementation with fatty acids in children with developmental coordination disorder," *Pediatrics*, vol. 115, no. 5, pp. 1360–1366, 2005.

[41] W. C. Heird and A. Lapillonne, "The role of essential fatty acids in development," *Annual Review of Nutrition*, vol. 25, pp. 549–571, 2005.

[42] A. Thapar and M. Rutter, "Do prenatal risk factors cause psychiatric disorder? Be wary of causal claims," *British Journal of Psychiatry*, vol. 195, no. 2, pp. 100–101, 2009.

[43] J. W. Anderson, B. M. Johnstone, and D. T. Remley, "Breast-feeding and cognitive development: a meta-analysis," *American Journal of Clinical Nutrition*, vol. 70, no. 4, pp. 525–535, 1999.

[44] N. B. Allen, P. M. Lewinsohn, and J. R. Seeley, "Prenatal and perinatal influences on risk for psychopathology in childhood and adolescence," *Development and Psychopathology*, vol. 10, no. 3, pp. 513–529, 1998.

[45] M. Robinson, W. H. Oddy, J. Li et al., "Pre- and postnatal influences on preschool mental health: a large-scale cohort study," *Journal of Child Psychology and Psychiatry and Allied Disciplines*, vol. 49, no. 10, pp. 1118–1128, 2008.

[46] D. M. Dignam, "Understanding intimacy as experienced by breastfeeding women," *Health Care for Women International*, vol. 16, no. 5, pp. 477–485, 1995.

[47] P. J. Rogers, K. M. Appleton, D. Kessler et al., "No effect of n-3 long-chain polyunsaturated fatty acid (EPA and DHA) supplementation on depressed mood and cognitive function: a randomised controlled trial," *British Journal of Nutrition*, vol. 99, no. 2, pp. 421–431, 2008.

[48] B. M. Ross, J. Seguin, and L. E. Sieswerda, "Omega-3 fatty acids as treatments for mental illness: which disorder and which fatty acid?" *Lipids in Health and Disease*, vol. 6, article 21, 2007.

[49] S. R. De Vriese, A. B. Christophe, and M. Maes, "Lowered serum n-3 polyunsaturated fatty acid (PUFA) levels predict the occurrence of postpartum depression: further evidence that lowered n-PUFAs are related to major depression," *Life Sciences*, vol. 73, no. 25, pp. 3181–3187, 2003.

[50] Y. W. Chen and S. C. Dilsaver, "Lifetime rates of suicide attempts among subjects with bipolar and unipolar disorders relative to subjects with other Axis I disorders," *Biological Psychiatry*, vol. 39, no. 10, pp. 896–899, 1996.

[51] U. Ramakrishnan, B. Imhoff-Kunsch, and A. M. Digirolamo, "Role of docosahexaenoic acid in maternal and child mental health," *American Journal of Clinical Nutrition*, vol. 89, no. 3, pp. 958S–962S, 2009.

[52] J. C. Browne, K. M. Scott, and K. M. Silvers, "Fish consumption in pregnancy and omega-3 status after birth are not associated with postnatal depression," *Journal of Affective Disorders*, vol. 90, no. 2-3, pp. 131–139, 2006.

[53] M. Makrides, C. T. Collins, and R. A. Gibson, "Impact of fatty acid status on growth and neurobehavioural development in humans," *Maternal and Child Nutrition*, vol. 7, no. 2, pp. 80–88, 2011.

[54] J. A. Dunstan, T. A. Mori, A. Barden et al., "Effects of n-3 polyunsaturated fatty acid supplementation in pregnancy on maternal and fetal erythrocyte fatty composition," *European Journal of Clinical Nutrition*, vol. 58, no. 3, pp. 429–437, 2004.

[55] M. Makrides, R. A. Gibson, A. J. McPhee et al., "Effect of DHA supplementation during pregnancy on maternal depression and neurodevelopment of young children: a randomized controlled trial," *Journal of the American Medical Association*, vol. 304, no. 15, pp. 1675–1683, 2010.

[56] S. M. Innis and R. W. Friesen, "Essential n-3 fatty acids in pregnant women and early visual acuity maturation in term infants," *American Journal of Clinical Nutrition*, vol. 87, no. 3, pp. 548–557, 2008.

[57] C. Furuhjelm, K. Warstedt, J. Larsson et al., "Fish oil supplementation in pregnancy and lactation may decrease the risk of infant allergy," *Acta Paediatrica, International Journal of Paediatrics*, vol. 98, no. 9, pp. 1461–1467, 2009.

[58] J. A. Dunstan, K. Simmer, G. Dixon, and S. L. Prescott, "Cognitive assessment of children at age 2 1/2 years after

maternal fish oil supplementation in pregnancy: a randomised controlled trial," *Archives of Disease in Childhood*, vol. 93, no. 1, pp. F45–F50, 2008.
[59] I. B. Helland, L. Smith, B. Blomen, K. Saarem, O. D. Saugstad, and C. A. Drevon, "Effect of supplementing pregnant and lactating mothers with n-3 very-long-chain fatty acids on children's iq and body mass index at 7 years of age," *Pediatrics*, vol. 122, no. 2, pp. e472–e479, 2008.
[60] M. Makrides, R. A. Gibson, A. J. McPhee et al., "Neurodevelopmental outcomes of preterm infants fed high-dose docosahexaenoic acid: a randomized controlled trial," *Journal of the American Medical Association*, vol. 301, no. 2, pp. 175–182, 2009.
[61] C. L. Jensen, R. G. Voigt, A. M. Llorente et al., "Effects of early maternal docosahexaenoic acid intake on neuropsychological status and visual acuity at five years of age of breast-fed term infants," *Journal of Pediatrics*, vol. 157, no. 6, pp. 900–905, 2010.
[62] C. L. Jensen, R. G. Voigt, T. C. Prager et al., "Effects of maternal docosahexaenoic acid intake on visual function and neurodevelopment in breastfed term infants," *American Journal of Clinical Nutrition*, vol. 82, no. 1, pp. 125–132, 2005.
[63] B. J. Manley, M. Makrides, C. T. Collins et al., "High-dose docosahexaenoic acid supplementation of preterm infants: respiratory and allergy outcomes," *Pediatrics*, vol. 128, no. 1, pp. e71–e77, 2011.
[64] L. Lauritzen, M. H. Jørgensen, S. F. Olsen, E. M. Straarup, and K. F. Michaelsen, "Maternal fish oil supplementation in lactation: effect on developmental outcome in breast-fed infants," *Reproduction Nutrition Development*, vol. 45, no. 5, pp. 535–547, 2005.
[65] N. Auestad, M. B. Montalto, R. T. Hall et al., "Visual acuity, erythrocyte fatty acid composition, and growth in term infants fed formulas with long chain polyunsaturated fatty acids for one year," *Pediatric Research*, vol. 41, no. 1, pp. 1–10, 1997.
[66] N. Auestad, D. T. Scott, J. S. Janowsky et al., "Visual, cognitive, and language assessments at 39 months: a follow-up study of children fed formulas containing long-chain polyunsaturated fatty acids to 1 year of age," *Pediatrics*, vol. 112, no. 3, part 1, pp. e177–e183, 2003.
[67] L. J. Whalley, H. C. Fox, K. W. Wahle, J. M. Starr, and I. J. Deary, "Cognitive aging, childhood intelligence, and the use of food supplements: possible involvement of n-3 fatty acids," *American Journal of Clinical Nutrition*, vol. 80, no. 6, pp. 1650–1657, 2004.
[68] S. L. Huffman, R. K. Harika, A. Eilander, and S. J. Osendarp, "Essential fats: how do they affect growth and development of infants and young children in developing countries? A literature review," *Maternal and Child Nutrition*, vol. 7, supplement 3, pp. 44–65, 2011.
[69] P. S. Crespo, N. T. Quirante, L. A.-E. Azuara, L. C. Gonza'lez, J. A. P Perera, and F. A. Lodeiro, "Ácidos grasos n-3 y n-6 en plasma al nacer y al año de edad y relación con el tipo de alimentación," *Anales de Pediatría*, vol. 68, pp. 570–575, 2008.
[70] R. V. Patin, M. R. Vítolo, M. A. Valverde, P. O. Carvalho, G. M. Pastore, and F. A. Lopez, "The influence of sardine consumption on the omega-3 fatty acid content of mature human milk," *Jornal de Pediatria*, vol. 82, no. 1, pp. 63–69, 2006.
[71] E. Oken, K. P. Kleinman, S. F. Olsen, J. W. Rich-Edwards, and M. W. Gillman, "Associations of seafood and elongated n-3 fatty acid intake with fetal growth and length of gestation: results from a US pregnancy cohort," *American Journal of Epidemiology*, vol. 160, no. 8, pp. 774–783, 2004.
[72] A. L. Brantsaeter, B. E. Birgisdottir et al., "Maternal seafood consumption and infant birth weight, length and head circumference in the Norwegian Mother and Child Cohort Study," *British Journal of Nutrition*, vol. 107, no. 3, pp. 436–444, 2012.
[73] C. D. Leite and G. C. Vicente, "Effects of flaxseed on rat milk creamatocrit and its contribution to offspring body growth," *Journal of Pediatrics*, vol. 88, no. 1, pp. 74–78, 2012.
[74] L. F. M. D. F. Cardozo, L. L. Soares, M. A. Chagas, and G. T. Boaventura, "Maternal consumption of flaxseed during lactation affects weight and hemoglobin level of offspring in rats," *Jornal de Pediatria*, vol. 86, no. 2, pp. 126–130, 2010.
[75] F. S. Fernandes, A. S. de Souza, M. das Graças Tavares do Carmo, and G. T. Boaventura, "Maternal intake of flaxseed-based diet (*Linum usitatissimum*) on hippocampus fatty acid profile: implications for growth, locomotor activity and spatial memory," *Nutrition*, vol. 27, no. 10, pp. 1040–1047, 2011.
[76] A. D. Stein, M. Wang, R. Martorell et al., "Growth to age 18 months following prenatal supplementation with docosahexaenoic acid differs by maternal gravidity in Mexico," *Journal of Nutrition*, vol. 141, no. 2, pp. 316–320, 2011.
[77] L. Lauritzen, C. Hoppe, E. M. Straarup, and K. F. Michaelsen, "Maternal fish oil supplementation in lactation and growth during the first 2.5 years of life," *Pediatric Research*, vol. 58, no. 2, pp. 235–242, 2005.

Obesity-Related Factors in Turkish School Children

Cihad Dündar[1] and Hatice Öz[2]

[1] *Department of Public Health, Faculty of Medicine, Ondokuz Mayıs University, 55139 Samsun, Turkey*
[2] *Provincial Directorate of Health, 55060 Samsun, Turkey*

Correspondence should be addressed to Cihad Dündar, chddundar@gmail.com

Academic Editors: F. J. Gómez-Pérez and I. Zakeri

Objective. To determine the prevalence of obesity and its risk factors in Turkish children. *Method*. This cross-sectional survey was conducted on students including 1271 boys and 1206 girls selected from 20 secondary schools in Samsun, Turkey. A predesigned questionnaire was used to elicit the information on individual characteristics. The height and weight of students were measured in their classroom. Obesity was defined as body mass index at or above the 95th percentile for age of the sex-specific CDC growth charts. *Result*. The mean age was 12.8 ± 0.9 years, and the prevalence of obesity was found at 10.3%. There were higher numbers of obese students in boys than in girls ($X^2 = 53.4$; $P < 0.001$). The prevalence of obesity was 10.0% and 16.8% in public and private school students, respectively. The percentage of obese children in students who skipped breakfast was found to be higher than that in the group that consumed 3 meals a day regularly. There was no difference at time spent in sedentary behavior except watching TV, and prevalence of obesity in the group of students watching television over 3 hours per day was higher than that in their counterparts ($X^2 = 13.6$; $P < 0.01$). The time of engagement in sports was lower in obese group statistically ($F = 8.9$; $P < 0.001$). *Conclusion*. In order to prevent childhood obesity, monitoring children's lifestyle by parents is necessary.

1. Introduction

The issue of being overweight and obese is becoming an increasingly prevalent problem in both the developed and developing world, and it is one of the most serious public health challenges of the 21st century [1]. In 2007, it was estimated that globally 22 million children under 5 years were overweight, with more than 75% of overweight and obese children living in low- and middle-income countries [2]. It is not only the scale of childhood obesity that is challenging, but also the speed at which the prevalence has increased. The greatest annual increases in obesity since 1970 in school children have been in North America and Western Europe [3].

Obesity, which is defined as the condition of excessive fat in the body, has significant health consequences. It is the result of undesirable weight gain caused when people consume more energy than they expend [4]. The explanation of the primary cause of being overweight and obese is not clear in adolescents, although dietary, genetic, and physical activity patterns must be important factors [5]. It is seen as a problem associated with adulthood; obesity during childhood is also becoming a concern. However, childhood obesity is an important public health issue with increasing prevalence and important consequences (comorbidities of obesity in childhood include type 2 diabetes, hypertension, dyslipidaemia, emotional and behavioural problems, asthma, and sleep apnea) [6].

Many survey data indicate that leisure activity is increasingly sedentary, due to the wide availability of entertainment such as television, videos, and computer games. This sedentary behavior is emerging as an important component of obesity and should be recognized as a behavior that is distinct from physical activity [7]. In addition, with increasing urbanization, there has been a decrease in the frequency and duration of physical activities of children, such as walking to school [8, 9].

The aim of this study is to determine the prevalence of obesity and the related factors in a representative sample of secondary school children living in the province of Samsun, the 15th high populated city of Turkey.

Table 1: Demographic characteristics of study group.

Characteristics	Boys ($n = 1271$) Mean ± Sd	Boys Range	Girls ($n = 1206$) Mean ± Sd	Girls Range	Total ($n = 2477$) Mean ± Sd	Total Range
Age, y	12.9 ± 1.0	11–14	12.8 ± 0.9	11–14	12.8 ± 0.9	11–14
Height, cm	155.2 ± 10.5	120.0–193.0	154.5 ± 7.5	128.0–177.0	154.9 ± 9.2	120.0–193.0
Weight, kg	48.6 ± 12.8	21.2–103.9	48.5 ± 11.3	22.8–97.6	48.5 ± 12.1	21.2–103.9
BMI, kg/m^2	19.9 ± 3.7	12.4–40.0	20.2 ± 3.9	11.9–40.5	20.1 ± 3.8	11.9–40.5

2. Methods

2.1. Samples and Survey Procedures. This cross-sectional regional survey was conducted on 2477 students selected from classes VI, VII and VIII in a total of 20 secondary schools in the province of Samsun in April 2009. This representative sample was selected from 24.691 students in 68 secondary schools by a multistage random sampling method according to school type (public or private), number of classes, and gender. In choosing the sample, the following weighing procedures were used. First, the number of private and public schools was determined according to their percentages in all secondary schools in central Samsun. Hereafter, the number of classes VI, VII and VIII in the different schools was determined according to their percentages in all secondary schools in central Samsun. Finally, the classrooms were chosen randomly. The participants filled out the predesigned questionnaires under the supervision of trained nurses. The height and weight of students were measured in the classrooms. For the measurements, the students were dressed in light indoor clothing and had bare feet or stockings. The subjects were weighed to the nearest 0.1 kg with an electronic scale (Bosch, PPW4010; Stuttgart, Germany) that was calibrated daily at the beginning of each working day. Height was measured to the nearest 0.1 cm with a stadiometer (Charder HM200P Portstad Portable Stadiometer, Stuttgart, Germany) in a vertical erect position, with parallel feet, and with the shoulders and bottom touching the wall. The nurses recorded birth date and measured height and weight twice; the averages were recorded. The height and weight data were used to calculate the BMI (kg/m^2) using the formula: weight (kg) divided by height (m) squared. The cut-off points of CDC growth charts and percentiles of the age- and gender-specific BMI were used to determine Turkish children's underweight, overweight, and obesity status [10]. Students who had BMI for age ≥85th and <95th percentile of the reference population were classified as overweight and BMI for age ≥95th percentile of reference population were classified as obese. Students who had BMI for age <5th percentile of the reference population were classified as underweight.

2.2. Sedentary Behaviour. Television, videos, and computers are well-recognized domains of sedentary behaviour, but other sedentary activities in which adolescents engage include studying, sitting around and talking with friends, travel by motor vehicles, hobbies, and crafts. The questionnaire was developed to measure a broad range of sedentary activities common amongst adolescents reported in the literature [9]. The students were asked to report the time usually spent watching television, videos, or playing video games; using a computer for fun or study; doing homework/study or reading for fun; talking on the telephone, sitting with friends or hanging out; travelling in a car, bus, or train, before and after school on a usual weekday and for each weekend.

Table 2: BMI categories by gender.

BMI categories	Boys n	Boys %	Girls n	Girls %
Underweight	26	2.0	45	3.7
Normal	753	59.2	845	70.1
Overweight	354	27.9	200	16.6
Obese	138	10.9	116	9.6
Total	1271	100.0	1206	100.0

$X^2 = 53.4$; $P < 0.001$.

2.3. Statistical Analysis. Data was analyzed using SPSS for Windows, Release 12.0 (SPSS, Chicago, Ill, USA). Logistic regression and Chi-square analysis were applied to determine the statistical significance of the difference in the prevalence of obesity between the groups with respect to gender, school type, and time spent in sedentary behaviour. The significance of differences was defined as $P < 0.05$.

The study was approved by Local Ethic Committee of Medical Research of Ondokuz Mayıs University, and written informed consent was obtained from each parent.

3. Results

The sample is composed of 2477 children, including 1271 boys (51.3%) and 1206 girls (48.7%), 11 to 14 years old, attending secondary schools in the province of Samsun. The mean age was 12.8 ± 0.9 years, and the prevalence of obesity was defined at 10.3% (Table 1).

As shown in Table 2, there were higher numbers of overweight and obese students in boys than in girls statistically ($X^2 = 53.4$; $P < 0.001$).

A total of 95.9% of students attended public schools, while 4.1% attended private schools. The prevalence of obesity was 10.0% and 16.8% in public and private school students, respectively. The difference was statistically significant ($X^2 = 4.9$; $P < 0.05$).

As presented in Table 3, 46.8% of students had eaten their 3 daily meals regularly every day. The proportion of obese students that consumed fewer than three meals was

Table 3: BMI categories by daily meal regularity.

BMI categories	Regular (3 times/day)		Irregular	
	n	%	*n*	%
Underweight	33	2.9	38	2.9
Normal	765	65.9	833	63.2
Overweight	273	23.5	281	21.4
Obese	89	7.7	165	12.5
Total	1160	100.0	1317	100.0

$X^2 = 16.2$; $P < 0.01$.

significantly higher than that of those who consumed meals regularly during the day ($X^2 = 16.2$; $P < 0.01$).

Further, the number of students who skipped breakfast was 731 (29.5%), and the prevalence of obesity in students who skipped breakfast was found to be higher than that in their counterparts ($X^2 = 9.1$; $P < 0.05$).

While underweight students reported that they spend 5.2 ± 4.2 hours doing sports a week, normal, overweight, and obese students reported that they spend 6.0 ± 4.7 hours, 5.8 ± 4.6 hours, and 4.3 ± 3.5 hours, respectively. The difference was highly significant ($F = 8.9$; $P < 0.001$).

As shown in Table 4, the time spent in sedentary behaviour was the same in all BMI groups.

The prevalence of obesity was found to be higher in the group that spent over 3 hours watching TV than in those that spent less time (Table 5).

Step-down multiple logistic regression using backward LR method was applied to determine the significant correlates of obesity in the study population. The final model showed that gender (boys: OR = 1.557; 95% CI 1.174–2.064), irregular meal habits (OR = 1.843; 95% CI 1.398–2.430), private school (OR = 2.230; 95% CI 1.384–3.593), and sport (OR = 0.900; 95% CI 0.867–0.934) were significantly associated with obesity among the study population. The area under the curve for this final model was derived by multivariate logistic regression and was found to be 89.7% suggesting a good fit of the model.

4. Discussion

Childhood obesity is rapidly increasing in Europe, with the highest prevalence rates (31–39%) of overweight children reported in Mediterranean countries and in the USA (30% of children and adolescents who age 5–17 years are overweight) [11]. In this study the overall prevalence of obesity in secondary school children aged 11 to 14 years was found to be 10.3% and the prevalence of overweight was 22.4%. The prevalence of obesity is lower than in the USA and Europe but has demonstrated an increase in BMI amongst adolescents in the last decade. By comparison, in 1998, the prevalence of obesity in school children aged 12 to 15 years was found to be 5.1% in the province of Samsun [12]. High consumption of foods rich in fat and calories and the sedentary lifestyle among communities in the East Mediterranean region, in combination with a shift from traditional food to more Westernized foods characterized by high fat, high cholesterol, high sodium, and fibre contents, seem to be playing an important role in the rise of the level of obesity.

In some recent researches it was found that, of the obese and overweight children, most belonged to high social class families, and that less belonged to middle and low social class families [13, 14]. In our study, the prevalence of obesity was 10.0% and 16.8% in public and private school students, respectively. Similar findings were reported from India, that is, 6% were in corporation schools and 24% in well-off schools [15].

Consistent with some reports [16–18], and contrary to others [19, 20], the prevalence of obesity was found significantly higher in boys than in girls. The population living in the province of Samsun, in Northern Turkey, has middle-upper socioeconomic status. While the higher prevalence of obesity in boys occurring in Western Turkey has a high socioeconomic status, the prevalence of obesity is higher in girls in Eastern Turkey who are from a low socioeconomic status. For example, the prevalence of obesity was found to be 0.9% in boys and 3.8% in girls, aged between 8 and 17 years, in Elazig, in Eastern Turkey; contrary to these low prevalence rates, Neyzi et al. found a higher prevalence of obesity as 11.2% in adolescent boys and 9.4% in adolescent school girls aged 9–17 years in Istanbul, in Western Turkey [21]. Similarly, the prevalence of being overweight and obese was found to be higher in boys than in girls in Brazilian [22], Canadian [23], and Australian [24] adolescents. Unlike these results, in the studies conducted on Tehrani [18] and Egyptian [25] adolescent students, the prevalence of being overweight among girl students was found higher than among boys. A potential explanation could be that girls who live in developed countries have more chance with outdoor activities and sports than those who live in undeveloped and in some developing countries. Since the difference in obesity cannot be explained by differences in socioeconomic status alone, additional research is required to clarify why these regional and gender differences exist.

The prevalence of obesity was found to be significantly higher in the group that ate their daily meals irregularly when compared to the group that consistently ate their 3 daily meals. Previous studies have shown an inverse association between meal frequency and the prevalence of obesity in children [26] while others failed to detect significant associations [27]. Some studies have suggested that skipping breakfast is associated with the overweight/obese status [28, 29]. Skipping breakfast was also found to be associated with increased BMI in the current study. Moreover, it should be taken into consideration that the regression analysis indicated that irregular meal consumption is seen as a predictor of being obese. This highlights the importance of promoting the consumption of breakfast and all other meals throughout adolescence.

Although some studies found a better pattern of eating habits in children engaged in sports compared with their nonactive peers [30], in a current study both meal frequency and skipping breakfast were not associated with physical activity. Furthermore, this data needs some further attention since a significant association was found between meal frequency and obesity which linked the breakfast skipping

Table 4: BMI categories by time spent in other sedentary behaviour.

BMI categories	Time spent (hours/week) PC games and internet*	Homework reading*	Hanging out*	Travel*	Cinema*
Underweight	5.7 ± 4.3	8.2 ± 6.4	4.1 ± 3.8	0.9 ± 0.6	0.9 ± 0.8
Normal	5.8 ± 3.1	7.8 ± 6.5	4.3 ± 3.1	1.3 ± 0.8	1.2 ± 0.6
Overweight	6.3 ± 4.2	8.1 ± 6.7	3.9 ± 2.5	1.4 ± 1.1	1.3 ± 0.3
Obese	6.1 ± 4.6	8.3 ± 7.4	3.7 ± 2.8	1.3 ± 0.9	1.2 ± 0.6

*$P > 0.05$.

Table 5: BMI categories by time spent in watching TV.

BMI categories	Duration (hours/day) <3 hours		≥3 hours	
	n	%	n	%
Underweight	40	2.7	31	3.2
Normal	1007	67.0	591	60.6
Overweight	323	21.5	231	23.7
Obese	132	8.8	122	12.5
Total	1502	100.0	975	100.0

$X^2 = 13.6$; $P < 0.01$.

behaviour among children in developed countries. Ekelund et al. [31] reported that they did not observe any association between TV viewing and physical activity, and the association between TV viewing and adiposity was independent of physical activity. This may suggest that TV viewing does not displace physical activity and that other factors, such as dietary behaviour and quality while viewing TV, may influence energy balance and thereby body weight. In Turkish adolescents, the prevalence of obesity was found to be higher in the group that spent more than 3 hours watching TV than in those that spent less time, and there was no difference in the time spent in sedentary behaviour among different BMI categories except the duration of watching TV. Some researchers reported that children who spent more time watching television per day had significantly greater BMI, compared with those watching less than 2 hours per day [7, 32]. One meta-analysis, which found that sedentary behaviour was not associated with physical activity or BMI, also suggests that future research needs to consider different types and levels of sedentary behaviours when examining associations between physical activity and obesity [33]. The relationship between BMI and physical activity may be moderated by sedentary activity. This may explain why some researchers did not find an association between BMI and physical activity in children and adolescents despite the postulated relationship between reduced energy expenditure and obesity.

In conclusion, the current data provides strong evidence that supports the idea that the amount of hours spent watching television and irregular meal consumption of adolescents are directly related to the risk of obesity. In order to prevent childhood obesity, it is the duty of parents to monitor their children's lifestyle choices by reducing the consumption of fast food, being involved in regular family meals, and limiting the number of hours spent by their children watching television. In addition, in order to avoid greater pressure on future healthcare-related issues caused by obesity-related disorders, it is imperative to develop effective prevention strategies, for either all children or simply those Turkish adolescents living in urban areas who tend to be at a higher risk of obesity.

Conflict of Interests

The authors declare no conflict of interests.

Acknowledgments

The authors wish to thank Dr. Eylem Işık Uyar and Nurse Nefise Özyurt for their precious collaboration during data collection.

References

[1] M. A. Cretikos, L. Valenti, H. C. Britt, and L. A. Baur, "General practice management of overweight and obesity in children and adolescents in Australia," *Medical Care*, vol. 46, no. 11, pp. 1163–1169, 2008.

[2] R. R. Kipping, R. Jago, and D. A. Lawlor, "Obesity in children. Part 1: epidemiology, measurement, risk factors, and screening," *British Medical Journal*, vol. 337, p. a1824, 2008.

[3] Y. Wang and T. Lobstein, "Worldwide trends in childhood overweight and obesity," *International Journal of Pediatric Obesity*, vol. 1, no. 1, pp. 11–25, 2006.

[4] P. M. Anderson and K. F. Butcher, "Childhood obesity: trends and potential causes," *Future of Children*, vol. 16, no. 1, pp. 19–45, 2006.

[5] M. C. Gulliford, D. Mahabirb, B. Rockeb, S. Chinna, and R. Ronaa, "Overweight, obesity and skinfold thicknesses of children of African or Indian descent in Trinidad and Tobago," *International Journal of Epidemiology*, vol. 30, no. 5, pp. 989–998, 2001.

[6] M. Westwood, D. Fayter, S. Hartley et al., "Childhood obesity: should primary school children be routinely screened? A systematic review and discussion of the evidence," *Archives of Disease in Childhood*, vol. 92, no. 5, pp. 416–422, 2007.

[7] S. L. Wong and S. T. Leatherdale, "Association between sedentary behavior, physical activity, and obesity: inactivity among active kids," *Preventing Chronic Disease*, vol. 6, no. 1, p. A26, 2009.

[8] N. F. Krebs, M. S. Jacobson, and American Academy of Pediatrics Committee on Nutrition, "Prevention of pediatric overweight and obesity," *Pediatrics*, vol. 112, no. 2, pp. 424–430, 2003.

[9] L. L. Hardy, S. L. Bass, and M. L. Booth, "Changes in sedentary behavior among adolescent girls: a 2.5-year prospective cohort

study," *Journal of Adolescent Health*, vol. 40, no. 2, pp. 158–165, 2007.

[10] M. De Onis, A. W. Onyango, E. Borghi, A. Siyam, C. Nishida, and J. Siekmann, "Development of a WHO growth reference for school-aged children and adolescents," *Bulletin of the World Health Organization*, vol. 85, no. 9, pp. 660–667, 2007.

[11] A. Archenti and L. Pasqualinotto, "Childhood obesity: the epidemic of the third millenium," *Acta Biomedica de l'Ateneo Parmense*, vol. 79, no. 2, pp. 151–155, 2008.

[12] R. Sancak, C. Dundar, M. Totan et al., "The prevalence of obesity and predisposal factors in students of secondary school and lycee," *Journal of Experimental and Clinical Medicine*, vol. 16, no. 1, pp. 19–24, 1999.

[13] I. El-Bayoumy, I. Shady, and H. Lotfy, "Prevalence of obesity among adolescents (10 to 14 Years) in Kuwait," *Asia-Pacific Journal of Public Health*, vol. 21, no. 2, pp. 153–159, 2009.

[14] L. Sevcikova, J. Novakova, J. Hamade et al., "Social factors and nutritional status of children and adolescents," *Epidemiology*, vol. 19, no. 6, pp. 186–187, 2008.

[15] S. Bhave, A. Bavdekar, and M. Otiv, "IAP national task force for childhood prevention of adult diseases: childhood obesity," *Indian Pediatrics*, vol. 41, no. 6, pp. 559–575, 2004.

[16] N. F. Chu, "Prevalence and trends of obesity among school children in Taiwan—the Taipei children heart study," *International Journal of Obesity*, vol. 25, no. 2, pp. 170–176, 2001.

[17] E. Köksal, M. Gezmen Karadağ, H Yıldıran et al., "Dietary glycemic index, glycemic load and anthropometric measurements in adolescents," *Turkiye Klinikleri Journal of Medical Sciences*, vol. 31, no. 4, pp. 960–968, 2011.

[18] B. Mohammadpour-Ahranjani, A. Rashidi, M. Karandish, M. R. Eshraghian, and N. Kalantari, "Prevalence of overweight and obesity in adolescent Tehrani students, 2000-2001: an epidemic health problem," *Public Health Nutrition*, vol. 7, no. 5, pp. 645–648, 2004.

[19] R. Kelishadi, M. Hashemi Pour, N. Sarraf-Zadegan et al., "Obesity and associated modifiable environmental factors in Iranian adolescents: Isfahan healthy Heart program—heart health promotion from childhood," *Pediatrics International*, vol. 45, no. 4, pp. 435–442, 2003.

[20] H. Whelton, J. Harrington, E. Crowley, V. Kelleher, M. Cronin, and I. J. Perry, "Prevalence of overweight and obesity on the island of Ireland: results from the North South Survey of Children's Height, Weight and Body Mass Index, 2002," *BMC Public Health*, vol. 7, article 187, 2007.

[21] N. Öner, U. Vatansever, A. Sari et al., "Prevalence of underweight, overweight and obesity in Turkish adolescents," *Swiss Medical Weekly*, vol. 134, no. 35-36, pp. 529–533, 2004.

[22] D. A. S. Silva, A. Pelegrini, J. M. F. de Lima e Silva, and E. L. Petroski, "Epidemiology of abdominal obesity among adolescents from a Brazilian state capital," *Journal of Korean Medical Science*, vol. 26, no. 1, pp. 78–84, 2011.

[23] I. Janssen, P. T. Katzmarzyk, W. F. Boyce, M. A. King, and W. Pickett, "Overweight and obesity in Canadian adolescents and their associations with dietary habits and physical activity patterns," *Journal of Adolescent Health*, vol. 35, no. 5, pp. 360–367, 2004.

[24] T. Olds, M. Wake, G. Patton et al., "How do school-day activity patterns differ with age and gender across adolescence?" *Journal of Adolescent Health*, vol. 44, no. 1, pp. 64–72, 2009.

[25] E. Salazar-Martinez, B. Allen, C. Fernandez-Ortega, G. Torres-Mejia, O. Galal, and E. Lazcano-Ponce, "Overweight and obesity status among adolescents from Mexico and Egypt," *Archives of Medical Research*, vol. 37, no. 4, pp. 535–542, 2006.

[26] A. M. Toschke, H. Küchenhoff, B. Koletzko, and R. Von Kries, "Meal frequency and childhood obesity," *Obesity Research*, vol. 13, no. 11, pp. 1932–1938, 2005.

[27] T. A. Nicklas, S. J. Yang, T. Baranowski, I. Zakeri, and G. Berenson, "Eating patterns and obesity in children—the Bogalusa Heart Study," *American Journal of Preventive Medicine*, vol. 25, no. 1, pp. 9–16, 2003.

[28] G. Barba, E. Troiano, P. Russo, and A. Siani, "Total fat, fat distribution and blood pressure according to eating frequency in children living in southern Italy: the ARCA project," *International Journal of Obesity*, vol. 30, no. 7, pp. 1166–1169, 2006.

[29] G. R. H. Sandercock, C. Voss, and L. Dye, "Associations between habitual school-day breakfast consumption, body mass index, physical activity and cardiorespiratory fitness in English schoolchildren," *European Journal of Clinical Nutrition*, vol. 64, no. 10, pp. 1086–1092, 2010.

[30] J. K. Croll, D. Neumark-Sztainer, M. Story, M. Wall, C. Perry, and L. Harnack, "Adolescents involved in weight-related and power team sports have better eating patterns and nutrient intakes than non-sport-involved adolescents," *Journal of the American Dietetic Association*, vol. 106, no. 5, pp. 709–717, 2006.

[31] U. Ekelund, S. Brage, K. Froberg et al., "TV viewing and physical activity are independently associated with metabolic risk in children: the European youth heart study," *PLoS Medicine*, vol. 3, no. 12, pp. 2449–2457, 2006.

[32] J. Giammattei, G. Blix, H. H. Marshak, A. O. Wollitzer, and D. J. Pettitt, "Television watching and soft drink consumption: associations with obesity in 11- to 13-year-old schoolchildren," *Archives of Pediatrics and Adolescent Medicine*, vol. 157, no. 9, pp. 882–886, 2003.

[33] H. Munakata, M. Sei, A. A. Ewis et al., "Prediction of Japanese children at risk for complications of childhood obesity: gender differences for intervention approaches," *Journal of Medical Investigation*, vol. 57, no. 1-2, pp. 62–68, 2010.

5

Heme Iron Content in Lamb Meat Is Differentially Altered upon Boiling, Grilling, or Frying as Assessed by Four Distinct Analytical Methods

Azin Pourkhalili,[1] Maryam Mirlohi,[2] and Ebrahim Rahimi[1]

[1] *Department of Food Science and Technology, Faculty of Agriculture, Islamic Azad University, Shahrekord Branch, Shahrekord 88137-33395, Iran*
[2] *Food Security Research Center, School of Nutrition and Food Science, Isfahan University of Medical Science, Isfahan 8174-73461, Iran*

Correspondence should be addressed to Maryam Mirlohi; m_mirlohi@hlth.mui.ac.ir

Academic Editors: K. Ebihara and D. Li

Lamb meat is regarded as an important source of highly bioavailable iron (heme iron) in the Iranians diet. The main objective of this study is to evaluate the effect of traditional cooking methods on the iron changes in lamb meat. Four published experimental methods for the determination of heme iron were assessed analytically and statistically. Samples were selected from lambs' loin. Standard methods (AOAC) were used for proximate analysis. For measuring heme iron, the results of four experimental methods were compared regarding their compliance to Ferrozine method which was used for the determination of nonheme iron. Among three cooking methods, the lowest total iron and heme iron were found in boiling method. The heme iron proportions to the total iron in raw, boiled lamb meat and grilled, were counted as 65.70%, 67.75%, and 76.01%, receptively. Measuring the heme iron, the comparison of the methods in use showed that the method in which heme extraction solution was composed of 90% acetone, 18% water, and 2% hydrochloric acid was more appropriate and more correlated with the heme iron content calculated by the difference between total iron and nonheme iron.

1. Introduction

Being a rich source of protein as well as having balanced component of most essential elements like vitamins and minerals, red meat plays an important role in human' diet especially in developing countries where the intakes of synthetic supplements and alternative fortified foods are less in diet. The importance of meat iron depends on its heme iron content with more bioavailability (from 15% to 35%) than that of the nonheme (2% to 20%) [1]. Based on official data reported in Iran, Iran is the sixth world's producer of lamb or mutton meat; annual consumption of red meat is estimated to be 12.3 kg per capita. Lamb meat is the most popular type of meat among Iranians. However, endemic anemia due to iron deficiency is highly prevalent [2].

It is proven that during cooking, as a heat-induced interaction, oxidation of myoglobin results in oxidative cleavage of porphyrin ring of heme, and some portions of heme iron are converted in to nonheme iron. However, studies have shown that the severity of the reaction is influenced by the applied cooking method as well as the type of meat. In this regard, the previous studies have not supported a similar result.

Turhan et al. studied the effect of cooking methods on total and heme iron contents of fish species. They showed significant differences between the cooking methods; the highest total and heme iron losses were observed in grilled fish [3]. While, according to Schricher and Miller, the highest heme iron loss was found in microwave-cooked and baked beef samples [4].

To determine the content of heme iron and nonheme iron in meat, one of them is usually measured and subtracted from the total iron in order to obtain the content of the another one. The measuring methods of heme iron and nonheme iron are performed in a completely different manner this may lead to different interpretations which result in variation among the reported studies. For heme iron measurement, the spectrophotometric method introduced by Hornsey is well referred in the literature [5]. However, there are some slight differences in the adopted experiments conducted by other researchers regarding the proportion of the samples to heme iron extraction solution as well as the composition of the solution used for heme iron extraction with respect to acetone, water, and hydrochloric acid. Variation in the applied methods might also be an alternative source of inconsistency among the results of previous studies.

Since the traditional ways of cooking lamb in Iran are boiling, frying, and grilling, the main objective of this study was to evaluate the effect of traditional cooking methods on the heme iron to nonheme iron conversion. In this regard, this study looked to the correlation between the results of four heme iron measurement methods and the results of its calculation based on non heme iron measurement.

2. Material and Methods

2.1. Sample Procedures. Five raw nonprepacked meat samples from sheep (Lori-Bakhtiari, 6 months) were purchased from selected butchery in Isfahan, Iran. Sections of longissimus dorsi meat from each sample were aseptically removed and placed in separate sterile plastic bags to prevent spilling and cross-contamination and were immediately transported to the laboratory in a cooler with ice packs. Muscle samples were trimmed of connective and adipose tissues and sliced into square cuts of 2.5 × 2.5 cm of thickness. The cuts were vacuum packed in four layers of polyethylene packagings and were stored frozen at −18 until analysis. Frozen samples were thawed 4-5 h at 4 ± 2°C before analysis. All the analyses were done in triplicate for each meat sample.

2.2. Cooking Methods. The meat samples were subjected to each of the cooking method (boiling, frying, and grilling), while the raw meat was sampled directly as an uncooked control. Internal temperatures were monitored using thermometer (thermometer ST-131 waterproof digital).

Boiling was performed at approximately 97°C (water temperature) for 90 min in stainless steel pan. The internal temperature during boiling was 93°C. The meat samples were pan fried in sunflower oil for 20 min. The internal temperature during frying was determined as 85°C. Grilled meats were prepared using burning stove. The cuts were placed at 10 cm above the flame for 10 min, turned by 2 min interval. The internal temperature was not exceeded at 86°C.

2.3. Proximate Composition. Proximate composition of raw and cooked lamb meat was done for moisture, fat, ash, protein, and loss weight content. Moisture contents of ground meat sample were determined by drying in an oven at 105°C until constant weight [6]. The fat content was determined by Folch method [7]. Ash content was determined as dried for 4 h at 125°C at heated temperature oven (500–550°C) for 6–8 h [8]. The protein was determined by micro-Kjeldahl procedure [9]. Loss weight was determined by weighting samples before and after cooking.

2.4. Total Iron. An accurately weighed 3 g sample was dried for 4 h at 125°C as heated temperature oven (500–550°C) for 6–8 h. The ash was digested in 5 mL of 2 M HNO_3 by boiling for about 2 min and then left to cool down to the room temperature. The cooled solution was filtered through Whatman filter paper (no.41) and made up to 25 mL with 2 M HNO_3. The samples were then analyzed for total iron by atomic absorption spectrophotometery (Model 2380, PerkinElmer, USA) at a wavelength of 248.3 nm [8].

2.5. Heme Iron. Heme iron was determined using four Hornsey modified methods [5].

Experiment A. Ground sample (10 g) was weighed into 50 mL centrifuge tubes. Then, 20 mL of acid-acetone mixture was added (40 mL of acetone, 9 mL of water, and 1 mL of concentrated hydrochloric acid). Each sample was homogenized for 30 s. Then, an additional 20 mL of acid-acetone mixture was added, and the samples were mixed thoroughly the tubes were then capped tightly and kept in the dark for 1 h. The extract was centrifuged at 2200 rpm for 10 min. The supernatant was filtered through glass microfiber filters (Whatman GF/A), and the absorbance was measured at 640 nm (Model 6105, Jenway Uv/Vis Spectrophotometer, UK) against a reagent blank [3].

Experiment B. Ground sample (10 g) was weighed into 50 mL centrifuge tubes. Then, 45 mL of acid-acetone mixture was added (45 mL of acetone, 4 mL of water, and 0.5 mL of concentrated hydrochloric acid). Each sample was homogenized for 30 s. The samples were mixed thoroughly the tubes were then capped tightly and kept in the dark for 1 h. Further steps were carried out as in experiment 1 [10].

Experiment C. Ground sample (5 g) was weighed into 50 mL centrifuge tubes. Then, 10 mL of acid-acetone mixture was added (40 mL of acetone, 8 mL of water, and 1 mL of concentrated hydrochloric acid). Each sample was homogenized for 30 s. Then, an additional 10 mL of acid-acetone mixture was added, and the samples were mixed thoroughly the tubes were then capped tightly and kept in the dark for 30 min. The extract was centrifuged at 3000 rpm for 20 min, and the supernatant was processed as in experiments 1 and 2 [11].

Experiment D. Freeze-dried meat sample (0.05 g) was weighted into 50 mL centrifuge tubes. Then, 20 mL of acid-acetone mixture was added (15.6 mL of acetone, 3.75 mL of water, and 0.65 mL of concentrated hydrochloric acid). Each sample was homogenized for 30 s. The extract was centrifuged at 2200 rpm for 10 min. the supernatant was processed as above in experiments 1 and 2 [12].

The absorbance was multiplied by 6800 and then divided by the sample weight to give the concentration of total pigments in the meat as μg hematin/g meat. The iron content was calculated with the factor of 0.0882 μg iron/μg hematin [3].

Table 1: Proximate composition of raw and cooked lamb (dry weight basis).

	Moisture (%)	Fat (%)	Ash (%)	Protein (%)	Loss weight (%)
Raw	73.60 ± 0.28*	33.51 ± 0.31	3.77 ± 0.03	63.40 ± 0.21	—
Boiled	60.50 ± 0.09	25.64 ± 0.74	1.84 ± 0.04	53.84 ± 0.48	46.80 ± 0.23
Fried	53.33 ± 2.25	58.10 ± 1.15	4.40 ± 0.01	59.45 ± 0.33	42.42 ± 0.45
Grilled	64.16 ± 0.75	34.16 ± 0.45	3.88 ± 0.04	60.05 ± 0.38	32.88 ± 1.05

*Data in the table are means of triplicate independent experiments.

2.6. Nonheme Iron. Nonheme iron was analyzed by the Ferrozine method described by Ahn et al. [13]. Briefly, 0.50 g of freeze-dried sample was dissolved in 3 mL of 0.1 M citrate phosphate buffer (pH 5.5) and 1 mL of 2% ascorbic acid in 0.2 M HCl and was left to stand at room temperature for 15 min before adding 2 mL of 11.3% trichloroacetic acid and then was centrifuged at 3000 rpm for 10 min. To 2 mL of the supernatant, 0.8 mL of 10% ammonium acetate and 0.2 mL Ferrozine reagent were added, and the absorbance was measured at 562 nm (Model 6105, Jenway Uv/Vis Spectrophotometer, UK) against a standard curve [14]. Using 1000 mg/L stock solution of $FeCl_3$, standard solutions were adjusted at 10, 25, 50, and 100 mg/L.

Standard curve was prepared by plotting the absorbance against the several concentrations of $FeCl_3$ standard solutions. The represented equation of $y = 0.0015x+$ was obtained with $r^2 = 0.92$.

All the chemical reagents was from (Merck-Germany) with the exception of Ferrozine reagent which was from (Sigma-USA).

2.7. Statistical Analysis. All data were tested using one-way ANOVA test and the pairwise comparison was performed using Tukey-Kramer multiple comparison test. The level of significance was established at $P = 0.05$. Spearman correlation was used to find the most correlated heme measuring method to non heme iron determination Ferrozin method. SPSS software was used for data analyzing.

3. Result and Discussion

The results of the proximate analyses are presented in Table 1. The highest and the lowest moisture losses were found to be 20% and 9% in the fried and grilled samples, respectively. Fat content increased in fried and grilled samples and decreased in boiled ones. Previously, it was reported that the lowest moisture loss happens through grilling [15]. Frying and boiling resulted in the highest and the lowest fatty material in the cooked lamb pieces, respectively, which could be explained by oil absorption in fried samples [16, 17].

During the cooking process, meat protein denaturation occurs, and subsequent reduction in water holding capacity of proteins causes moisture loss and an increase in total dry matter and yields higher concentration of other components in the cooked meat. However, a portion of fat is melted and runs out with cooking juice; hence, the remained fatty material in the cooked meat is the outcome of the both above processes which completely depends on the cooking method. The ash content increased by grilling and frying up to 2.91% and 16.71% from that of the ash in raw sample, respectively, but it was reduced by 51.2% in the boiled samples [18].

The results of total iron, nonheme iron and heme iron determination are presented in Table 2, where heme iron was measured using four tested experiments, all derived from the Hornsey method [5]. Total iron was decreased after cooking by 52.28%, 33.37%, and 30.44% of its primary concentration in raw sample by boiling, frying, and grilling, respectively. The difference between raw, boiled, and fried samples was significant ($P < 0.05$). The least total iron change occurred in grilled samples. Instead, boiling caused noticeable iron loss. Although the decrease in total iron due to cooking was previously reported by others, the result obtained in the present study was in contrast to the result found by Turhan et al. in which the highest total iron loss happened in grilling (52.60%) [3]. Such difference may be due to different type of examined meats (fish and lamb) as well as different time and temperature profile applied in that study.

Reporting the iron concentration on the wet base gave rise to different results. An increase in the total iron in some of the cooked samples was observed (data is not shown). Such increase could be explained by decrease in the moisture content of the cooked samples due to protein denaturation and reduction in water holding capacity [12]. It was shown that cooking (baking) caused an increase in the total iron content in beef and lamb meat by 73% and 43%, respectively. Likewise, similar results were reported for beef by Purchas et al. when wet-based changes took in to account [14].

Nonheme iron also decreased after heat treatment (Table 2) in all the examined samples. Since the total iron underwent basic changes, variation in nonheme iron can be better explained by its ratio to the total iron in each treated sample which is presented in Table 3. In that setting, the highest non heme iron was observed in boiled ones. Because during a boiling treatment the temperature does not exceed 100°C, it is considered as mild cooking method, but long processing time (90 minutes) in our study alongside water vapor pressure may induce more non heme formation in boiled samples than that of fried and grilled counterparts.

Increase in the non heme iron concentration after cooking was reported by others [4, 14].

The presented results of heme iron determination in Table 2 showed that the slight differences in the four Hornsey derived heme iron measuring methods examined in this study have great impact on the obtained results. Using method D, the determined heme iron concentration

TABLE 2: Total iron, nonheme iron, and heme iron, measured by four distinct methods in raw and cooked lamb (μg/g) (dry weight basis).

	Total iron	Nonheme iron	Heme iron A	Heme iron B	Heme iron C	Heme iron D
			*44.62 ± 1.38[ad]	38.92 ± 2.49[ad]	73.67 ± 14.19[ad]	73.31 ± 31.4[a]
Raw	67.91 ± 8.07[a]	21.19 ± 2.89[a]	**40.98 49.14	36.44 41.41	60.88 95.02	31.2 99.6
			***6.93	6.38	19.26	42.81
			21.96 ± 1.08[bc]	21.42 ± 6.61[bc]	41.37 ± 7.09[b]	62.67 ± 32.6[a]
Boiled	32.41 ± 13.63[b]	17.36 ± 1.68[a]	20.51 23.09	14.91 30.65	30.87 56.51	26.98 85.16
			4.92	30.85	17.13	36.51
			32.57 ± 6.39[acd]	31.36 ± 2.00[acd]	65.94 ± 9.62[acd]	82.01 ± 18.48[a]
Fried	45.25 ± 6.35[b]	14.98 ± 3.96[a]	22.91 43.95	28.42 33.40	54.34 80.84	54.57 93.56
			19.63	6.37	14.59	22.53
			35.91 ± 6.97[ad]	33.74 ± 3.85[ad]	72.19 ± 22.33[acd]	82.0 ± 40.4[a]
Grilled	47.24 ± 16.22[ab]	15.48 ± 4.30[a]	26.12 48.30	30.38 37.94	44.82 96.87	46.8 125.9
			19.40	11.41	30.95	49.29

Within the columns, the values with different letter are significantly different ($P < 0.05$).
*Mean ± standard error.
**Minimum–Maximum range.
***Coefficient of variation.

exceeded the total iron content of the given samples. Using method C, the same result was observed. Bi variable Spearman correlation between the results of each heme iron measuring method and the calculated heme iron after non heme iron subtraction from that of the total iron was performed. The results showed that, using methods A and B, there was a significant correlation between the two sets of heme iron data mentioned above ($P = 0.003$ and $P = 0.014$). But, it was not the case for the two other methods (C and D). For the methods tested, A, B, C, and D, r^2 was obtained as 0.997, 0.986, 0.9, and 0.5, respectively. Therefore, comparing to other examined heme iron measuring methods, the method adopted by Turhan et al. in which heme extraction solution included more water and less acetone gave better results. Also, it was found in the present study that the experiments time length reduction had great impact on the accuracy of the results. This was considered in the given experiment [3].

Pigmentation and subsequent turbidity of the heme containing extraction solution is the main source of error for its spectrophotometric measurement. The higher proportion of acetone to other components of the extraction solution adversely affected the stability of the given solution. Therefore, the less acetone content in the heme extraction solution in method A could be regarded as one of the reasons that this method resulted in less pigmentation and provided more stable results comparing to other tested experiments.

Despite the sufficient number of repeated measurements, coefficients of variations obtained in the spectrophotometric measurements of heme iron by all tested methods analytically were not considered as proper values, which indicate a vast variation among the repeated measurements. It was particularly observable in the cooked meat samples and was more troublesome for the samples in which heat-induced Millard reaction and caramelization developed more complex colored substances.

Using the four experiments, boiled samples persistently showed to have the least heme iron content (Table 2). Based on the both reliable methods (A and B) in this study, heme iron concentration decreased in the all heat-treated samples; however, significant reduction occurred in boiling ($P > 0.05$). This is in accordance with the result of Turhan et al. [3] that stated that heme iron in fish reduced to 40.06%, 27.87%, 54.45% and 69.70% in baking, grilling, microwave, and boiling, respectively. In another study, it was illustrated that the heme iron content of meat decreased after heat treatment [19]. But, increase in the heme iron concentration through cooking (on the wet bases) was reported by about 53.48%, 33.92%, and 61.93% of the raw sample's heme iron concentration for beef, lamb, and turkey meat, respectively [12].

In Table 3, proportions of heme iron and non heme iron to the total iron in each set of samples are shown. Here, heme iron was obtained by method A. Nonheme iron was separately measured, using Ferrozine method. A logical adverse trend is observable between the presented data which confirms the primary result of this study stating that method A can be regarded as the most reliable and reproducible mean of heme iron spectrophotometric determination.

4. Conclusion

The results of this study showed that among the traditional cooking methods currently employed in Iran, grilling has the lowest impact on the total iron reduction and heme iron to nonheme iron conversion in lamb meat. In contrast, boiling has the most deteriorative effect on the nutritional value of lamb meat regarding the iron content and the relevant changes. This reduction could be critical when iron bioavailability is of concern in a society. Moreover, comparing the results derived from Hornsey's heme iron determination

Table 3: Percentage of heme iron and nonheme iron to total iron in raw and cooked lamb meat.

	Heme iron (%)*	Nonheme iron (%)**
Raw	65.70	31.20
Boiled	67.75	53.56
Fried	71.97	33.10
Grilled	76.01	32.76

*Heme iron determined by method A.
**Nonheme iron determined by Ferrozine method.

method, the one modified by Turhan et al., would bring about more accurate results which are well correlated with the results of Ferrozin nonheme iron method.

References

[1] L. K. Mahan and S. Escott-Stump, *Krouses Food, Nutrition, & Diet Theropy*, World of nutrition, Tehran, Iran, 2005.

[2] N. Rokni, *Meat Science & Technology*, University of Tehran, Tehran, Iran, 2003.

[3] S. Turhan, N. S. Ustun, and T. B. Altunkaynak, "Effect of cooking methods on total and heme iron contents of anchovy (*Engraulis encrasicholus*)," *Food Chemistry*, vol. 88, no. 2, pp. 169–172, 2004.

[4] B. Schricker and D. Miller, "Effects of cooking and chemical treatment on heme and nonheme iron in meat," *Journal of Food Science*, vol. 48, no. 4, pp. 1340–1343, 1983.

[5] H. Hornsey, "The colour of cooked cured pork. I.—Estimation of the Nitric oxide-Haem Pigments," *Journal of the Science of Food and Agriculture*, vol. 7, no. 8, pp. 534–540, 2006.

[6] AOAC, *Official Methods of Analysis of the Association of the Official Analysis Chemists*, Association of Official Analytical Chemist, Arlington, Va, USA, 15th edition, 1990.

[7] J. Folch, M. Lees, and G. H. Sloane-Stanley, "A simple method for the isolation and purification of total lipides from animal tissues," *The Journal of Biological Chemistry*, vol. 226, no. 1, pp. 497–509, 1957.

[8] S. Turhan, T. B. Altunkaynak, and F. Yazici, "A note on the total and heme iron contents of ready-to-eat doner kebabs," *Meat Science*, vol. 67, no. 2, pp. 191–194, 2004.

[9] AOAC, *Official Methods of Analysis of the Association of the Official Analysis Chemists*, Association of Official Analytical Chemist, Arlington, Va, USA, 16th edition, 1995.

[10] A. Ramos, M. C. Cabrera, M. del Puerto, and A. Saadoun, "Minerals, haem and non-haem iron contents of rhea meat," *Meat Science*, vol. 81, no. 1, pp. 116–119, 2009.

[11] N. Soltanizadeh, *Phisicochemical and Microbiological Character of Camel Meat Sausage, in Agriculture*, Isfahan technology university, Isfahan, Iran, 2007.

[12] G. Lombardi-Boccia, B. Martinez-Dominguez, and A. Aguzzi, "Total heme and non-heme iron in raw and cooked meats," *Journal of Food Science*, vol. 67, no. 5, pp. 1738–1741, 2002.

[13] D. Ahn, F. Wolfe, and J. Sim, "Three methods for determining nonheme iron in turkey meat," *Journal of Food Science*, vol. 58, no. 2, pp. 288–291, 1993.

[14] R. W. Purchas, D. C. Simcock, T. W. Knight, and B. H. P. Wilkinson, "Variation in the form of iron in beef and lamb meat and losses of iron during cooking and storage," *International Journal of Food Science and Technology*, vol. 38, no. 7, pp. 827–837, 2003.

[15] C. M. M. Alfaia, S. P. Alves, A. F. Lopes et al., "Effect of cooking methods on fatty acids, conjugated isomers of linoleic acid and nutritional quality of beef intramuscular fat," *Meat Science*, vol. 84, no. 4, pp. 769–777, 2010.

[16] M. Candela, I. Astiasarán, and J. Bello, "Deep-fat frying modifies high-fat fish lipid fraction," *Journal of Agricultural and Food Chemistry*, vol. 46, no. 7, pp. 2793–2796, 1998.

[17] I. S. Saguy and D. Dana, "Integrated approach to deep fat frying: engineering, nutrition, health and consumer aspects," *Journal of Food Engineering*, vol. 56, no. 2-3, pp. 143–152, 2003.

[18] J. Weber, V. C. Bochi, C. P. Ribeiro, A. D. M. Victório, and T. Emanuelli, "Effect of different cooking methods on the oxidation, proximate and fatty acid composition of silver catfish (*Rhamdia quelen*) fillets," *Food Chemistry*, vol. 106, no. 1, pp. 140–146, 2008.

[19] C. Chen, A. M. Pearson, J. I. Gray et al., "Some factors influencing the nonheme iron content of meat and its implications in oxidation," *Journal of Food Science*, vol. 49, no. 2, pp. 581–584, 1984.

Energy Requirement and Food Intake Behaviour in Young Adult Intact Male Cats with and without Predisposition to Overweight

Brigitta Wichert,[1] Julia Trossen,[1] Daniel Uebelhart,[2] Marcel Wanner,[1] and Sonja Hartnack[3]

[1] *Institute of Animal Nutrition, Vetsuisse Faculty, University of Zurich, Winterthurerstraße 260, 8057 Zurich, Switzerland*
[2] *Department of Rheumatology and Institute of Physical Medicine, University Hospital Zurich, Gloriastraße 25, 8091 Zurich, Switzerland*
[3] *Section of Epidemiology, Vetsuisse Faculty, University of Zurich, Winterthurerstraße 270, 8057 Zurich, Switzerland*

Correspondence should be addressed to Brigitta Wichert, bwichert@vetphys.uzh.ch

Academic Editor: Anna Brzozowska

Obesity is a common problem in cats. In the experimental cat family of the institute of animal nutrition besides a "normal" lean phenotype, cats with predisposition to an overweight phenotype are present. To investigate energy requirements and food intake behaviour of intact male cats of different phenotypes, six "normal" lean cats (GL) and six cats disposed to overweight (GO) were used. At the beginning of the experiment, all cats had an ideal body condition score of 5. To reach this the GO cats had to pass a weight-loss program. Energy requirements of the cats were determined using respiration chambers, whereas the amount and frequency of food intake was measured with a feeding station recording the data automatically. Energy requirement at weight constancy of the GO cats was even on fat-free mass (FFM) significantly ($P = 0.02$) lower (162.6 kJ/kg FFM/d) than that of the "normal" lean cats (246 kJ/kg FFM/d). The GO cats also showed a higher food intake 34.5 ± 1.5 g dry matter/kg body weight$^{0.67}$ compared to the GL cats (24.0 ± 2.1 g dry matter/kg body weight$^{0.67}$)($P = 0.001$). In conclusion quantifiable differences in food intake and behaviour in cats predisposed to overweight compared to "normal" lean cats were found.

1. Introduction

Obesity is an increasing problem in cats. In recent studies, the prevalence of feline obesity in different countries has ranged from 6% to 52% [1, 2]. Obesity is the result of a higher energy intake in comparison to the energy requirement. This can be caused by an increased energy intake, decreased energy expenditure, or both. Multiple factors like castration, highly palatable food, cats keeping indoors, and genetic factors are related to obesity [2–4]. In several human and rodent studies, a genetic background was supported [5–7]. Recently also in cats a genetic association with overweight has been described in the experimental cat population of the Institute of Animal Nutrition of the Vetsuisse Faculty of Zurich [8]. However, to our knowledge, nothing is known about energy expenditure or food intake behaviour of intact cats developing overweight. An increase in food intake can be due to a higher meal frequency or a higher food intake per meal. The cat as a hunter of small prey animals has to eat about twelve small prey animals, corresponding to twelve meals in 24 hours [9]. A similar meal frequency of about 12–20 meals per day was observed in the studies of Mugford and Thorne [10], Kane et al. [11], and Peachey and Harper [12]. However, Horwitz et al. [13] described that meal size was influenced by daytime as well as palatability and protein content of food. In contrast to this, the speed of food intake was more connected to food structure.

The aim of the present study was to quantify the difference in energy expenditure or food intake behaviour in intact male cats with and without predisposition to overweight.

2. Material and Methods

2.1. Cats. The study population consisted of six intact male cats displaying a phenotype lean (group GL) and six intact male cats with a phenotype overweight (group GO) aged 1.3 ± 0.06 years. Classification into phenotype lean/overweight was based on body condition score (BCS) measured

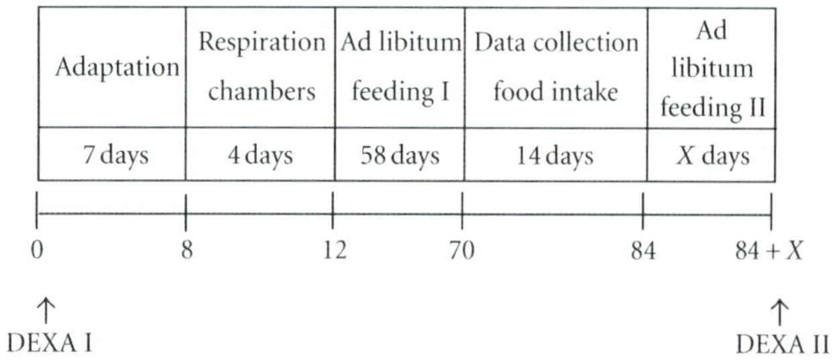

FIGURE 1: Experimental study design of the five experimental phases including measurements in the respiration chambers, measurements of food intake as well as dual energy X-ray absorptiometry measurements.

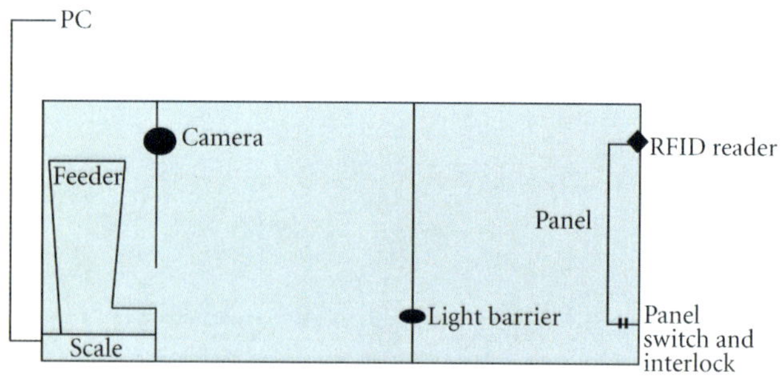

FIGURE 2: Design of the automatically cat food station: documenting food intake per meal, meal frequency, visits of the station without eating, and the time of entering the station. The cats were recognized by their implanted microchip.

TABLE 1: Chemical composition (%) of the commercial dry cat food used during the whole experiment.

Ingredients	Content
Crude protein	32%
Crude fat	21%
Crude fiber	2%
Crude ash	6%
Nitrogen-free extracts	31%
Dry matter	92%
Gross energy	22.9 kJ

at month eight according to Laflamme [14]. All cats were reared under the same conditions, clinically healthy, and intact male European Shorthair cats. They originated from a larger breeding project with a focus on segregation of lean and overweight phenotypes in the cat-breeding family of the Institute of Animal Nutrition at the Vetsuisse Faculty, Zurich [8]. Ethical approval for animal experimentation was obtained from the Swiss veterinary authorities (license number 180/2009).

2.2. Study Design. The experimental study design comprised five different phases (Figure 1). Before starting the experiment, all cats of group GO passed through a weight loss program until reaching a BCS of 5. After that the cats of group GO were fed to maintain a constant body weight (BW) for at least 4 weeks. The cats of group GL were fed ad libitum during the whole experiment.

2.2.1. Adaptation Period (Duration 7 Days). The cats of group GO were fed to maintain a constant bodyweight (BW). During the adaptation period, cats were adapted to a commercial dry cat food (Table 1) and special cat toilettes allowing for separate collection of faeces and urine [15].

2.2.2. Respiration Chamber Period (Duration 5 Days). Cats were kept individually for 22.5 hours per day in the respiration chambers (1.4 m × 1.0 m × 0.9 m). After one day for adaptation, on a daily basis, O_2 consumption and CO_2 production were determined with reference to body weight, body weight$^{0.67}$, and fat-free mass [16]. On a daily basis, faeces and urine were collected separately, and food intake was measured. From these data nitrogen, carbon and energy balances were calculated.

An equalized energy balance at weight constancy is named energy requirement in the text although energy consumption in respiration chambers mostly is lower compared to that under usual living conditions, as activity is limited.

2.2.3. Ad Libitum Feeding Phase I (Duration 58 Days). During this period cats were kept in groups of two cats each in an indoor-outdoor enclosure.

2.2.4. Automatic Food Station Phase (Duration 14 Days). During this phase, food intake per meal, frequency of meals, visits of the station without eating, and the time of entering the station were recorded. The intake of metabolisable energy (ME) was calculated using the ME-content of the dry food determined during the respiration measurement. Additionally, each action of the cats was documented using a camera. The automatic feeding station (Figure 2) recognized the cats by their implanted chip and assured that there was only one cat each inside the station with help of a light barrier that recognized movements in the feeding station. For the function of the feeding station as well as the documentation of the data, special software was developed (Gruber Informatik AG, Bergdietikon, Switzerland).

2.2.5. Ad Libitum Feeding Phase II (Duration Variable; Min 4 Weeks, Max 27 Weeks). During this period two cats were kept together in an indoor-outdoor enclosure and fed until a constant body weight was obtained for at least four weeks.

2.3. Measurements and Analysis

2.3.1. Body Weight and Body Fat. During the measurements in the respiration chamber, the cats were weighed daily, during other phases weekly. As shown in Figure 1, before respiration measurements and at the end of the second ad libitum feeding phase after four weeks of weight constancy, body fat content and lean body mass (=fat-free mass (FFM)) were determined by dual X-ray absorptiometry (DEXA).

Table 2: Mean of body weight (BW), body fat mass (total (g), and (%)) fat-free body mass (total (g), and (%)) and body weight (g) of the cats of the groups GL (lean phenotype) and GO (overweight phenotype); DEXA I: first DEXA measurement before the adaptation period; DEXA II: second DEXA measurement at the end of the second phase of ad libitum feeding after four weeks of weight constancy.

	GL		GO	
	DEXA I	DEXA II	DEXA I	DEXA II
Body weight ± SE (g)	5063 ± 251[aA]	4992 ± 267[aA]	5036 ± 261[aA]	6487 ± 324[bB]
Fat mass ± SE (g)	380 ± 51[aA]	336 ± 81[aA]	199 ± 39[aB]	893 ± 94[bB]
Fat mass ± SE (%)	7 ± 1[aA]	7 ± 1[aA]	5 ± 1[aB]	14 ± 1[bB]
Fat free mass ± SE (g)	4543.0 ± 214.4[aA]	4656.2 ± 196.9[aA]	4768.8 ± 262.2[aA]	5429.7± 251.6[bB]
Fat free mass ± SE (%)	89.8 ± 0.8[aA]	90.7 ± 1.4[aA]	92.0 ± 0.8[aB]	83.8 ± 1.0[bB]

Different letters show significant differences ($P < 0.05$), capital letters show group differences, whereas small letters show differences within one group.

Table 3: Differences between both phenotypes estimated with a linear mixed model approach (group means and standard errors of the estimated effect due to phenotype; GL: lean phenotype, GO: overweight phenotype).

	Phenotype GL mean	Phenotype GO mean	S.E.	P value
O_2 L/kg $BW^{0.67}$/d	19.67	17.31	1.05	0.026
O_2 L/kg BW/d	11.71	10.26	0.64	0.035
O_2 L/kg FFM/d	12.88	10.87	0.8	0.022
CO_2 L/kg $BW^{0.67}$/d	16.66	14.75	0.64	0.008
CO_2 L/kg BW/d	9.59	8.74	0.4	0.046
CO_2 L/kg FFM/d	10.57	9.25	0.46	0.01

For the DEXA measurement in the sternal recumbency, a Hologic QDR 4500 Discovery machine (Bedford, MA, USA) was used. QDR System software Version 12.4 and the Infant Whole Body scan type were used. The machine's lower body fat-measuring limit was approximately 4%. For data analyses, the global mode (includes the whole body with extremities and head) was used. The cats were sedated with medetomidine 0.05 mg/kg BW and butorphanol 0.2 mg/kg BW.

2.3.2. Statistical Analyses. The objective of the statistical analysis was to test the hypothesis of difference in "normal" lean cats and cats predisposed to overweight. For comparisons between two groups at the same time point or two time points within the same group, non-parametric tests (Wilcoxon rank sum and Wilcoxon signed rank) were performed with the software NCSS 2007 version 7.1.20 (Kaysville, Utah, USA). Statistical significance was set at $P \leq 0.05$. To estimate a potential effect of phenotype overweight versus lean during repeated measurements in the respiration chamber, linear and linear mixed effects models were used with the software R version 2.11.1 [17] and the packages nlme [18] and lmtest [19]. P values for linear models were derived from likelihood ratio tests. In order to account for potential correlation of measurements within cats, cat was used as random effect. Model selection was based on (AIC Akaike's information criterion) with a lower AIC indicating a better model fit and visual checking of the random effects residuals. Highly influential or leverage data points were determined using Cook's distance. Results are given in marginal means of effect sizes and their corresponding standard errors (S.E.).

3. Results

3.1. Body Weight and Fat Content. At the beginning of the adaptation period, there was no statistical difference in body weight between groups, but in body fat content (fat mass in g $P = 0.02$, fat mass in % $P = 0.03$) with group GO having a lower fat content (Table 2). Statistical differences between both groups were found at the end of the second ad libitum phase, with the group GO having a statistically significant higher body weight ($P = 0.013$) and body fat content (fat mass in g $P = 0.005$, fat mass in % $P = 0.005$) compared to group GL. Whereas the measurements in group GL did not differ significantly in between the first and the second measurement, in group GO statistical significant differences were found (body weight $P = 0.02$, body fat mass in g $P = 0.005$, body fat mass in % $P = 0.005$).

3.2. Respiration Measurements. Using a linear mixed model approach, significant differences in O_2 consumption as well as CO_2 production between both phenotypes, with phenotype GO having lower values were found (Table 3).

Two highly influential data points, which corresponded to the first measurements of O_2 consumption in each group and were assumed to be atypical, have been removed.

Based on pooled samples (four sampling days taken together for each cat), energy requirements at weight constancy for both groups was estimated with a linear regression approach with retained energy as independent and ME intake as dependent variable, additionally separately for each group. In this calculation the estimated intercept corresponds to the energy requirement at weight constancy of 246 (S.E. 22.6) kJ/BW FFM in group GL and 162.6 (S.E. 14.3) kJ/BW FFM in group GO. The estimated mean effect on energy value of eaten diet intake of group GO compared to GL was a reduction of 83.6 (S.E. 26.4) kJ/BW FFM ($P = 0.022$). The interaction between group effect and retained energy was significant ($P = 0.01$), indicating that the association between ME uptake and retained energy was significantly different between the two groups. The corresponding regression coefficients (indicating the increase in ME uptake per one unit increase in retained energy) were 0.73 (S.E. 0.14) for group GL and 1.2 (S.E. 0.12) for group GO. If ME uptake and retained energy were referred to $BW^{0.67}$, energy requirement was calculated to be 351 (S.E. 34.2) kJ/$BW^{0.67}$ in group GL and 261 (s.e. 29.8) kJ/$BW^{0.67}$ in group GO. The interaction between group effect and retained energy was not significant. The corresponding regression coefficients were 0.9 (S.E. 0.15) for group GL and 1.25 (S.E. 0.17) for group GO.

3.3. Food Intake Measurements. During the ad libitum feeding using the automatic feeding station, the cats of the obese phenotype (GO) showed a significantly ($P = 0.001$) higher food intake than the cats of group GL. It corresponded to an ME intake of 422 ± 37 kJ/kg $BW^{0.67}$ in group GL and 622 ± 27 kJ/kg $BW^{0.67}$ in group GO. Also the meal size differed significantly between the two groups, but the stay in the cat food station did not (Table 4). The meal frequency with 9.5 ± 0.3 times/24 hours in group GL and 7.2 ± 0.2 times/24 hours in group GO did not differ significantly ($P = 0.17$).

4. Discussion

In this experimental study a significant association between phenotype overweight versus lean in the following measured variables became evident: body weight and body fat, O_2 consumption, CO_2 production, energy requirement, food intake in g and in energy value of eaten diet, and meal size, but not duration of stay or frequency. The cats of group GL showed a constant body weight during the whole study time, despite ad libitum feeding. In contrast, cats from group GO started gaining body weight soon after the beginning of ad libitum feeding. Despite similar BCS and body weight in both groups initially, group GO had a significantly lower body fat content than the animals of group GL. This could be due to a misinterpretation of abdominal skin as abdominal fat as this is one important criteria in the body condition scoring system after Laflamme [14]. At the end of the second ad libitum phase, after four weeks of weight constancy, only the cats with phenotype GO showed a significant increase in body fat, and they had a significantly higher body fat content than the cats of group GL. This difference supported the assumed different phenotypes [8] and was expected as a weight regain after a weight-loss program of overweight individuals is a known effect in pets [20, 21].

Although kept under similar conditions, with a similar potential for activity, the measurements taken in the respiration chamber indicate a significantly lower metabolic activity of the cats with phenotype GO compared to phenotype GL. Due to the availability of pooled samples to estimate energy requirements only one data point for each animal could be used in a linear regression approach. This potentially lowered the power to detect a significant difference between the two groups with regard to their energy requirements if referred to $BW^{0.67}$. The estimated intercepts still indicate a potential higher energy requirement in group GL compared to group GO. Although not significant, the estimated regression coefficients, corresponding to the association between ME and retained energy, might indicate a different relationship between ME and retained energy in both groups. If the energy requirements were referred to fat-free body mass, a significant difference between both groups was found. This finding indicates that referring energy requirements to fat-free body mass might be more appropriate than to $BW^{0.67}$. With regard to the significant difference in energy requirements between the cats of phenotype overweight and lean, it might have happened in this study design, that the weight-loss program affected the energy expenditure of the group GO, since energy restriction in cats and dogs can result in a decrease in relative energy expenditure [21–23]. The potential effect due to the weight-loss program in cats of phenotype GO might have been persisted during the following different phases explaining part of the differences found. A potential way to circumvent the potential influence of a weight-loss program would be to evaluate energy requirements earlier in life, before a distinct phenotype becomes evident (and a weight-loss program necessary to assure a similar BCS in both groups). Also a higher amount of less metabolically active fat tissue has been assumed to cause lower-energy requirements in overweight cats compared to their lean counterparts [24, 25]. This can be excluded, however, for the cats of the present study, since the calculation of energy requirements based on fat-free mass confirmed the observed differences between the cats of the different phenotypes. It can be speculated that the difference in energy requirements also based on FFM, the possibly different relationship between ME and retained energy, and in O_2 consumption and CO_2 production were influenced by differences in activity of the cats of the two groups.

In the group GO, a significantly higher food intake either in g and in terms of energy value of diet and meal size became obvious during the measurements in the automatic cat feeding station. But duration of stay or frequency was not associated with phenotype.

Increased food intake and reduced energy expenditure in cats soon after castration has been described [20, 24]. The cats in the present study were intact males in their young adulthood originating from the same cat population and reared under similar conditions. Ad libitum access to feed led to an increase in body weight and a body condition score indicative of overweight within a couple of weeks in the group predisposed to overweight but not in the normal lean group (GL). In obesity mouse models, decreased energy expenditure and increased food intake have been associated

Table 4: Mean food intake, duration of single stays, food intake/min of stay, meal size, and meal frequency in the cat food station of the cats of group GL (lean phenotype) and GO (overweight phenotype), different letters show significant differences ($P < 0.05$).

	Group GL	Group GO
Food intake mean ± SE (g DM/kg $BW^{0.67}$/d)	24.0 ± 2.1^A	34.5 ± 1.5^B
Duration of stay mean ± SE (min/d)	3.3 ± 0.2^A	4.4 ± 0.5^A
Food intake mean ± SE g/min of stay	2.6 ± 0.1^A	3.7 ± 0.1^B
Meal Size mean ± SE (g/d)	8.6 ± 0.5^A	16.6 ± 1.8^B
Meal frequency mean ± SE/d	9.5 ± 0.3^A	7.2 ± 0.2^A

with mutations in the leptin system [26]. Also in obesity of humans some mutations influencing the eating behaviour are known [5, 27–30].

In humans a disordered energy balance with decreased energy expenditure and increased appetite after a weight reduction program in comparison to "normal" lean humans was observed [31]. The data of the present study support the assumption that the feeling of satiety is affected in the cats of the GO group, predisposed to overweight, since food intake, but not meal frequency or stay was significantly different between both groups. Meal frequency of all cats of the present study was in agreement with the observed frequencies by Mugford and Thorne [10], Kane et al. [11], and Peachey and Harper [12]. Because of this homogenous behaviour, rank order as cause of the differences in food intake could be excluded. This was also documented by the fact that the program did not recognize one cat of each group more often without entering the cat food station at the end. It could be concluded that the cats higher in ranking did not block the entrance of the cat food station for the other cat for a longer time. Apparently all cats followed their natural eating behaviour.

In conclusion, in the present study, the differences in food intake and energy expenditure in young intact male cats with and without predisposition to overweight could be quantified. The results indicate that in the cats showing an overweight phenotype the regulation of food intake differs from that of the "normal" lean cats. To specify the influence of energy expenditure without any weight-loss program, further investigation at earlier age in cats of the named experimental cat family is needed.

Acknowledgments

The authors thank Biomill SA for providing the cat food for the experiments. The authors also thank Ines Mittner, Barbara Schneider, and Maja Bollhalder for the laboratory analyses.

References

[1] K. Russell, R. Sabin, S. Holt, R. Bradley, and E. J. Harper, "Influence of feeding regimen on body condition in the cat," *Journal of Small Animal Practice*, vol. 41, no. 1, pp. 12–17, 2000.

[2] L. Colliard, B. M. Paragon, B. Lemuet, J. J. Bénet, and G. Blanchard, "Prevalence and risk factors of obesity in an urban population of healthy cats," *Journal of Feline Medicine and Surgery*, vol. 11, no. 2, pp. 135–140, 2009.

[3] A. J. German, "The growing problem of obesity in dogs and cats," *Journal of Nutrition*, vol. 136, no. 7, pp. 1940S–1946S, 2006.

[4] E. Kienzle and R. Bergler, "Human-animal relationship of owners of normal and overweight cats," *Journal of Nutrition*, vol. 136, no. 7, pp. 1947–1950, 2006.

[5] Y. Zhang, R. Proenca, M. Maffei, M. Barone, L. Leopold, and J. M. Friedman, "Positional cloning of the mouse obese gene and its human homologue," *Nature*, vol. 372, no. 6505, pp. 425–432, 1994.

[6] H. H. M. Maes, M. C. Neale, and L. J. Eaves, "Genetic and environmental factors in relative body weight and human adiposity," *Behavior Genetics*, vol. 27, no. 4, pp. 325–351, 1997.

[7] R. J. F. Loos and C. Bouchard, "Obesity—is it a genetic disorder?" *Journal of Internal Medicine*, vol. 254, no. 5, pp. 401–425, 2003.

[8] T. Haering, B. Wichert, G. Dolf, and B. Haase, "Segregation analysis for overweight in an experimental cat population," *Journal of Heredity*, vol. 102, supplement 1, pp. S28–S31, 2011.

[9] National Research Council (NRC), *Nutrient requirements of Dogs and Cats*, National Academic Press, Washington, DC, USA, 2006.

[10] R. A. Mugford and C. Thorne, "Comparative studies of meal patterns in pet and laboratory housed dogs and cats," in *Nutrition of the Dog and Cat*, R. S. Anderson, Ed., pp. 3–14, Pergamon Press, Oxford, UK, 1980.

[11] E. Kane, Q. R. Rogers, and J. G. Morris, "Feeding behavior of the cat fed laboratory and commercial diets," *Nutrition Research*, vol. 1, no. 5, pp. 499–507, 1981.

[12] S. E. Peachey and E. Jean Harper, "Aging does not influence feeding behavior in cats," *Journal of Nutrition*, vol. 132, no. 6, pp. 1735S–1739S, 2002.

[13] D. Horwitz, Y. Soulard, and A. Junien-Castagna, "The feeding behaviour of the cat," in *Encyclopedia of Feline Clinical Nutrition*, P. Pibot, V. Biourge, and D. Elliott, Eds., pp. 439–473, Royal Canin, 2008.

[14] D. Laflamme, "Development and validation of a body condition score system for cats: a clinical tool," *Feline Practice*, vol. 25, no. 5-6, pp. 13–17, 1997.

[15] L. Schade, *Untersuchungen zum Energiestoffwechsel von trächtigen Katzen*, thesis, Zürich, Switzerland, 2006.

[16] B. Wichert, L. Schade, S. Gebert et al., "Energy and protein needs of cats for maintenance, gestation and lactation," *Journal of Feline Medicine and Surgery*, vol. 11, no. 10, pp. 808–815, 2009.

[17] R Development Core Team, *R: A language and environment for statistical computing*, R Foundation for Statistical Computing, Vienna, Austria, 2010.

[18] J. Pinheiro, D. Bates, S. DebRoy, D. Sarkar, and R Core Team, "nlme: Linear and Nonlinear Mixed Effects Models," R package version 3.1-96, 2009.

[19] A. Zeileis and T. Hothorn, "Diagnostic checking in regression relationships," *R News*, vol. 2, no. 3, pp. 7–10, 2002.

[20] M. L. Kanchuk, R. C. Backus, C. C. Calvert, J. G. Morris, and Q. R. Rogers, "Weight gain in gonadectomized normal and lipoprotein lipase-deficient male domestic cats results from increased food intake and not decreased energy expenditure," *Journal of Nutrition*, vol. 133, no. 6, pp. 1866–1874, 2003.

[21] C. Villaverde, J. J. Ramsey, A. S. Green, D. K. Asami, S. Yoo, and A. J. Fascetti, "Energy restriction results in a mass-adjusted decrease in energy expenditure in cats that is maintained after weight regain," *Journal of Nutrition*, vol. 138, no. 5, pp. 856–860, 2008.

[22] J. J. Ramsey and K. Hagopian, "Energy expenditure and restriction of energy intake: could energy restriction alter energy expenditure in companion animals?" *Journal of Nutrition*, vol. 136, no. 7, pp. 1958S–1966S, 2006.

[23] D. Nagaoka, Y. Mitsuhashi, R. Angell, K. E. Bigley, and J. E. Bauer, "Re-induction of obese body weight occurs more rapidly and at lower caloric intake in beagles," *Journal of Animal Physiology and Animal Nutrition*, vol. 94, no. 3, pp. 287–292, 2010.

[24] M. J. Fettman, C. A. Stanton, L. L. Banks et al., "Effects of neutering on body weight, metabolic rate and glucose tolerance of domestic cats," *Research in Veterinary Science*, vol. 62, no. 2, pp. 131–136, 1997.

[25] E. Kienzle, G. Edtstadtler-Pietsch, and R. Rudnick, "Retrospective study on the energy requirements of adult colony cats," *Journal of Nutrition*, vol. 136, no. 7, pp. 1973S–1975S, 2006.

[26] P. Magni, M. Motta, and L. Martini, "Leptin: a possible link between food intake, energy expenditure, and reproductive function," *Regulatory Peptides*, vol. 92, no. 1–3, pp. 51–56, 2000.

[27] L. A. Tartaglia, M. Dembski, X. Weng et al., "Identification and expression cloning of a leptin receptor, OB-R," *Cell*, vol. 83, no. 7, pp. 1263–1271, 1995.

[28] K. S. Graham and R. L. Leibel, "Yellow mice, red hair, and childhood obesity: the melanocortinergic pathway in energy homeostasis," *Journal of Pediatrics*, vol. 139, no. 2, pp. 177–181, 2001.

[29] S. Carnell, C. M. A. Haworth, R. Plomin, and J. Wardle, "Genetic influence on appetite in children," *International Journal of Obesity*, vol. 32, no. 10, pp. 1468–1473, 2008.

[30] W. F. Mathes, S. A. Kelly, and D. Pomp, "Advances in comparative genetics: influence of genetics on obesity," *British Journal of Nutrition*, vol. 106, pp. S1–S10, 2011.

[31] M.-A. Cornier, "Is your brain to blame for weight regain?" *Physiology and Behavior*, vol. 104, no. 4, pp. 608–612, 2011.

7

Development, Characterization, and Optimization of Protein Level in Date Bars Using Response Surface Methodology

Muhammad Nadeem,[1] Salim-ur-Rehman,[2] Faqir Muhammad Anjum,[2] Mian Anjum Murtaza,[1] and Ghulam Mueen-ud-Din[1]

[1] *Institute of Food Science and Nutrition, University of Sargodha, Sargodha, Pakistan*
[2] *National Institute of Food Science and Technology, University of Agriculture, Faisalabad, Pakistan*

Correspondence should be addressed to Muhammad Nadeem, mnadeemb@yahoo.com

Academic Editors: M. Allman-Farinelli and D. Engeset

This project was designed to produce a nourishing date bar with commercial value especially for school going children to meet their body development requirements. Protein level of date bars was optimized using response surface methodology (RSM). Economical and underutilized sources, that is, whey protein concentrate and vetch protein isolates, were explored for protein supplementation. Fourteen date bar treatments were produced using a central composite design (CCD) with 2 variables and 3 levels for each variable. Date bars were then analyzed for nutritional profile. Proximate composition revealed that addition of whey protein concentrate and vetch protein isolates improved the nutritional profile of date bars. Protein level, texture, and taste were considerably improved by incorporating 6.05% whey protein concentrate and 4.35% vetch protein isolates in date bar without affecting any sensory characteristics during storage. Response surface methodology was observed as an economical and effective tool to optimize the ingredient level and to discriminate the interactive effects of independent variables.

1. Introduction

The food bars are snacks of good sensory and nutritional characteristics due to their high carbohydrates, proteins, lipids, and minerals contents. Snack foods such as potato chips, extruded products, chocolates bars available in market cannot meet the requirement of balanced diet [1]. These are unhealthyofferings for the consumers especially school going children. Increasing demand from consumers for nutritious snacks, has provoked the food manufacturers to develop food bars that provide nutrition and convenience [2].

School-going children need nutritious foods due to their enhance body development requirements. Food consumed by them should be rich in vitamins, minerals and balanced regarding major nutrients like carbohydrates, proteins and fats. The options available for the children to buy wholesome and nourishing food products are very limited. This gap needs to be filled by developing products that conform to emerging trends of nutraceutical and functional foods [1]. The products that are developed by utilizing dried fruit, processed legumes, and cereals along with nuts would be an attractive snack food for the school going children and for those people working outside their homes and are becoming more dependent on snacks for the supply of part of their daily nutritional requirements [3]. At the moment, the imported fruit bars are available at super stores only in the big cities. Some popular brands are Kellog's Nutri Grain, Nature Velley, and so forth. The market price for these bars is exorbitant and ranged from rupees 85–130 per 35–45 g bar. This price is out of reach for target children (low and middle income families). In principle, the cost of indigenously developed product should be below rupees 10. which will suit the target consumer. Quality and price are key factor for the development of a competitive product. To achieve this objective, economical and underutilized food sources with good nutritional value should be explored. Dates and Indian vetch (*Lathyrus sativus* L.) are good options in this regard as these are abundantly produced but are underutilized.

Date flesh contains substantial amount of carbohydrates (73.5%) along with ash (1.5%), protein (2.3%), lipids (0.2%), vitamins, and fifteen mineral elements [4]. The polysaccharides from date fruit have been used as a functional constituent and provide bioactive compounds in the formulation of drugs [5]. Dates and dried fruit have high concentration of polyphenols with excellent nutritional value that enrich lipoprotein in plasma and protect it from oxidation [6]. These have also been identified as having antioxidant and antimutagenic properties and help in controlling cardiovascular diseases [7].

Similarly, among the grains, corn has high total antioxidant activity followed by wheat, oat, and rice [8]. Whole grains and legumes are also rich sources of protein and dietary fiber. Due to their health benefits, these food stuffs have lured the scientists and technologists for the development of functional foods which is an emerging trend in the new millennium [9]. Indian vetch (*Lathyrus sativus* L.) is one of the cheapest legumes rather least investigated potential source of protein. It is high in good quality protein (28.70 g/100 g) and lysine content with agreeable taste, so it can be used in innovative food product developments. The elimination of antinutritional and toxic factors from said legume makes it a good candidate for supplementation in wheat flour [10]. Its flour can be utilized in different products after detoxification for enrichment in bread [11], chapatti [12], doughnuts [13], and pizza cheese [14]. The primary source of legume protein for supplementation can be utilized in various forms such as flour, concentrates, isolates, or textured vegetables protein [15, 16].

Dates have an edge over other sweet confections, as they not only give natural sugars, sucrose, and fructose but also have an excellent amount of dietary fibers, especially, when they are blended with cereals and legumes [5, 17, 18]. The high moisture content of fresh dates may be absorbed by cereal and legume flours, thus providing suitable matrix to date bar and thereby, boost its storability [19, 20]. Moreover, nutritional properties of dates, nuts, cereals, and legumes may be complementary to each other. Vital nutritional attributes like vitamins and minerals have good bioavailability in natural forms as compared to the conventional processed products.

Response surface methodology (RSM) is reported to be an effective measure for optimizing a process, when the independent variables, for example, protein sources, are hypothesized to possess a sovereign or cumulative effect on the desired responses [21]. Considering the aforementioned essentials, this project was designed to produce a nourishing date bar with commercial value. The present project was planned to assess the suitability of vetch protein isolate and whey protein supplementation in date bar by applying physicochemical tests and to optimize the protein level of date bars by using RSM.

2. Materials and Methods

2.1. Procurement of Raw Materials. Commercially available dates (Karblain), roasted gram and corn, peanuts, almonds, whey protein concentrate and Indian vetch, common salt, and cardamom were purchased from local market of Faisalabad. Analytical grade chemicals were purchased from Sigma Aldrich (Seelze, Germany) and Lab-Scan (Dublin, Ireland) available in the local market.

Table 1: Date bars formulation.

Ingredients	Quantity
Date paste	100 g
Composite flour	20 g
Peanuts	10 g
Almonds	10 g
Whey protein concentrate	As per Table 3
Vetch protein isolate	As per Table 3
Salt	0.5 g
Cardamom	1 g
Butylated hydroxytoluene (BHT)	0.002%

2.2. Pretreatment of Raw Materials. Dates were pitted, washed, and dried. Pitted dates were steamed for 3 minutes. These were then dried. Peanuts and almonds were shelled, skin removed, and crushed to form grits. Roasted corn and gram were ground to form flour. Butylated hydroxytoluene (BHT) and potassium sorbate were also ground separately with Merlin classic machine to fine powder.

2.3. Development of Bars. After preparation of raw materials, dates were passed through mincing machine to make paste. Other ingredients (roasted gram flour and corn flour, peanuts, almonds, whey protein concentrate and vetch protein isolates, common salt, cardamom, potassium sorbate, and butylated hydroxytoluene) were mixed thoroughly to distribute uniformly and to make a blend (Table 1). After mixing, sheeting was done, which was cut into bars of 2.5 cm width, 1 cm height, and 7 cm in length. Each bar of approximately 25 g was packed individually in aluminum foil. The quantity of date paste, roasted gram flour and corn flour, peanuts, almonds, common salt, cardamom, potassium sorbate, and butylated hydroxytoluene remained constant except two variables, that is, whey protein concentrate and vetch protein isolate in different proportions (Tables 2 and 3) according to the model created by applying RSM, and control bars were prepared without the addition of protein isolates. The process flow chart is given as follows (Figure 1).

2.4. Experimental Design for Protein Level Optimization. RSM was used to optimize the levels of independent variables, that is, vetch protein isolate and whey protein concentrate and their effect on dependent variables. In this study, a response surface box Behnken design was used. Maximum and minimum levels of independent variables were searched out by conducting early trials.

Fourteen date bar treatments were created using response surface design with 2 variables having 3 levels. Total 9 different formulations were produced and runs 4, 5, 8, 9,

Table 2: Level of independent variables (%).

Level of independent variable (%)	−1.0	0.0	1.0
Whey protein Concentrate	3	6	9
Vetch protein isolate	2	4	6

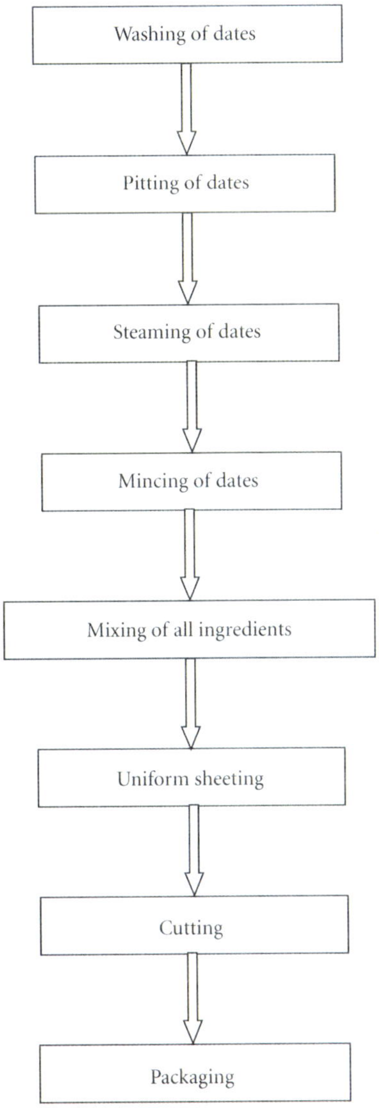

Figure 1: Process flow chart for date bars.

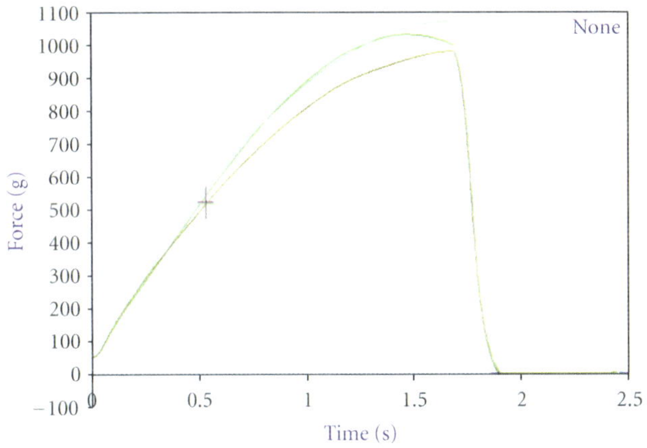

Figure 2: Representative graph of bend test of date bars.

and 13 correspond to centre point replicates. The complete experiment design for coded and actual levels is presented in Table 3.

2.5. Physicochemical Analysis of Date Bars. Date bars were stored at ambient temperature (25 ± 5°C). During storage period, these bars were evaluated for physico-chemical characteristics.

2.5.1. Texture Analysis. Texture of date bars was determined at different storage intervals according to the method as described by researchers [22] with some modifications by using a texture analyzer (Model TA-XT2.Plus.Stable Microsystems, Surrey, UK) with 5 kg load cell. The Texture Expert program version 4.0.9.0 was used for data analysis. Textural determinations (hardness and fracturability) were made by using a 3 points bending rig (HDP/3PB) for a bend test (Table 4). The bars were bent in order to check different structural characteristics present inside or on the surface. Samples for bending were placed centrally under the 3 points bending rig secured on heavy duty platform (HDP/90). Both the load cell and probes were calibrated before test. Hardness and fracturability measurement of samples by bending involved plotting force (g) and distance (mm) versus time (second). The maximum force (g) was used as an index of hardness (firmness) and distance (mm) as fracturability for the bend test (Figure 2).

2.5.2. Proximate Analysis. Proximate composition such as moisture, ash, crude protein, crude fat, and crude fiber of date bars was determined and expressed on dry-matter basis [23].

2.5.3. Sensory Analysis. Taste of date bars were evaluated at room temperature (i.e., 25 ± 5°C) in a sensory evaluation laboratory by a penal of ten untrained judges on 9-point Hedonic Scale [24].

2.6. Statistical Analysis. Results were statistically analyzed by using analysis of variance technique. Level of significance within means was calculated by using the Duncan Multiple Range Test [25]. Minitab (ver. 14.1) statistical software (Minitab Inc., PA, USA) was used for optimization studies.

TABLE 3: Experimental design for date bars formulation (independent variables).

Sr. number	Standard order	Run order	Pt type	Blocks	Whey protein Concentrate (%)	Vetch protein isolate (%)
1	1	1	1	1	3.00	2.00
2	2	2	1	1	9.00	2.00
3	5	3	0	1	6.00	4.00
4	6	4	0	1	6.00	4.00
5	7	5	0	1	6.00	4.00
6	3	6	1	1	3.00	6.00
7	4	7	1	1	9.00	6.00
8	13	8	0	2	6.00	4.00
9	14	9	0	2	6.00	4.00
10	11	10	−1	2	6.00	6.8284
11	9	11	−1	2	10.2426	4.00
12	8	12	−1	2	1.7574	4.00
13	12	13	0	2	6.00	4.00
14	10	14	−1	2	6.00	1.1715

TABLE 4: TA-XT2 settings for comparison of hardness and fracturability of date bars by bend test with 3 points bend rig.

Mode	Measure force in compression
Option	Return To Start
Pretest speed	1.0 mm/s
Test speed	3.0 mm/s
Posttest speed	10.0 mm/s
Distance	5 mm
Trigger force	Auto −50 g
Tare mode	Auto
Data acquisition rate	500 pps

3. Results

Date bars were developed using selected raw materials and protein levels were optimized by applying RSM. Bars, thus, prepared were analyzed for their physicochemical properties.

3.1. Physicochemical Analysis of Date Bars

3.1.1. Proximate Composition of Date Bars. Proximate analysis includes determination of moisture, crude protein, crude fat, crude fiber, ash, and NFE of date bar samples. The means regarding moisture, crude protein, crude fat, crude fiber, ash, and NFE are given in Table 5. The moisture content of date bar sample ranges from 15.56 ± 0.02 to 18.70 ± 0.02%, crude protein 7.41 ± 0.01 to 14.96 ± 0.01%, crude fat 5.55 ± 0.02 to 8.37 ± 0.01%, crude fiber 3.58 ± 0.01 to 3.91 ± 0.02%, ash 2.30 ± 0.01 to 2.91 ± 0.02%, and NFE 70.85 ± 0.02 to 81.12 ± 0.07%. There was a significantly increasing trend in crude protein, crude fat and ash content, with the addition of whey protein concentrate and vetch protein isolate. Minimum crude protein, crude fat and ash contents were recorded in control bar (T_0) while maximum crude protein content was recorded in T_6 (14.96 ± 0.01%) and crude fat and ash content in T_7 (8.37 ± 0.01%, 2.91 ± 0.02%, resp.).

3.2. Optimization of Protein Levels in Date Bars Using RSM.

Dates provide appreciable amount of carbohydrates and other nutrients but are deficient in protein. In order to improve the protein level in date bars, economical and underutilized protein sources have been explored. The date bars were prepared by using the best formulation, incorporating whey protein concentrate and vetch protein isolate at variable levels. RSM was applied to estimate the responses of independent variables that is, whey protein concentrate (X) and vetch protein isolate (Y) during storage. Second-order polynomial model was fitted for independent variables. The regression equations and coefficients were determined by using multiple regression analysis of storage's data regarding different parameters.

3.2.1. Hardness (Firmness) of Date Bars. The responses for hardness from central composite design (CCD) were fitted with second order polynomial equations (Table 6). The statistical analysis by applying analysis of variance technique to the full regression of model indicated nonsignificant effect ($P > 0.05$) of variables. However, linear terms of variable (X) are observed to negatively change the hardness of bars at all storage intervals, whereas quadratic terms of vetch protein isolate (Y) have a positive effect. The interaction of these two terms (XY) was found negative over all storage intervals. The coefficients of determination (90.6%) assured that models are adequately fitted. Both independent variables contribute toward increase in firmness, that is, upto 2468.56 g in date bars at 0 to 90 days storage intervals (Figures 3 and 4).

3.2.2. Fracturability of Date Bars. The models were developed for fracturability of date bars as affected by independent variables during 90 days storage (Table 7). The effect of linear terms of X and Y are statistically significant ($P < 0.05$) for

TABLE 5: Mean values for moisture, crude protein, crude fat, crude fiber, ash, and NFE in date bars (%)*.

Treatment	Moisture	Crude protein	Crude fat	Crude fiber	Ash	NFE
T_0	15.56 ± 0.02j	7.41 ± 0.01j	5.55 ± 0.02j	3.58 ± 0.01ef	2.30 ± 0.01g	81.12 ± 0.07a
T_1	16.34 ± 0.01h	9.80 ± 0.02h	6.37 ± 0.02g	3.65 ± 0.02de	2.64 ± 0.02f	77.53 ± 0.01b
T_2	16.63 ± 0.01g	10.49 ± 0.01g	8.03 ± 0.02b	3.84 ± 0.02ab	2.84 ± 0.01abc	74.79 ± 0.02e
T_3	17.23 ± 0.01e	12.16 ± 0.01e	7.20 ± 0.02e	3.74 ± 0.01c	2.80 ± 0.02bcd	74.09 ± 0.01f
T_4	18.20 ± 0.01c	13.76 ± 0.01c	6.16 ± 0.02h	3.56 ± 0.02f	2.66 ± 0.02ef	73.85 ± 0.05g
T_5	18.42 ± 0.01b	14.48 ± 0.01b	7.87 ± 0.01c	3.91 ± 0.02a	2.87 ± 0.02ab	70.85 ± 0.02j
T_6	18.70 ± 0.02a	14.96 ± 0.01a	7.07 ± 0.02f	3.70 ± 0.01cd	2.77 ± 0.02cd	71.48 ± 0.03i
T_7	17.41 ± 0.01d	12.63 ± 0.02d	8.37 ± 0.01a	3.88 ± 0.02ab	2.91 ± 0.02a	72.20 ± 0.04h
T_8	16.86 ± 0.02f	11.64 ± 0.02f	6.04 ± 0.01i	3.60 ± 0.03ef	2.61 ± 0.02f	76.10 ± 0.06d
T_9	16.18 ± 0.01i	9.30 ± 0.02i	7.38 ± 0.02d	3.79 ± 0. 02bc	2.75 ± 0.01de	76.77 ± 0.02c

Means with different letters in each column differ highly significantly $P < 0.01$*: dry weight basis.

TABLE 6: Regression coefficients for the models representing as a function of variations in the independent variables for hardness (firmness) of date bars and their respective R^2.

Terms of model equations	Days 0	15	30	45	60	75	90
Constant	115.34	468.85	−204.7	31.03	−1022.0	−150.2	−564.9
X	76.45	64.90	234.2	259.22	503.0	447.7	531.0
Y	87.03	182.37	535.8*	561.53	890.0	607.1	870.2
$X \times X$	−6.46	−9.55	−20.3	−22.47	−41.0	−33.9	−41.5
$Y \times Y$	−12.29	−28.92	−61.7*	−72.79	−105.0	−72.8	−110.2
$X \times Y$	−2.45	7.08	−7.8	−4.50	−6.0	−9.9	4.4
R^2	90.6%	59.3%	85.6%	60.7%	63.3%	54.9%	57.6%

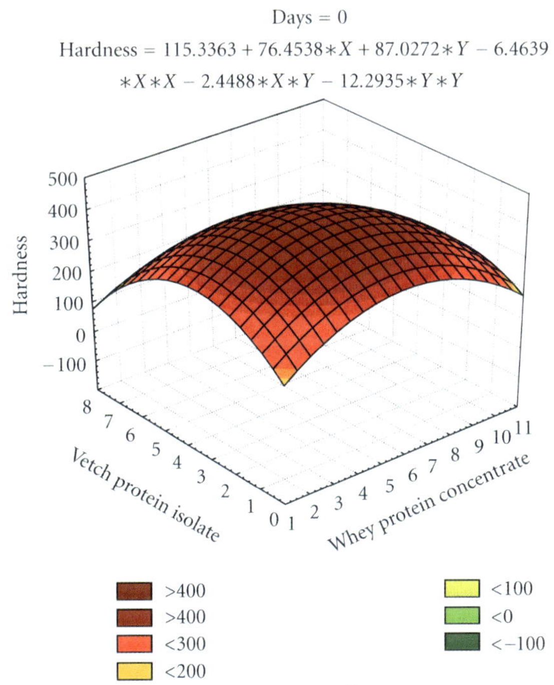

FIGURE 3: Effect of independent variables (X, Y) on hardness (firmness) in date bars during storage (at 0 day).

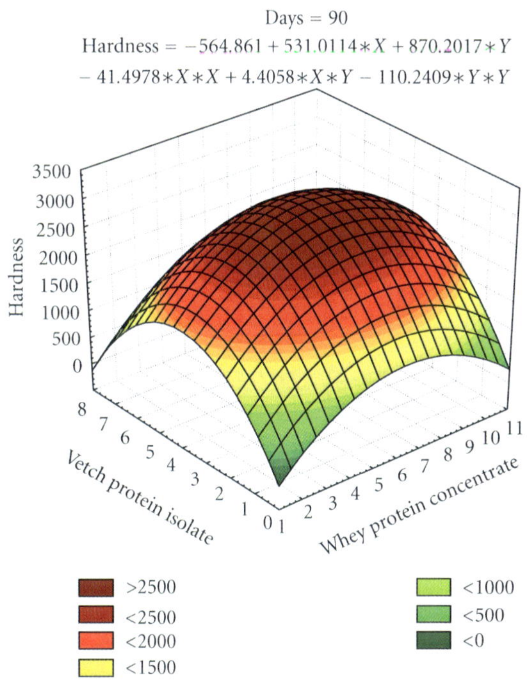

FIGURE 4: Effect of independent variables (X, Y) on hardness (firmness) in date bars during storage (at 90 days).

TABLE 7: Regression coefficients for the models representing as a function of variations in the independent variables for fracturability of date bars and their respective R^2.

Terms of model equations	Days						
	0	15	30	45	60	75	90
Constant	70.5340**	69.6997**	69.2231**	70.1477**	71.0520**	72.5183**	74.7418**
X	0.0908	0.4879*	0.7661	0.5701*	0.5857*	0.4703*	0.3155*
Y	0.0816	0.7057*	1.2051	1.0154*	0.9146*	0.5800*	0.3175
$X \times X$	−0.0008	−0.0340*	−0.0622	−0.0332*	−0.0349*	−0.0281*	−0.0349*
$Y \times Y$	0.0070	−0.0741*	−0.1312	−0.0922*	−0.0736*	−0.0350	−0.0342
$X \times Y$	−0.0062	0.0067	0.0075	−0.0167	−0.0271	−0.0254	0.0167
R^2	93.9%	96.5%	81.8%	96.4%	94.8%	93.7%	95.1%

*significant ($P < 0.05$); **highly significant ($P < 0.01$) X: whey protein concentrate Y: vetch protein isolate.

TABLE 8: Regression coefficients for the models representing as a function of variations in the independent variables for taste of date bars and their respective R^2.

Terms of model equations	Day						
	0	15	30	45	60	75	90
Constant	4.6671***	3.8671***	3.9293***	3.1233**	3.6379***	3.6232***	3.1879***
X	0.3809*	0.4360**	0.3691***	0.3743	0.2760**	0.2617*	0.3010*
Y	0.9118**	0.9915***	1.0390***	1.2077**	0.7514**	0.6640**	0.6015**
$X \times X$	−0.0277*	−0.0243**	−0.0264***	−0.0250	−0.0208**	−0.0257**	−0.0208*
$Y \times Y$	−0.0875**	−0.0921**	−0.1094***	−0.1250**	−0.0843**	−0.0890**	−0.0593**
$X \times Y$	−0.0166	−0.0291*	−0.0167**	−0.0208	0.0000	0.0166	−0.0083
R^2	89.9%	95.0%	98.8%	89.4%	95.2%	94.2%	89.6%

*significant ($P < 0.10$); **significant ($P < 0.05$); ***significant ($P < 0.01$)
X: whey protein concentrate
Y: vetch protein isolate.

fracturability of date bars during storage. The X^2 quadratic terms are found significant at 15, 45, 60, 75, and 90 days storage intervals whereas the quadratic terms for Y^2 are found significant at 15, 45, and 60 days. The interaction of two variables (XY) shows nonsignificant effect during at all storage intervals. The coefficients of determination (96.5%) assured that models are well fitted. The independent variables contribute towards increase in fracturability in date bars at 0 to 90 days storage intervals (Figure 5).

3.2.3. Taste of Date Bars. The coefficients of determination (R^2) for these models (R^2 = 89.9%, 95.0%, 98.8%, 89.4%, 95.2%, 94.2%, and 89.6% resp.) exhibit the adequacy of models and showed that it covers more variability in data (Table 8). The effect of linear terms of X and Y for taste of date bars is significant during storage. The X^2 and Y^2 quadratic terms are also found significant during storage interval of 90 days. The interaction of two variables (XY) shows significant effect on taste at 15 and 30 days of storage intervals. Independent variables (whey protein concentrate and vetch Protein isolate, that is, 5.75% and 4.36%, resp.) have well contributed towards achieving good score for taste of date bars. The scores for taste decline during 90 days storage intervals. However, during the entire storage period, the taste of date bars is found acceptable (Figure 6).

4. Discussion

As the dates are not a good source of protein; so, whey protein and vetch protein isolate has been used for the development of date bars. Addition of whey protein concentrate and vetch protein isolate in appropriate proportions has improved nutritional status as well as physical and chemical properties of date bars. The protein content increased to 7.55% in date bars. Similar results were observed by some other research workers who observed an increase in protein level in date bars from 10.7 to 12.1% with the addition of soy protein isolate, single-cell proteins, almonds, and skim milk powder. Moreover, it has improved the chemical scores of essential amino acids in date bars [26, 27] The protein content of bars can also be increased by fortification of peanut flour, soy flour [28], mesquite cotyledon [1, 29, 30], and black and red beans [31]. Although, fortification of date bars with these sources increases protein, fiber, and ash contents and it also improves minerals such as Ca, Mg, Na, K, P, Zn, and essential amino acids without affecting their sensory acceptability. In the present research work, ash content increases to the tune of 0.60% with the addition of whey protein concentrate.

Fat is an important constituent of bars which does not only provide energy but also increases the palatability. Moreover, it acts as binder along with sweeteners in agglutination of the ingredients of food bar which are responsible to

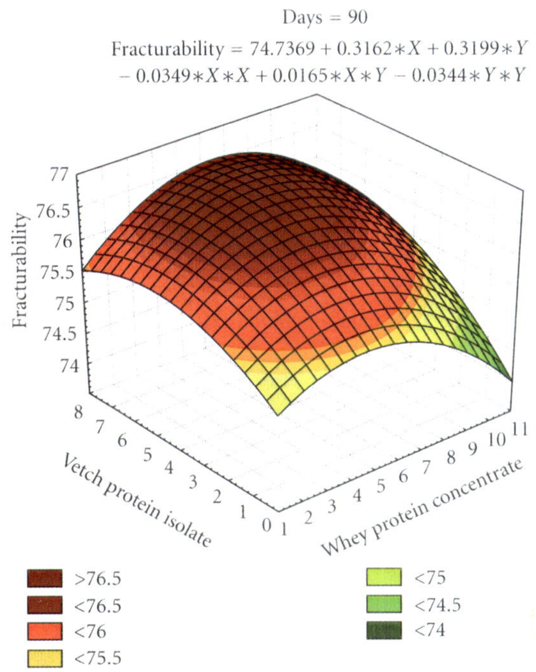

Figure 5: Effect of independent variables (X, Y) on fracturability in date bars during storage (at 90 days).

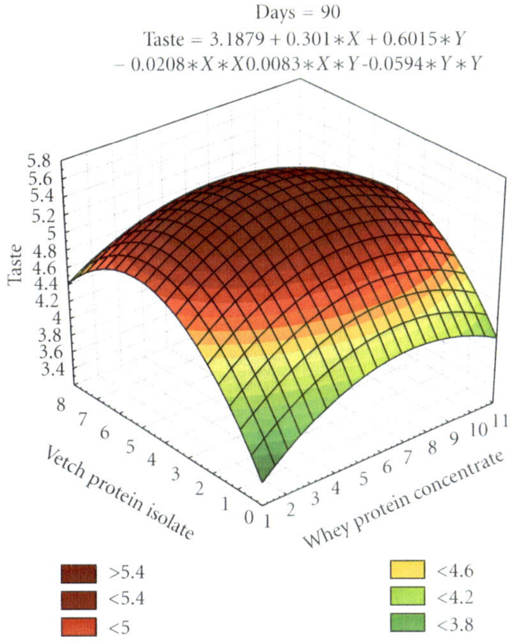

Figure 6: Effect of independent variables (X, Y) on taste in date bars during storage (at 90 days).

impart firmness and compactness to texture of food bars [32]. During this study, fat content has been increased in the date bars (2.82%) with the supplementation of whey protein concentrate.

Optimization of ingredients in the food's formulation is necessary for the development of a product. The optimization of protein and fat levels can also optimize level of carbohydrates of food bars [33]. A candy bar fortified with soy protein contained 58.7% carbohydrates, 12.4% protein, and 9% fat [29]. Similarly, the addition of legume flours increases protein, fat, fiber, ash, minerals, and vitamins in chocolate bars [34]. In the present scanario, high-energy fortified date bars have been developed with an excellent profile of protein, carbohydrate, and fat. These date bars provide good amount of nutrients that can meet the terms of daily nutritional requirements an individual [35]. These can be incorporated in manu of school going children, working people, sportmen, emergency situation, as snack food and nutritional servings. The soy-based candy bar containing 14% protein, 22% fat, and 65% carbohydrates could provide 375.2 kcal/100 g [29].

In optimization study, the effect of levels of independent variables; protein sources of dependent variables such as hardness, fracturability, and taste for date bars was optimized. The second-order polynomial models were fitted for independent variables:

$$Z = \beta 0 + \beta 1X + \beta 2Y + \beta 11X^2 + \beta 22Y^2 + \beta 12XY. \quad (1)$$

In this equation: Z = dependent variable to be measured, $\beta 0$ = regression coefficient for treatment effect, $\beta 1$ = regression coefficient for $X, \beta 2$ = regression coefficient for Y, X = coded level of whey protein concentrate, Y = coded level of vetch protein isolate.

A number of techniques is available to find out the best levels of input variables, which in turn optimize their responses [36]. The most straight forward way to undertake is to draw the surface or contour plots of the fitted models. In this study, during data analysis, surface plots were drawn with the help of computer software, Statistica. Three levels, each of whey protein concentrate and vetch protein isolate at different rates were used. The levels were coded as −1, 0 and +1. The relationship between coded (X) and experimental levels (x) of whey protein concentrate and vetch protein isolate is given as

$$X_1 = \frac{x_1 - 6}{6}, \qquad X_2 = \frac{x_2 - 4}{4}. \quad (2)$$

Whereas X_1 and X_2 are the coded values for whey protein concentrate and vetch protein isolate, respectively. RSM is employed to check the worth of many factors and their complex interaction through multiple regression analysis [37]. This methodology is now gaining significance in food research studies by optimizing the ingredients level [38], composite flours [39], product improvers [40], and process conditions for product development like temperature, pressure, humidity, pH, and so forth [41, 42]. To optimize the protein levels in date bars, response optimizing function of statistical program Minitab (ver. 14.1) was used. For the optimization process, maximum taste and firm texture were targeted.

The texture in terms of hardness and fracturability is a feature of prime importance in date bar quality parameters. The surface plots (Figures 3–5) depicted that the maximum hardness (2887.31 g) and fracturability (74.70 mm) were achieved by adding 5.39% and 6.89% whey protein

TABLE 9: Cost analysis of date bars.

Ingredients	Rate (Rs./Kg)	Quantity (g/100 g bar)	Quantity (g/25 g bar)	Ingredient cost (Rs.)
Dates	120	70	17.50	2.10
Peanuts	140	6.25	1.56	0.20
Almonds	320	6.25	1.56	0.50
Composite flour	50	12.5	3.13	0.15
Other ingredients	250	5	1.25	0.30
Packing material	0.20/bar	—	1	0.20
Over head charges (10%)				0.35
Per bar (25 g)		Total cost (100 Kcal)		3.80

1 date bar (25 g) = Rs 3.80. PKR
1 US Dollar = 88Rs. = 23 date bars.

concentrate and 3.69% and 4.24% vetch protein isolate, respectively. In a previous study, response surface methodology was applied to optimize the baking parameters of chapatti, that is, thickness, baking time, and temperature of chapatti. It was found that thickness of chapatti had negative effect on hardness, and cohesiveness, whereas baking time and temperature had positive effects on the hardness and chewiness of the chapatties [43]. Similar results were also observed by researchers working on different types of bars. The bars containing whey protein isolate has shown soft texture throughout storage period which might be due to formation of continuous matrix of protein and sugars, whereas texture became hard in case of bars prepared with calcium caseinate which might happened due to the migration of water molecule from protein towards sugars after 10–18 h of preparation [44].

The proteins from different sources may not behave like protein-fortified food bars. Similarly, mango bars with soy protein has higher hardness and springiness. The bars which were fortified with coconut powder have relatively less hardness which might be due to less protein content [45]. Protein bars containing added protein, fat, sugars, and minimum amount of water (water activity in the range of 6.0–6.5) indicated that fracturability force increased and continued with passage of time. During this period, rate of chemical reaction might be decreased and protein particles have crowded together resulting in precipitation of soluble protein due to moisture migration. These observations suggested that the role of chemical reaction is less as compared to variation in microstructure caused by moisture migration in hardening of protein bars [46].

The functions of added protein are to keep the ingredients of snack bars intact, set the structure, increase the strength, and contribute to water holding capacity and Maillard browning. The whey protein has considerable viscosity, gel strength, and water holding properties which may contribute to bar firmness during shelf life [47–49]. Moreover, the increase in firmness of bars might be due to the migration of moisture between the carbohydrates (such as starches, pectins, sugars, and maltodextrin) and the proteins [48].

Figure 6 depicts 5.5 as maximum score for the taste of date bars at 90 days storage. This value has been selected as target value for taste attribute. The optimized levels for two variables were found as 6.37% (X) and 4.64% (Y). When these values are put in regression model for taste at 90 days, the calculated value attained is 5.5 as well.

It is obvious from the results that each aspect of independent variables suggests different optimized levels. The response optimization function of Minitab program was commissioned to reach a cumulative result. For the target values of taste and texture, the optimized variable levels were as follows:

whey protein concentrate (X) = 6.05% vetch protein isolate (Y) = 4.35%.

5. Conclusion

Physico-chemical properties and sensory characteristics for date bars were evaluated to assess the suitability of supplementation of protein from two different sources such as plant source (vetch protein isolate) and animal source (whey protein concentrate). The results for proximate composition revealed that addition of whey protein concentrate and vetch protein isolates has significantly elevated the nutritional status of date bars. It has been found that the protein level could considerably be improved by incorporating 6.05% whey protein concentrate and 4.35% vetch protein isolates in date bar without affecting any sensory characteristics (taste) during storage. Response surface methodology was observed as the best tool to discriminate the interactive effects of independent variables.

These date bars can be commercialized and become a source of foreign exchange. The cost of production of these bars is given in Table 9. The studies revealed that the potential exists to produce an economical date bars. The outcomes derived from present research work would be supportive for the scientists, researchers and stakeholders dealing with food for better understanding of storage stability of date bars.

References

[1] A. M. Estevez, B. Escobar, and V. Ugarte, "Use of mesquite cotyledon (*Prosopis chilensis*) in manufacturing of cereal bars," *Archivos Latinoamericanos de Nutrición*, vol. 50, pp. 148–151, 2000.

[2] M. Izzo and K. Niness, "Formulating nutrition bars with inulin and oligofructose," *Cereal Foods World*, vol. 46, no. 3, pp. 102–106, 2001.
[3] N. Rosa, R. A. C. C. Jauregui, E. M. Maria, E. S. Pinto, and A. G. A. Jose, "Acceptability of snacks produced by the extrusion of amaranth and blends of chickpea and bovine lung," *International Journal of Food Science & Technology*, vol. 38, pp. 795–798, 2003.
[4] W. Al-Shahib and R. J. Marshall, "The fruit of the date palm: its possible use as the best food for the future?" *International Journal of Food Sciences and Nutrition*, vol. 54, no. 4, pp. 247–259, 2003.
[5] A. Puri, R. Sahai, and L. Kiran, "The anti-cancer activity of polysaccharide prepared from Libyan dates," *Journal of Ethnopharmacology*, vol. 71, pp. 89–92, 2000.
[6] J. A. Vinson, L. Zubik, P. Bose, N. Samman, and J. Proch, "Dried fruits: excellent in vitro and in vivo antioxidants," *Journal of the American College of Nutrition*, vol. 24, no. 1, pp. 44–50, 2005.
[7] P. K. Vayalil, "Antioxidant and antimutagenic properties of aqueous extract of date fruit (*Phoenix dactylifera* L. Arecaceae)," *Journal of Agricultural and Food Chemistry*, vol. 50, no. 3, pp. 610–617, 2002.
[8] K. K. Adom and R. H. Liu, "Antioxidant activity of grains," *Journal of Agricultural and Food Chemistry*, vol. 50, no. 21, pp. 6182–6187, 2002.
[9] Y. Xu, "Perspectives on the 21st century development of functional foods: bridging Chinese medicated diet and functional foods," *International Journal of Food Science and Technology*, vol. 36, no. 3, pp. 229–242, 2001.
[10] S. Sharma, U. Bajwa, and H. P. S. Nagi, "Rheological and baking properties of cowpea and wheat flour blends," *Journal of the Science of Food and Agriculture*, vol. 79, pp. 657–662, 1999.
[11] S. A. Lodhi, Salim-Ur-Rehman, and N. Huma, "Effect of supplementation of detoxified matri flour with wheat flour on the quality of pan bread," *Pakistan Journal of Scientific and Industrial Research*, vol. 46, no. 3, pp. 207–210, 2003.
[12] S. Ur-Rehman, A. Paterson, S. Hussain, I. A. Bhatti, and M. A. Raza Shahid, "Influence of detoxified Indian vetch (*Lathyrus sativus* L.) on sensory and protein quality characteristics of composite flour chapatti," *Journal of the Science of Food and Agriculture*, vol. 86, no. 8, pp. 1172–1180, 2006.
[13] S. U. Rehman, A. Paterson, S. Hussain, M. Anjum Murtaza, and S. Mehmood, "Influence of partial substitution of wheat flour with vetch (*Lathyrus sativus* L) flour on quality characteristics of doughnuts," *LWT—Food Science and Technology*, vol. 40, no. 1, pp. 73–82, 2007.
[14] S. Rehman, J. R. Piggott, M. M. Ahmad, S. Hussain, N. Ahmad, and P. Owusu-Darko, "Preparation and evaluation of pizza cheese made from blend of vetch-bovine milk," *International Journal of Food Science and Technology*, vol. 43, no. 5, pp. 770–778, 2008.
[15] A. Wondimu and N. G. Malleshi, "Development of weaning foods based on malted, popped, and roller-dried barley and chickpea," *Food and Nutrition Bulletin*, vol. 17, no. 2, pp. 169–176, 1996.
[16] A. Khurram, S. U. Rehman, U. A. Bajwa, B. E. Bajwa, and K. Jabbar, "Preparation and evaluation of texturized vegetables meat from legumes," *International Journal of Agriculture and Biology*, vol. 4, pp. 523–525, 2003.
[17] Anonymous, "Islamabad: Pakistan 5th largest producer of dates," 2002, http://archives.dawn.com/dawnftp/72.249.57.55/dawnftp/fixed/arch/arch_2002.html.
[18] M. Al-Farsi, C. Alasalvar, A. Morris, M. Baron, and F. Shahidi, "Compositional and sensory characteristics of three native sun-dried date (*Phoenix dactylifera* L.) varieties grown in Oman," *Journal of Agricultural and Food Chemistry*, vol. 53, no. 19, pp. 7586–7591, 2005.
[19] W. H. Barreveld, "Date Palm Product," FAO Agriculture Services Bulletin no. 101, Food and Agriculture Organization of the United Nation, Rome, Italy, 1993.
[20] I. A. Ahmed and R. K. Robinson, "The ability of date extracts to support the production of aflatoxins," *Food Chemistry*, vol. 66, no. 3, pp. 307–312, 1999.
[21] B. Martínez, F. Rincón, M. V. Ibáñez, and P. Abellán, "Improving the nutritive value of homogenized infant foods using response surface methodology," *Journal of Food Science*, vol. 69, no. 1, pp. SNQ38–SNQ43, 2004.
[22] M. S. Rahman and S. A. Al-Farsi, "Instrumental texture profile analysis (TPA) of date flesh as a function of moisture content," *Journal of Food Engineering*, vol. 66, no. 4, pp. 505–511, 2005.
[23] AOAC, *Official Methods of Analysis*, Association of Official Analytical Chemists, Arlington, Va, USA, 15th edition, 2000.
[24] D. G. Land and R. Shepherd, "Scaling and ranking methods," in *Sensory Analysis of Foods*, J. R. Piggott, Ed., pp. 155–185, Elsevier, New York, NY, USA, 1988.
[25] R. G. D. Steel, J. H. Torrie, and D. A. Dickey, *Principles and Procedures of Statistics. A Biometrical Approach*, McGraw Hill, New York, NY, USA, 3rd edition, 1997.
[26] J. K. Khalil, "Date bars fortified with soy or yeast proteins and dry skim milk," in *Dates of Saudi Arabia*, W. N. Sawaya, Ed., pp. 143–165, Safir Press, Riyadh, Saudi Arabia, 1986.
[27] S. Al-Hooti, J. S. Sidhu, J. Al-Otaibi, H. Al-Ameeri, and H. Qabazard, "Date bars fortified with almonds, sesame seeds, oat flakes and skim milk powder," *Plant Foods for Human Nutrition*, vol. 51, no. 2, pp. 125–135, 1997.
[28] W. N. Sawaya, H. A. Khatchadourian, J. K. Khalil, and A. S. Mashadi, "Processing of three major Saudi Arabian date cultivars into Jam," *Journal of Food Science and Technology*, vol. 20, pp. 149–152, 1983.
[29] E. Wittig de Penna, A. Bunger, M. Sansur, L. López, and R. Santana, "Development of soy-based protein candy bars for athletes," *Archivos latinoamericanos de nutrición*, vol. 43, no. 3, pp. 241–247, 1993.
[30] B. A. Escobar, A. M. A. Estévez, A. L. Tepper, and M. R. Aguayo, "Nutritional characteristics of cereal and peanut bars," *Archivos Latinoamericanos de Nutricion*, vol. 48, no. 2, pp. 156–159, 1998.
[31] G. Maurer, G. Fukuda, and S. Nielsen, "Development of bean-based granola bars and cereal," *Cereal Foods World*, vol. 50, no. 1, pp. 27–32, 2005.
[32] B. Escobar, A. M. Estevez, M. Vasquez, E. Castillo, and E. Yanez, "Cereal bars with peanut and puffed amaranthus: chemical and stability in accelerated storage," *Archivos Latinoamericanos de Nutrición*, vol. 44, pp. 10–36, 1994.
[33] J. A. Bower and R. Whitten, "Sensory characteristics and consumer liking for cereal bar snack foods," *Journal of Sensory Studies*, vol. 15, no. 3, pp. 327–345, 2000.
[34] U. N. Onwuka and K. S. Abasiekong, "Production and evaluation of chocolate bars from roasted and unroasted African breadfruit, and bambara groundnut flours," *Journal of Food Processing and Preservation*, vol. 30, no. 5, pp. 534–548, 2006.
[35] E. W. de Penna, A. Infante, A. Suarez, L. Lopez, R. Santana, and H. Torti, "Development of an energy food for athletes," *Archivos Latinoamericanos de Nutrición*, vol. 42, pp. 331–344, 1992.

[36] G. E. P. Box and N. R. Draper, *Empirical Model-Building and Response Surface*, John Wiley & Sons, New York, NY, USA, 1986.
[37] C. Montgomery, G. C. Runger, and N. F. Hubele, *Engineering Statistics*, John Wiley & Sons, New York, NY, USA, 2001.
[38] C. Collar, P. Andreu, J. C. Martínez, and E. Armero, "Optimization of hydrocolloid addition to improve wheat bread dough functionality: a response surface methodology study," *Food Hydrocolloids*, vol. 13, no. 6, pp. 467–475, 1999.
[39] T. A. Shittu, A. O. Raji, and L. O. Sanni, "Bread from composite cassava-wheat flour: I. Effect of baking time and temperature on some physical properties of bread loaf," *Food Research International*, vol. 40, no. 2, pp. 280–290, 2007.
[40] C. Collar, E. Santos, and C. M. Rosell, "Assessment of the rheological profile of fibre-enriched bread doughs by response surface methodology," *Journal of Food Engineering*, vol. 78, no. 3, pp. 820–826, 2007.
[41] K. Katina, R. L. Heiniö, K. Autio, and K. Poutanen, "Optimization of sourdough process for improved sensory profile and texture of wheat bread," *LWT—Food Science and Technology*, vol. 39, no. 10, pp. 1189–1202, 2006.
[42] L. Flander, M. Salmenkallio-Marttila, T. Suortti, and K. Autio, "Optimization of ingredients and baking process for improved wholemeal oat bread quality," *LWT—Food Science and Technology*, vol. 40, no. 5, pp. 860–870, 2007.
[43] D. N. Yadav, P. E. Patki, C. Mahesh, G. K. Sharma, and A. S. Bawa, "Optimisation of baking parameters of chapati with respect to vitamin B 1 and B2 retention and quality," *International Journal of Food Science and Technology*, vol. 43, no. 8, pp. 1474–1483, 2008.
[44] S. M. Loveday, J. P. Hindmarsh, L. K. Creamer, and H. Singh, "Physicochemical changes in a model protein bar during storage," *Food Research International*, vol. 42, no. 7, pp. 798–806, 2009.
[45] M. A. Mir and N. Nath, "Sorption isotherms of fortified mango bars," *Journal of Food Engineering*, vol. 25, no. 1, pp. 141–150, 1995.
[46] S. M. Loveday, J. P. Hindmarsh, L. K. Creamer, and H. Singh, "Physicochemical changes in intermediate-moisture protein bars made with whey protein or calcium caseinate," *Food Research International*, vol. 43, no. 5, pp. 1321–1328, 2010.
[47] M. E. R. Ortiz, E. S. Martín-Martínez, and L. P. M. Padilla, "Rheological and thermal properties of extruded mixtures of rice starch and isolated soy protein," *Starch/Staerke*, vol. 60, no. 10, pp. 577–587, 2008.
[48] P. A. Shaun, *Mechanisms of nutrition bar hardening: effect of hydrolyzed whey protein and carbohydrate source*, Master of Science, Utah State University, Logan, Utah, USA, 2008.
[49] S. Uthayakumaran, M. Newberry, M. Keentok, F. L. Stoddard, and F. Bekes, "Basic rheology of bread dough with modified protein content and glutenin-to-gliadin ratios," *Cereal Chemistry*, vol. 77, no. 6, pp. 744–749, 2000.

8

The Effects of Body Acupuncture on Obesity: Anthropometric Parameters, Lipid Profile, and Inflammatory and Immunologic Markers

Hamid Abdi,[1,2] Baixiao Zhao,[1] Mahsa Darbandi,[2] Majid Ghayour-Mobarhan,[2,3] Shima Tavallaie,[2] Amir Ali Rahsepar,[3,4] Seyyed Mohammad Reza Parizadeh,[2] Mohammad Safariyan,[2] Mohsen Nemati,[2] Maryam Mohammadi,[2] Parisa Abbasi-Parizad,[2] Sara Darbandi,[2] Saeed Akhlaghi,[2] and Gordon A. A. Ferns[5]

[1] *Departments of Acupuncture Therapy, Beijing University of Chinese Medicine, Beijing 100029, China*
[2] *Biochemistry and Nutrition Research Center, Faculty of Medicine, Mashhad University of Medical Sciences (MUMS), Mashhad, Iran*
[3] *Cardiovascular Research Center, Faculty of Medicine, Mashhad University of Medical Sciences, Mashhad 9196773117, Iran*
[4] *Young Researchers Club, Mashhad Branch, Islamic Azad University, Mashhad 9187147578, Iran*
[5] *Institute for Science and Technology in Medicine, Keele University, Thornburrow Drive, Hartshill, Stoke-on-Trent, ST4 7QB, UK*

Correspondence should be addressed to Majid Ghayour-Mobarhan, ghayourm@mums.ac.ir

Academic Editor: Francesco Giallauria

A randomized controlled clinical trial in 196 obese subjects was performed to examine the effectiveness of body acupuncture on body weight loss, lipid profile and immunogenic and inflammatory markers. Subjects received authentic (cases) or sham (controls) acupuncture for 6 weeks in combination with a low-calorie diet. In the following 6 weeks, they received the low-calorie diet alone. Subjects were assessed at the beginning, 6 and 12 weeks later. Heat shock protein (Hsps)-27, 60, 65, 70 antibody titers and high sensitivity C-reactive protein (hs-CRP) levels were also assessed. A significant reduction in measures of adiposity and improvement in lipid profile were observed in both groups, but the levels of anti-Hsp-antibodies decreased in cases only. A reduction in anthropometric and lipid profile in cases were sustained in the second period, however, only changes in lipid profile were observed in the control group. Anti-Hsp-antibodies and hs-CRP levels continued to be reduced in cases but in controls only the reduction in hs-CRP remained. Changes in anthropometric parameters, lipid profile, and anti-Hsp-antibodies were more evident in cases. Body acupuncture in combination with diet restriction was effective in enhancing weight loss and improving dyslipidemia.

1. Introduction

Obesity is becoming increasingly common in the general population and is associated with several other conditions such as hypertension, diabetes, dyslipidemia, and cardiovascular disease [1]; these are also increasing in their prevalence. The general principles for the treatment of obesity are to achieve weight loss, to maintain this reduction in body weight following this loss, and to finally reduce the risk factors for obesity. There are several different modalities for treatment of obesity one of which is acupuncture. It would be desirable to control obesity by safe and effective treatment modalities, and among the different methods acupuncture is one of the most popular complementary treatments. Acupuncture is performed by stimulating particular points on the skin called acupoints. Among several methods used for acupoints stimulation [2], needling is one of the most common methods, and stimulation can either be manual or electrical (electroacupuncture). Acupuncture has been used in the treatment of several diseases including obesity [3–5] and also immune-related diseases, such as allergic disorders, autoimmune diseases, and immunodeficiency-syndromes [6–8].

Heat shock proteins (Hsps) are highly conserved proteins expressed by several cell types following exposure to environmental stresses. Over the past 2 decades, there has been an increasing interest in the relationship between Hsps and cardiovascular disease, and particularly whether an autoimmune response may be implicated by formation of anti-Hsp antibodies [9]. In this regard, most of the studies have focused on the relation between cardiovascular disease and Hsp/anti-Hsp-60, -65, -70 while there is recent evidence that supports the role of Hsp/anti-Hsp27 in cardiovascular events (reviewed by Ghayour-Mobarhan et al.) [9]. Wick et al. [10] propose that autoimmunity to Hsps (formation of anti-Hsp antibodies) may contribute to the progression of atherosclerosis [11, 12]. Serum C-reactive protein (CRP) is a feature of systemic inflammation [13] and is positively associated with measures of adiposity such as body mass index (BMI) and waist circumferences (WCs) as demonstrated by 2 large cross-sectional studies [14, 15]. While obesity is related to higher levels of CRP [16], following weight loss reduction in CRP levels has been also reported [17, 18].

There are several studies which have evaluated the effect of acupuncture in the management of obesity. However, most studies have methodological limitations, including small sample size and inadequately controlled study design [19]. To our knowledge, the effect of acupuncture during body weight loss has not been evaluated with respect to inflammatory and immunological markers such as hs-CRP and anti-HSP antibodies. Thus, we aimed to perform a randomized controlled clinical trial in patients suffering from obesity to examine its effectiveness in body weight loss, changing the lipid profile, and inflammatory and immunological markers by body acupuncture.

2. Material and Methods

2.1. Study Design and Subjects. Two hundred and twenty overweight and obese subjects were recruited from the nutrition clinic, Quem hospital, Mashhad, Iran. In this study, overweight was defined as a BMI of 25 to <30, and a BMI of ≥30 was defined as obesity. They neither had received any other weight control measures nor had any medical and/or drug history within the last 3 months before their participation in the study. Participants were informed about the study both verbally and by written information sheets. Volunteers were given time to discuss the study and were encouraged to ask questions. Those who had exclusion criteria such as diabetes, hypertension, heart disease, endocrine abnormalities, and pregnancy. Finally, 196 subjects were enrolled into the study after checking for the inclusion and exclusion criteria. These subjects were randomized into 2 groups of case and control of body acupuncture (each group had 98 subjects). The subjects were aged between 18 and 55 years and had a body mass index (BMI) between 25 and 45 kg/m^2. Each patient gave informed written consent to participate in the study, which was approved by the Mashhad University of Medical Science Ethics Committee.

Anthropometric and biochemical assessments were measured before and after treatment. The participants were asked to follow an isocaloric diet (wash-out diet) for 2 weeks before starting the trial to match the two groups for initial diet, and a low-calorie diet for 6 weeks. The low-calorie diet consisted of 1000 kcal deficit per day, less than the individual daily energy expenditure. The resting energy expenditure was calculated using the equation of Harris Benedict [20] and was used to determine the amount of food per day for each participant. The wash-out diet and the 6-week dietary program for each participant were planned by a nutritionist based on the participant's energy expenditure. The diet was prescribed and the participant's compliance was checked every week.

Hypercholesterolemia was defined using a serum total-cholesterol concentration ≥200 mg/dL or treatment with lipid-lowering drugs, diabetes by fasting plasma glucose level ≥126 mg/dL on ≥2 occasions or treatment with antidiabetic drugs, and hypertension by blood pressures ≥140/90 mmHg on ≥2 occasions or if patients were on treatment with antihypertensive medications [21].

2.2. Acupuncture Treatment in Cases. Eight acupuncture points on the abdomen, including Tianshu (ST-25) both sides, Weidao (GB-28) both sides, Zhongwan (REN-12) Shuifen (REN-9) Guanyuan (REN-4) Sanyinjiao (SP-6), and additional Points are Quchi (LI-11) and Fenlong (ST-40) for excess mood (patients with higher energy), and Qihai (REN-6) and Yinlingqau (SP-9) for deficiency mood (patients with lower energy) on both lower legs were selected. In the authentic body-acupuncture group, acupuncture needling with manipulation and use the normal electric lines of the electric acupuncture machine (Ying Lee, KWD 808) to 4 needles on the abdomen, two needles (ST-25) and (GB-28) on each side, was applied for 20 minutes.

In this group, the stainless steel acupuncture needles (3.8 cm long) were inserted to a depth of approximately 2.5 cm after skin sterilization. The needles in the lower legs were manipulated by rotating them back and forth until the subjects had the sensation of *De-Xi*, a term used in acupuncture to describe a feeling of heaviness in the area surrounding the locus of insertion. The needles in the abdomen were applied with electricity. The needles were connected to an electrical stimulator. Electricity was generated as an output of programmed pulse voltage, 30–40 Hz, dense-disperse wave, 390 μS square pulse, and at a maximal tolerable intensity, 500 Ω (12–23 V) (a strong but not painful sensation to the patient). Each acupuncture treatment lasted for 20 minutes. All subjects were asked to receive two treatment sessions per week for a total of 6 weeks. After that all patients in both groups received no acupuncture treatment for next 6 weeks, but were still given advice to keep going on their diet control. All needling was done by a specialized acupuncturist.

In sham acupuncture group, for points on the RN meridian, 0.3 cm laterally to the real location was used, and needling was very superficially as much as possible. Other points are located 0.5 cm up and 0.5 cm laterally to the real location and needling was also very superficially. Disconnected electric lines of the acupuncture machine were applied to 4 needles, each side two needles (ST-25) and (GB-28), for 20 minutes was also used. No major adverse effects were observed in any of patients.

2.3. Anthropometric Measurements. For all patients, body weight (BW), BMI, and body fat mass were measured by body composition analyzer BC-418 (TANITA, Japan) according to a standard protocol [22]. Height and body weight were measured with the subjects dressed in light clothing after an overnight fasting. The body weight of each subject was measured with a standard scale to an accuracy of ±0.1 kg, and height was measured to an accuracy of ±0.1 cm. Hip circumference (HC) was measured at the levels of the major trochanters through the pubic symphysis, and waist circumference (WC) was measured midway between the lateral lower rib margin and the iliac crest with the scale to the nearest ±0.1 cm. The body mass index (BMI) was calculated as weight (kg) divided by height squared (m^2).

2.4. Collection of Blood Samples. Blood samples were taken from each patient for analysis after a 12-hour fasting, 3 times during the study (at the beginning, 6 and 12 weeks later). Following venepuncture, blood samples were collected into Vacutainer tubes and centrifuged at 10,000 g for 15 min at 4°C. Hemolyzed samples were excluded from analysis. After separation, aliquots of serum were frozen at −80°C until analysis.

2.5. Routine Biochemical Analysis and Serum Anti-HSP-27, 60, 65, 70 Antibody Titers. A full-fasted lipid profile comprising total cholesterol, triglycerides, high-density lipoprotein cholesterol (HDL-C), and low-density lipoprotein-cholesterol (LDL-C) were determined for each subject. Serum lipid and fasting blood sugar (FBS) concentrations were measured enzymatically with the use of commercial kits. hs-CRP was measured by a PEG-enhanced immunoturbidimetry method with an Alycon analyzer (ABBOTT, Chicago, Ill, USA). Serum HSP27, 60, 65, 70 antibody titers were measured using an in-house ELISA assay, as we have explained before [11, 23].

2.6. Statistical Analysis. SPSS software (version 16, Chicago, Ill, USA) was used to perform the statistical analysis. Data were checked for normality. Values were expressed as mean ± SEM or, in the case of nonnormally distributed data (like triglyceride), as median and interquartile range. Data that were normally distributed were analyzed using Student's t-test. Data found to be nonnormally distributed were analyzed using the nonparametric Mann-Whitney test. For comparison between two related samples, the paired t-test (normally distributed data) and the Wilcoxon signed ranks test (non-normally distributed data) were used. For multiple comparisons of parameters Bonferroni corrections were used. A two-sided P value of <0.05 was considered statistically significant.

TABLE 1: Comparison between clinical and biochemical characteristics of participants.

Group	Real (n = 79)	Sham (n = 82)
Age (year)	36.88 ± 0.98	37.41 ± 1.01
Weight (kg)	84.10 ± 1.67	85.02 ± 1.75
Height (cm)	161.08 ± 0.83	160.79 ± 0.92
Body fat (%)	37.00 ± 0.69	37.08 ± 0.79
BMI (Kg/m^2)	32.30 ± 0.52	32.74 ± 0.59
WC (cm)	102.39 ± 1.28	100.74 ± 1.36
HC (cm)	113.76 ± 1.03	114.98 ± 1.18
WC/HC ratio	0.90 ± 0.1	0.87 ± 0.008
FBS (mg/dL)	84.48 ± 1.46	87.76 ± 2.58
TC (mg/dL)	173.54 ± 4.13	171.96 ± 4.11
TG (mg/dL)	112.48 ± 6.24	123.58 ± 5.8
HDL-C (mg/dL)	42.60 ± 0.99	41.65 ± 1.06
LDL-C (mg/dL)	108.19 ± 3.44	107.46 ± 3.05
DBP (mmHg)	73.33 ± 1.71	75.95 ± 1.67
SBP (mmHg)	107.91 ± 1.92	107.38 ± 1.77
Anti-HSP27 antibody	0.37 (0.32–0.41)	0.35 (0.33–0.41)
Anti-HSP60 antibody	0.74 (0.68–0.86)	0.72 (0.69–0.78)
Anti-HSP65 antibody	0.81 (0.73–0.90)	0.81 (0.78–0.83)
Anti-HSP70 antibody	0.59 (0.55–0.67)	0.61 (0.57–0.66)
hs-CRP (mg/dL)	1.78 (1.15–3.06)	1.79 (0.99–3.39)

BMI: body mass index; WC: waist circumference; HC: hip circumference; FBS: fasting blood sugar; TC: total cholesterol; TG: triglycerides; HDL-C: high-density lipoprotein cholesterol; LDL-C: low-density lipoprotein cholesterol, DBP: diastolic blood pressure, SBP: systolic blood pressure, Anti-Hsp antibody: Anti-heat shock protein, hs-CRP: high-sensitivity C-reactive protein. Values are expressed as mean ± SEM, or median and interquartile range. Chi-square test (for qualitative variable), independent sample t-test (for normally distributed data), and Mann-Whitney test (for non-normally distributed data) were used for comparison 2 groups.

3. Results

3.1. Demographic Data. One hundred and ninety-six participants fulfilled the inclusion criteria. Then, they were divided into 2 groups (cases and controls) including 98 subjects. By the end of the study 35 subjects withdrew for personal reasons and 161 participants completed the study (Figure 1). The analysis showed that sex, age, basal levels of anthropometric parameters, lipid profiles, and also levels of anti-Hsp27 antibodies and hs-CRP were not significantly different between case and control groups ($P > 0.05$) at baseline. Clinical and biochemical characteristics of participants have been summarized in Table 1.

3.2. Comparison at First 6 Weeks (First Period). In the authentic acupuncture body group, in the first period of intervention including both acupuncture and low-calorie diet, in authentic acupuncture subjects significant reduction in body weight ($P < 0.001$), body fat percentage ($P < 0.001$), BMI ($P < 0.001$), WC ($P < 0.001$), HC ($P < 0.001$), total cholesterol ($P < 0.001$), triglyceride ($P < 0.001$), HDL-C ($P < 0.05$), and LDL-C ($P < 0.001$) was observed. In the sham body acupuncture group, after 6 weeks of intervention, body weight ($P < 0.001$), body fat percentage ($P < 0.001$),

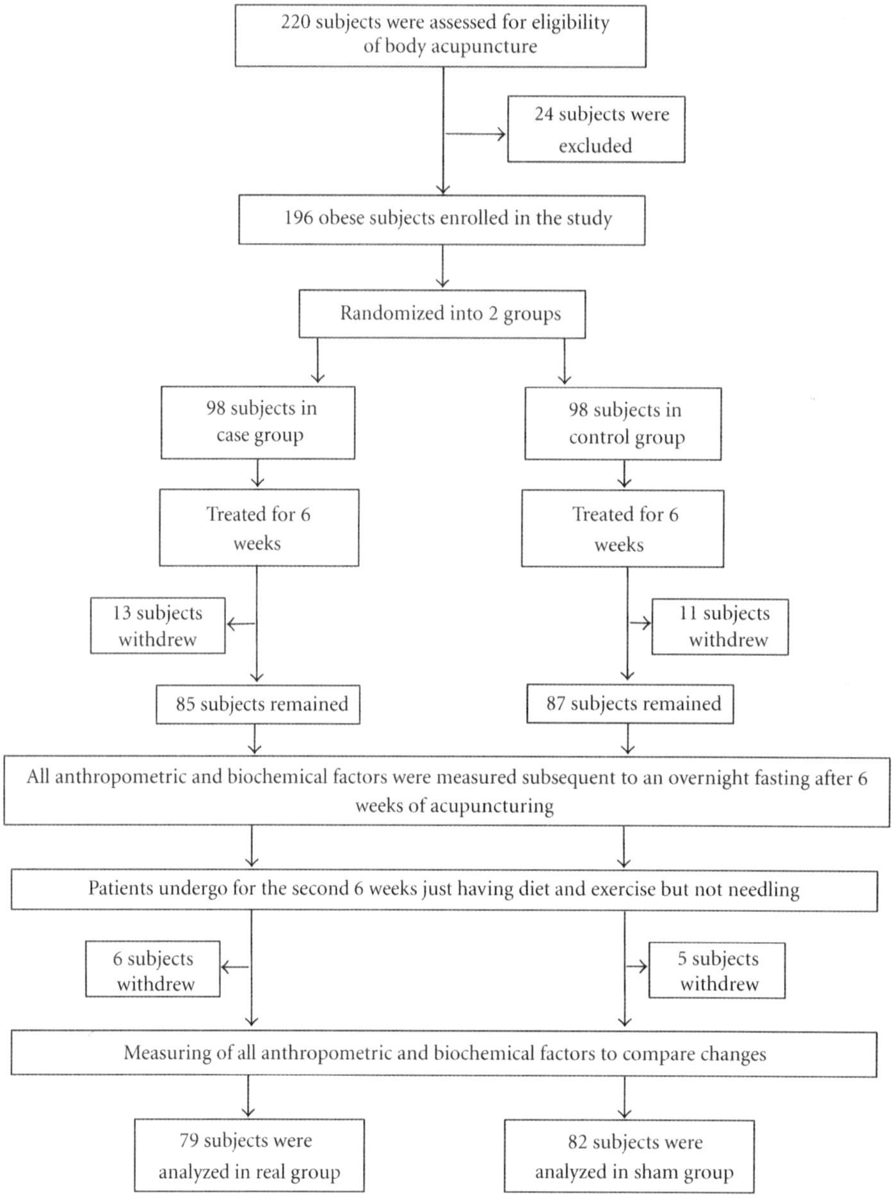

FIGURE 1: Trial profile and design.

BMI ($P < 0.001$), WC ($P < 0.001$), HC ($P < 0.001$), total cholesterol ($P < 0.01$), HDL-C ($P < 0.001$), and LDL-C ($P < 0.01$) were reduced significantly. Interestingly in the first period of study, all immunological (anti-Hsp antibodies) but not inflammatory (hs-CRP) factors decreased significantly in cases but not in controls ($P < 0.001$), however, just anti-HSP60 antibodies where reduced statistically ($P < 0.05$). Table 2 summarizes the levels of different parameters.

In the control group, significant changes were observed for triglyceride ($P < 0.01$), HDL-C ($P < 0.001$), and LDL-C ($P < 0.05$). The same as the first period of the study, all immunological and inflammatory factors including anti-Hsp antibodies and hs-CRP levels continued their reduction significantly in authentic group ($P < 0.001$), while in controls no statistically changes were seen for these parameters except for hs-CRP ($P < 0.001$) (Table 2).

3.3. Comparison at Second 6 Weeks (Second Period). In the authentic acupuncture group, in the second period of intervention including just low-calorie diet, significant changes were found in body weight ($P < 0.001$), BMI ($P < 0.01$), WC ($P < 0.001$), HC ($P < 0.001$), triglyceride ($P < 0.01$), HDL-C ($P < 0.001$), and LDL-C ($P < 0.001$).

3.4. Comparison the Whole Period of the Study. After 12 weeks of study, in cases of acupuncture body group, significant changes were found in body weight ($P < 0.001$), BMI ($P < 0.001$), WC ($P < 0.001$), HC ($P < 0.001$), total-cholesterol ($P < 0.001$), triglyceride ($P < 0.001$), HDL-C ($P < 0.001$), and LDL-C ($P < 0.001$) (Table 2). In the control

TABLE 2: Comparison of clinical and biochemical characteristics of participants of body group.

Variable	Real group			Sham group		
	1st sample	2nd sample	3rd sample	1st sample	2nd sample	3rd sample
Weight (kg)	84.10 ± 1.67	81.23 ± 1.68$^{\alpha}$	81.27 ± 2.41$^{\alpha,\beta}$	85.02 ± 1.75	82.81 ± 1.81$^{\alpha}$	84.96 ± 2.56$^{\alpha}$
Body fat (%)	37.00 ± 0.69	36.03 ± 0.7$^{\alpha}$	37.91 ± 1.91	37.08 ± 0.79	36.54 ± 0.84$^{\alpha}$	36.35 ± 1.01$^{\alpha}$
BMI (Kg/m^2)	32.30 ± 0.52	31.17 ± 0.53$^{\alpha}$	30.98 ± 0.62$^{\alpha,\beta}$	32.74 ± 0.59	31.87 ± 0.61$^{\alpha}$	31.73 ± 0.74$^{\alpha}$
WC (cm)	102.39 ± 1.28	95.12 ± 1.2$^{\alpha}$	92.90 ± 1.43$^{\alpha,\beta}$	100.74 ± 1.36	96.66 ± 1.26$^{\alpha}$	97.16 ± 1.31$^{\alpha}$
HC (cm)	113.76 ± 1.03	106.59 ± 0.93$^{\alpha}$	105.84 ± 1.19$^{\alpha,\beta}$	114.98 ± 1.18	111.10 ± 1.15$^{\alpha}$	110.40 ± 1.48$^{\alpha}$
WC/HC ratio	0.90 ± 0.1	0.89 ± 0.01	0.087 ± 0.01	0.87 ± 0.008	0.87 ± 0.007	0.88 ± 0.008
FBS (mg/dL)	84.48 ± 1.46	87.46 ± 1.33	87.27 ± 3.1	87.76 ± 2.58	89.64 ± 3.40	90.03 ± 3.37
TC (mg/dL)	173.54 ± 4.13	148.18 ± 3.92$^{\alpha}$	137.98 ± 3.71$^{\alpha,\beta}$	171.96 ± 4.11	162.23 ± 3.72$^{\alpha}$	157.15 ± 3.82$^{\alpha}$
TG (mg/dL)	112.48 ± 6.24	92.51 ± 4.40$^{\alpha}$	87.69 ± 4.55$^{\alpha,\beta}$	123.58 ± 5.8	122.97 ± 5.68	108.76 ± 6.37$^{\alpha,\beta}$
HDL-C (mg/dL)	42.60 ± 0.99	38.51 ± 0.88$^{\alpha}$	54.33 ± 2.96$^{\alpha,\beta}$	41.65 ± 1.06	38.16 ± 0.94$^{\alpha}$	53.05 ± 3.01$^{\alpha,\beta}$
LDL-C (mg/dL)	108.19 ± 3.44	91.34 ± 3.48$^{\alpha}$	74.50 ± 3.60$^{\alpha,\beta}$	107.46 ± 3.05	99.92 ± 2.89$^{\alpha}$	93.27 ± 3.12$^{\alpha,\beta}$
Anti-HSP27	0.37 (0.32–0.41)	0.33 (0.29–0.37)$^{\alpha}$	0.31 (0.28–0.34)$^{\alpha,\beta}$	0.35 (0.33–0.41)	0.36 (0.32–0.39)	0.36 (0.33–0.41)
Anti-HSP60	0.74 (0.68–0.86)	0.73 (0.62–0.80)$^{\alpha}$	0.70 (0.62–0.77)$^{\alpha,\beta}$	0.72 (0.69–0.78)	0.73 (0.68–0.78)$^{\alpha}$	0.73 (0.67–0.78)
Anti-HSP65	0.81 (0.73–0.90)	0.80 (0.73–0.86)$^{\alpha}$	0.77 (0.70–0.83)$^{\alpha,\beta}$	0.81 (0.78–0.83)	0.80 (0.77–0.84)	0.80 (0.77–0.84)
Anti-HSP70	0.59 (0.55–0.67)	0.56 (0.52–0.64)$^{\alpha}$	0.54 (0.50–0.60)$^{\alpha,\beta}$	0.61 (0.57–0.66)	0.60 (0.57–0.65)	0.61 (0.56–0.66)
hs-CRP (mg/dL)	1.78 (1.15–3.06)	1.3 (1.3–3.0)	0.8 (0.23–1.4)$^{\alpha,\beta}$	1.79 (0.99–3.39)	1.3 (1.3–3.2)	1.10 (0.33–2.00)$^{\alpha,\beta}$

R: Real; S: Sham; BMI: Body mass index; WC: waist circumference; HC: Hip circumference; FBS: Fasting blood sugar; TC: total cholesterol; HDL-C: high-density lipoprotein cholesterol; LDL-C: low-density lipoprotein cholesterol; DBP: diastolic blood pressure; SBP: systolic blood pressure. Values are expressed as mean ± SEM, or median and interquartile range. $^{\alpha}$means significant changes in comparison with first sample and $^{\beta}$means significant changes in comparison with second sample.

group, body weight ($P < 0.001$), body fat percentage ($P < 0.001$), BMI ($P < 0.001$), HC ($P < 0.001$), total cholesterol ($P < 0.001$) and triglycerides ($P < 0.01$), HDL-C ($P < 0.01$), and LDL-C ($P < 0.001$) changed significantly. Overall, immunological and inflammatory factors including anti-Hsp27 antibodies and hs-CRP levels decreased significantly ($P < 0.001$) in the authentic but not control group, except the hs-CRP levels which also significantly reduced in control subjects ($P < 0.001$) (Table 2).

3.5. Comparison between Changes in the First and Second Periods of Study. In the acupuncture group, changes in the first (acupuncture and low-calorie diet) versus second (only low-calorie diet) period was significantly different for body weight ($P < 0.001$), BMI ($P < 0.001$), WC ($P < 0.001$), HC ($P < 0.001$), total cholesterol ($P < 0.001$), triglycerides ($P < 0.01$), HDL-C ($P < 0.001$), and hs-CRP ($P < 0.05$). In all above parameters except HDL-C and hs-CRP, the changes were more significant in the first period when compared with second one. In acupuncture control group, body weight ($P < 0.01$), WC ($P < 0.001$), HC ($P < 0.05$), HDL-C ($P < 0.001$), and anti-Hsp27 ($P < 0.05$) were significantly different. All above changes were more significant for the first period of study compared with second period except the HDL-C (Table 3).

3.6. Comparison of the Changes in Different Parameters between the Case and Control Groups. For anthropometric parameters, acupuncture was more effective for reducing body weight in all 3 periods of the study ($P < 0.05$), BMI in the first period of the study ($P < 0.05$), WC in all 3 periods of the study ($P < 0.05$), and HC in the first and whole period of the study ($P < 0.001$). For lipid profile, total-cholesterol in the first and whole periods ($P < 0.05$), triglycerides in the first period ($P < 0.01$), and LDL-C in the first and whole period of the study were significantly and more effectively reduced by authentic body acupuncture.

With regards to immunological markers, authentic body acupuncture was more effective as we observed that anti-Hsp27 antibodies were significantly reduced in the all 3 periods of the study when, compared with control acupuncture ($P < 0.001$). The same results were observed for other anti-Hsps ($P < 0.001$). However, the marker of inflammation, hs-CRP was not significantly changed between cases and controls ($P > 0.05$).

4. Discussion

In the first period of the study, a significant reduction in anthropometric and lipid profile was observed in both cases and controls, but the levels of anti-Hsp antibodies were found to fall in cases but not controls. In the second period which provides evidence for the ability of acupuncture to produce a sustained reduction in anthropometric and lipid profile, whilst in the control group, only changes in lipid profile were sustained. As before, anti-Hsp antibodies and

Table 3: Comparison of changes in clinical and biochemical characteristics of body acupuncture.

Variable	Real group				Sham group				
	1st period	2nd period	Whole period	P value 1 v. 2	1st period	2nd period	Whole period	P value 1 v. 2	P value R. v. S.
Weight (kg)	2.98 ± 0.22	1.22 ± 0.18	4.15 ± 0.37	0.000	2.21 ± 0.23	0.29 ± 0.29	2.40 ± 0.60	0.001	1st P: 0.019 2nd P: 0.006 3rd P: 0.012
Body fat (%)	0.90 ± 0.18	−1.39 ± 1.72	−0.38 ± 1.70	0.177	0.77 ± 0.20	0.43 ± 0.40	1.22 ± 0.35	0.507	1st P: 0.632 2nd P: 0.326 3rd P: 0.377
BMI (Kg/m^2)	1.16 ± 0.09	0.29 ± 0.10	1.47 ± 0.14	0.000	0.86 ± 0.10	0.47 ± 0.27	1.24 ± 0.16	0.221	1st P: 0.038 2nd P: 0.523 3rd P: 0.294
WC (cm)	7.05 ± 0.60	1.76 ± 0.40	8.93 ± 0.79	0.000	4.07 ± 0.52	−0.50 ± 0.93	3.97 ± 0.92	0.000	1st P: 0.000 2nd P: 0.020 3rd P: 0.000
HC (cm)	7.16 ± 0.40	1.63 ± 0.37	8.70 ± 0.56	0.000	3.76 ± 0.56	1.17 ± 0.68	5.49 ± 0.64	0.011	1st P: 0.000 2nd P: 0.538 3rd P: 0.000
WC/HC ratio	0.007 ± 0.006	0.003 ± 0.004	0.015 ± 0.008	0.384	0.006 ± 0.005	−0.01 ± 0.008	−0.005 ± 0.008	0.106	1st P: 0.926 2nd P: 0.064 3rd P: 0.095
FBS (mg/dL)	−2.70 ± 1.39	−0.70 ± 3.43	−3.61 ± 2.98	0.611	−2.08 ± 1.74	2.83 ± 2.03	0.45 ± 1.58	0.170	1st P: 0.780 2nd P: 0.388 3rd P: 0.237
TC (mg/dL)	25.35 ± 2.60	7.52 ± 2.99	32.62 ± 3.59	0.000	10.98 ± 3.58	6.80 ± 3.44	18.51 ± 4.46	0.456	1st P: 0.001 2nd P: 0.873 3rd P: 0.014
TG (mg/dL)	19.97 ± 3.55	5.73 ± 2.52	25.97 ± 5.53	0.003	1.48 ± 5.85	17.19 ± 6.84	21.82 ± 7.57	0.530	1st P: 0.002 2nd P: 0.200 3rd P: 0.357
HDL-C (mg/dL)	4.02 ± 0.97	−16.07 ± 2.88	−12.12 ± 3.12	0.000	3.97 ± 0.99	−13.15 ± 2.80	−10.64 ± 3.11	0.000	1st P: 0.974 2nd P: 0.471 3rd P: 0.739
LDL-C (mg/dL)	17.17 ± 2.23	15.19 ± 2.96	31.85 ± 3.13	0.734	9.03 ± 2.55	7.22 ± 2.80	15.34 ± 3.29	0.581	1st P: 0.017 2nd P: 0.054 3rd P: 0.000
Anti-HSP27 Antibody	0.03 (0.01–0.06)	0.02 (0.0–0.04)	0.05 (0.02–0.08)	0.083	0.01 (−0.01–0.02)	−0.01 (−0.02–0.01)	0.0 (−0.01–0.02)	0.028	1st P: 0.000 2nd P: 0.000 3rd P: 0.000 1st P: 0.000

Table 3: Continued.

Variable	Real group				Sham group				
	1st period	2nd period	Whole period	*P* value 1 v. 2	1st period	2nd period	Whole period	*P* value 1 v. 2	*P* value R. v. S.
Anti-HSP60 Antibody	0.03 (0.02–0.05)	0.02 (0.01–0.05)	0.06 (0.04–0.09)	0.114	0.01 (−0.007–0.02)	0.0 (−0.01–0.02)	0.01 (−0.01–0.02)	0.264	2nd *P*: 0.000 3rd *P*: 0.000 1st *P*: 0.003
Anti-HSP65 Antibody	0.02 (−0.01–0.05)	0.03 (0.01–0.05)	0.05 (0.03–0.08)	0.370	0.01 (−0.01–0.02)	0.005 (−0.01–0.017)	0.01 (−0.01–0.02)	0.569	2nd *P*: 0.000 3rd *P*: 0.000 1st *P*: 0.000
Anti-HSP70 Antibody	0.02 (0.01–0.04)	0.02 (0.01–0.04)	0.05 (0.03–0.07)	0.936	0.01 (−0.01–0.02)	−0.005 (−0.02–0.01)	0.0 (−0.01–0.02)	0.096	2nd *P*: 0.000 3rd *P*: 0.000 1st *P*: 0.790
hs-CRP (mg/dL)	0.0 (−0.63–0.94)	0.90 (0.15–1.7)	1.06 (0.18–1.47)	0.024	0.0 (−0.58–0.75)	0.8 (0.1–1.60)	0.62 (0.13–1.39)	0.226	2nd *P*: 0.691 3rd *P*: 0.256

R: real; S: sham; BMI: body mass index; WC: waist circumference; HC: hip circumference; FBS: fasting blood sugar; TC: total cholesterol; HDL-C: high-density lipoprotein cholesterol; LDL-C: low-density lipoprotein cholesterol, DBP: diastolic blood pressure, SBP: systolic blood pressure. Values are expressed as mean ± SEM, or median and interquartile range. Paired *t*-test and Wilcoxon signed ranked test were used for comparison between first and second periods for normally and nonnormally distributed data, respectively. Independent sample *t*-test (for normally distributed data) and Mann-Whitney test (for non-normally distributed data) were used for comparison 2 groups.

hs-CRP levels continued to fall in cases while no significant changes were observed in controls except hs-CRP. When the whole period of the study was assessed, the reduction in anthropometric, lipid profile and also hs-CRP levels were observed in both cases and controls, but the changes in anti-Hsp antibodies were only statistically significant in the group treated with authentic acupuncture. In addition, the analysis showed that changes in most of the parameters were more significant in the first period of the study when acupuncture were accompanied with diet restriction, compared with second period consisting of diet restriction only. Moreover, changes in anthropometric parameters, lipid profile, and anti-Hsp antibodies were more significant in cases in comparison with the control group. However, the changes in hs-CRP level were not significantly different. Changes in anthropometric and lipid profile in the first, second, and whole period of the study have been summarized in Figure 2.

Consistent with our results, indicating the greater efficacy of body acupuncture therapy for reduction of anthropometric parameters in cases when compared with controls, there are other studies reporting similar findings. Hsu et al. [4] performed a randomized crossover trial in obese women and found that anthropometric parameters changed significantly by electroacupuncture when compared with sit-up exercise. The same results have been found by other studies [3, 5]. However, there are some studies that have reported no significant effect of acupuncture in the treatment of obesity, but it should be noted that these studies were performed by auricular acupuncture therapy [24–26].

It is thought that acupuncture exerts its effects on weight loss through different mechanisms. In terms of traditional medicine, it is believed that acupuncture alters levels of central nervous system by stimulating peripheral nerves at acupoints. Signals are then carried by stimulated nerve resulting in changes in satiety and mood. These mechanisms have been reviewed by Lacey et al. [2]. Acupuncture appears to be able to improve mood by increasing the release of neurotransmitters [27] and suppress appetite by the serotonin and endorphin-induced decreases in stress and depression [28, 29], whereas this effect was not seen by exercise and diet. In addition, it has been shown that application of electroacupuncture at Zusanli (ST-36) and Neiting (ST-44) of the rat caused the increase in the electrical activity of ventral-medical hypothalamus in the obese rat, leading to activation of the satiety center [30]. Waist circumference is related to the subcutaneous fat tissue of the abdomen, and higher effects of body acupuncture in lipolitic activity and enhancing lipid metabolisms could be attributed to the direct effects of body acupuncture in redistribution, lyses of fat tissue [5], and reducing waist circumferences.

Concerning the effects on lipid profile in both cases and controls, positive changes (increase in levels of HDL-C and decrease in other parameters including triglycerides, total-cholesterol and LDL-C) were observed, however, the changes were significantly different between 2 groups being higher for acupuncture body group, indicating that whilst diet had important effects on the lipid profile but the combination of diet restriction and acupuncture therapy, leads to a further improvement in lipid profile levels. Moreover, Li and Wang [31] have reported significant changes in total and LDL cholesterol in during acupuncture therapy when compared with control subjects. In other study, it was reported that a significant decrease of triglyceride, total cholesterol, LDL-C but no changes in HDL-C in acupuncture group when compared with controls [32]. In several studies, a similar pattern of changes in triglyceride, total-cholesterol, LDL-C, and HDL-C changed has been reported as our study following acupuncture [19, 33, 34], however, 2 of these studies did not find any changes for HDL-C [19, 32], this may be explained by application of different acupoints. It has been suggested that these changes in lipid metabolism may be caused by increase in the serum betaendorphin levels [32].

Reduction in anti-Hsp antibodies in all periods of the study was significant only in authentic group in comparison with controls. Moreover, in the first period of the study when acupuncture combined with diet restriction, this finding was more prominent. To our knowledge, no study has evaluated the effects of acupuncture therapy on these antibodies. However, in a study, it has been reported that dietary constituents are associated with immune response to Hsps in dyslipidemic patients [23]. Our results indicate that acupuncture therapy may have direct effects on immune system and modulates the function of our immunity. As previously noted, these anti-Hsp antibodies have a potential pathologic role in atherogenesis and may progress further inflammatory processes.

Moreover, as reviewed by Cabyoglu et al. [35], acupuncture is able to increase the levels of encephalin, endomorphin-1, beta endorphin, serotonin, and dopamine and has immunomodulator effects on immune system and lipolitic effects on metabolism. These may be caused by the direct impression of body acupuncture on the adipose tissue of the abdomen. As the results show, body acupuncture was more effective in reduction of waist and hip circumferences, which means the greater losing of adipose tissue of the abdomen, leading to production of less inflammatory markers for the stimulation of the immune system. This role is suggested to be explained by the interaction between the autonomic nervous system (ANS) and the immune functions and the brain as the communicator between 2 systems [36]. By communicating with brain the inflammatory cytokine stimulate neural outflow via the ANS [36], leading to release of acetylcholine via parasympathetic nerve (vagus) endings, resulting to neuroimmune reflex and suppressing the release of inflammatory cytokines [36]. However, it should be noted that this could be a part of the mechanism of how acupuncture works, as we know despite the auricle that vagus nerve is superficial and can be stimulated by acupuncture leading to release of acetylcholine via parasympathetic nerve (vagus) endings, during body acupuncture vagus nerve does not stimulate directly and it should be some other explanatory mechanism.

In addition, reductions in hs-CRP levels were seen in different periods of the study in both groups, interestingly, the analysis showed that changes in hs-CRP levels were not different between cases and control, implying this notion that hs-CRP changed independent of the effects of

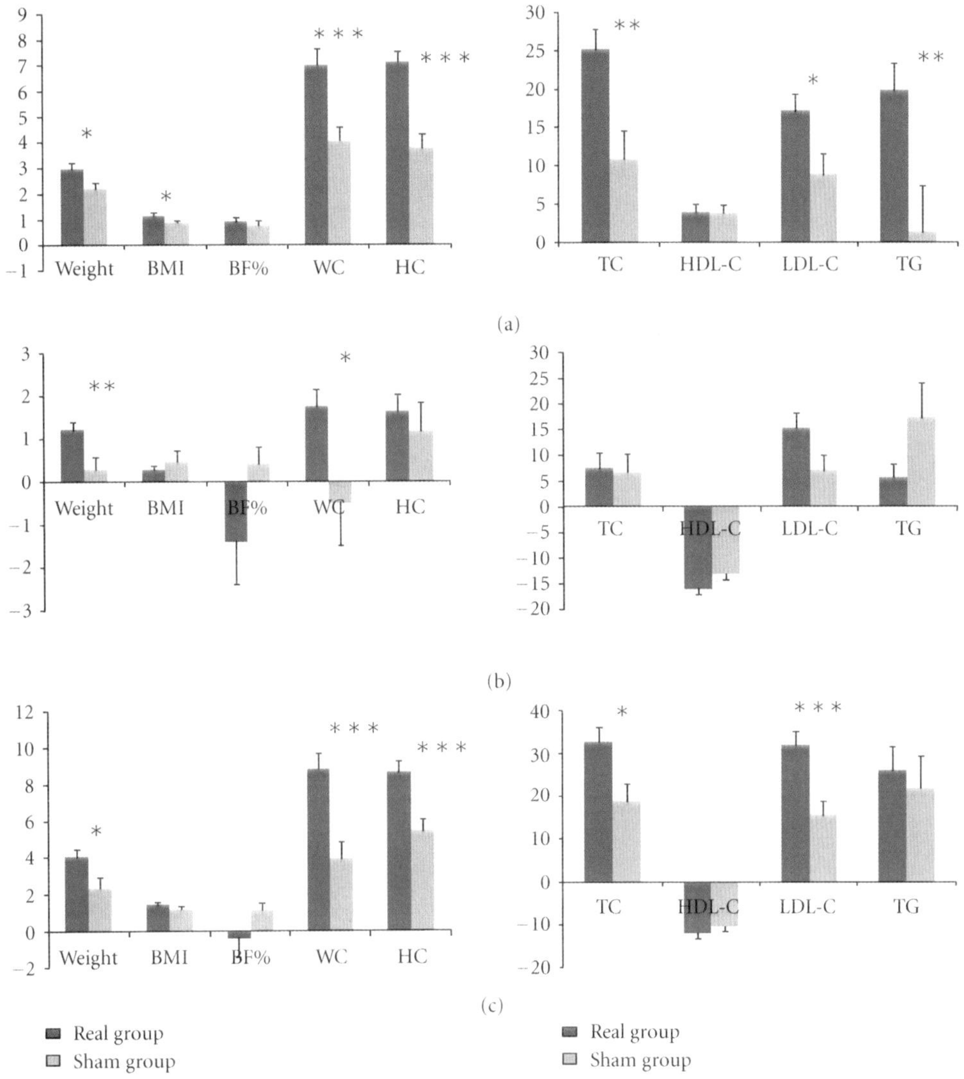

FIGURE 2: Changes of anthropometric parameters and lipid profile in real and sham groups. BMI: body mass index, BF%: body fat percentage, WC: waist circumferences, HC: hip circumferences, TC: total cholesterol, HDL-C: high density lipoprotein-cholesterol, LDL-C: low density lipoprotein-cholesterol, TG: triglycerides. (a), (b) and (c) means first, second and whole period of the study, respectively, $^{*}P < 0.05$, $^{**}P < 0.01$, and $^{***}P < 0.001$, respectively.

acupuncture. There are evidences that demonstrate the fact that elevated CRP levels are closely related to obesity [16]. It has been also suggested that adipose tissue releases the proinflammatory cytokines [37], so it is logical that weight loss is associated with decrease in CRP levels. Other studies have found the same result as ours about the reduction in CRP levels following weight loss [17, 18]. Although there are no studies assessing the role of acupuncture on hs-CRP changes during weight loss, but there are some studies which have evaluated the changes in hs-CRP levels in rheumatologic diseases. Similar to our results in patients with rheumatologic problems, some studies reported the inability of acupuncture to reduce the hs-CRP levels [38, 39] and some other not [40].

In conclusion, body acupuncture in combination with diet restriction was found to be effective for weight loss and also reduction of the obesity-associated risks factors, such as dyslipidemia. However, these effects can be achieved by other modalities but due to lack of adverse events and continued effects after the therapy, acupuncture could be used as a proffered or synergic treatment option for obesity control. Moreover, it was found that it has immunomodulatory but not anti-inflammatory effects on immune system by regulation of the levels of anti-Hsp antibodies.

Abbreviations

BMI: Body mass index
WC: Waist circumference
HC: Hip circumference
FBS: Fasting blood sugar
TC: Total cholesterol

TG:	Triglycerides
HDL-C:	High-density lipoprotein cholesterol
LDL-C:	Low-density lipoprotein cholesterol
DBP:	Diastolic blood pressure
SBP:	Systolic blood pressure
Anti-Hsp antibody:	Antiheat shock protein and
hs-CRP:	High-sensitivity C-reactive protein.

Acknowledgments

The authors are particularly grateful to the patients and their family members who volunteered to participate in this study. This work was supported by Iranian Ministry of Health and Education, Mashhad University of Medical Science (MUMS), Iran and Beijing University of Chinese Medicine, China. The Grant number of this study was 86058 in medical research council of Mashhad University of Medical Science (MUMS). B. Zhao and H. Abdi Both contributed equally as the first author.

References

[1] "Clinical guidelines on the identification, evaluation, and treatment of overweight and obesity in adults—the evidence report," *National Institutes of Health Obesity Research*, vol. 6, supplement 2, pp. 51S–209S, 1998.

[2] J. M. Lacey, A. M. Tershakovec, and G. D. Foster, "Acupuncture for the treatment of obesity: a review of the evidence," *International Journal of Obesity*, vol. 27, no. 4, pp. 419–427, 2003.

[3] M. S. Lee, J. Hwan Kim, H. J. Lim, and B. C. Shin, "Effects of abdominal electroacupuncture on parameters related to obesity in obese women: a pilot study," *Complementary Therapies in Clinical Practice*, vol. 12, no. 2, pp. 97–100, 2006.

[4] C. H. Hsu, K. C. Hwang, C. L. Chao, J. G. Lin, S. T. Kao, and P. Chou, "Effects of electroacupuncture in reducing weight and waist circumference in obese women: a randomized crossover trial," *International Journal of Obesity*, vol. 29, no. 11, pp. 1379–1384, 2005.

[5] C. H. Hsu, K. C. Hwang, C. L. Chao, H. H. Chang, and P. Chou, "Electroacupuncture in obese women: a randomized, controlled pilot study," *Journal of Women's Health*, vol. 14, no. 5, pp. 434–440, 2005.

[6] W. Biernacki and M. D. Peake, "Acupuncture in treatment of stable asthma," *Respiratory Medicine*, vol. 92, no. 9, pp. 1143–1145, 1998.

[7] S. Joos, C. Schott, H. Zou, V. Daniel, and E. Martin, "Immunomodulatory effects of acupuncture in the treatment of allergic asthma: a randomized controlled study," *Journal of Alternative and Complementary Medicine*, vol. 6, no. 6, pp. 519–525, 2000.

[8] H. Lee, J. Y. Lee, Y. J. Kim et al., "Acupuncture for symptom management of rheumatoid arthritis: a pilot study," *Clinical Rheumatology*, vol. 27, no. 5, pp. 641–645, 2008.

[9] M. Ghayour-Mobarhan, A. A. Rahsepar, S. Tavallaie, S. Rahsepar, and G. A. A. Ferns, "The potential role of heat shock proteins in cardiovascular disease: evidence from in vitro and in vivo studies," *Advances in Clinical Chemistry*, vol. 48, pp. 27–72, 2009.

[10] G. Wick, G. Schett, A. Amberger, R. Kleindienst, and Q. Xu, "Is atherosclerosis an immunologically mediated disease?" *Immunology Today*, vol. 16, no. 1, pp. 27–33, 1995.

[11] M. Ghayour-Mobarhan, A. Sahebkar, S. M. R. Parizadeh et al., "Antibody titres to heat shock protein 27 are elevated in patients with acute coronary syndrome," *International Journal of Experimental Pathology*, vol. 89, no. 3, pp. 209–215, 2008.

[12] Q. Xu, S. Kiechl, M. Mayr et al., "Association of serum antibodies to heat-shock protein 65 with carotid atherosclerosis: clinical significance determined in a follow-up study," *Circulation*, vol. 100, no. 11, pp. 1169–1174, 1999.

[13] I. Atar, O. Gulmez, A. Atar et al., "The effects of prior beta-blocker therapy on serum C-reactive protein levels after percutaneous coronary intervention," *Clinical Cardiology*, vol. 28, no. 5, pp. 243–246, 2005.

[14] S. Mora, I. M. Lee, J. E. Buring, and P. M. Ridker, "Association of physical activity and body mass index with novel and traditional cardiovascular biomarkers in women," *Journal of the American Medical Association*, vol. 295, no. 12, pp. 1412–1419, 2006.

[15] M. Visser, L. M. Bouter, G. M. McQuillan, M. H. Wener, and T. B. Harris, "Elevated C-reactive protein levels in overweight and obese adults," *Journal of the American Medical Association*, vol. 282, no. 22, pp. 2131–2135, 1999.

[16] I. Lemieux, A. Pascot, D. Prud'homme et al., "Elevated C-reactive protein: another component of the atherothrombotic profile of abdominal obesity," *Arteriosclerosis, Thrombosis, and Vascular Biology*, vol. 21, no. 6, pp. 961–967, 2001.

[17] J. W. Anderson, E. C. Konz, and D. J. A. Jenkins, "Health advantages and disadvantages of weight-reducing diets: a computer analysis and critical review," *Journal of the American College of Nutrition*, vol. 19, no. 5, pp. 578–590, 2000.

[18] A. E. Hak, C. D. A. Stehouwer, M. L. Bots et al., "Associations of C-reactive protein with measures of obesity, insulin resistance, and subclinical atherosclerosis in healthy, middle-aged women," *Arteriosclerosis, Thrombosis, and Vascular Biology*, vol. 19, no. 8, pp. 1986–1991, 1999.

[19] Q. Sun and Y. Xu, "Simple obesity and obesity hyperlipemia treated with otoacupoint pellet pressure and body acupuncture," *Journal of Traditional Chinese Medicine*, vol. 13, no. 1, pp. 22–26, 1993.

[20] M. Siervo, V. Boschi, and C. Falconi, "Which REE prediction equation should we use in normal-weight, overweight and obese women?" *Clinical Nutrition*, vol. 22, no. 2, pp. 193–204, 2003.

[21] F. Crea, A. Gaspardone, F. Tomai et al., "Risk factors in schoolchildren associated with a family history of unheralded myocardial infarction or uncomplicated stable angina in male relatives," *Journal of the American College of Cardiology*, vol. 23, no. 6, pp. 1472–1478, 1994.

[22] L. Manneras, S. Cajander, M. Lönn, and E. Stener-Victorin, "Acupuncture and exercise restore adipose tissue expression of sympathetic markers and improve ovarian morphology in rats with dihydrotestosterone-induced PCOS," *The American Journal of Physiology*, vol. 296, no. 4, pp. R1124–R1131, 2009.

[23] M. Ghayour-Mobarhan, S. A. New, D. J. Lamb et al., "Dietary antioxidants and fat are associated with plasma antibody titers to heat shock proteins 60, 65, and 70 in subjects with dyslipidemia," *The American Journal of Clinical Nutrition*, vol. 81, no. 5, pp. 998–1004, 2005.

[24] D. B. Allison, K. Kreibich, S. Heshka, and S. B. Heymsfield, "A randomised placebo-controlled clinical trial of an acupressure device for weight loss," *International Journal of Obesity*, vol. 19, no. 9, pp. 653–658, 1995.

[25] R. Mazzoni, E. Mannucci, S. M. Rizzello, V. Ricca, and C. M. Rotella, "Failure of acupuncture in the treatment of obesity:

a pilot study," *Eating and Weight Disorders*, vol. 4, no. 4, pp. 198–202, 1999.

[26] M. S. Mok, L. N. Parker, S. Voina, and G. A. Bray, "Treatment of obesity by acupuncture," *The American Journal of Clinical Nutrition*, vol. 29, no. 8, pp. 832–835, 1976.

[27] J. S. Han and L. Terenius, "Neurochemical basis of acupuncture analgesia," *Annual Review of Pharmacology and Toxicology*, vol. 22, pp. 193–220, 1982.

[28] H. Akil, S. J. Watson, E. Young, M. E. Lewis, H. Khachaturian, and J. M. Walker, "Endogenous opioids: biology and function," *Annual Review of Neuroscience*, vol. 7, pp. 223–255, 1984.

[29] Z. Wenhe and S. Yucun, "Change in levels of monoamine neurotransmitters and their main metabolites of rat brain after electric acupuncture treatment," *International Journal of Neuroscience*, vol. 15, no. 3, pp. 147–149, 1981.

[30] M. Zhao, Z. Liu, and J. Su, "The time-effect relationship of centralaction in acupuncture treatment for weight reduction," *Journal of Traditional Chinese Medicine*, vol. 20, no. 1, pp. 26–29, 2000.

[31] L. Li and Z. Y. Wang, "Clinical therapeutic effects of body acupuncture and ear acupuncture on juvenile simple obesity and effects on metabolism of blood lipids," *Zhongguo Zhen Jiu*, vol. 26, pp. 173–176, 2006.

[32] M. T. Cabioglu and N. Ergene, "Electroacupuncture therapy for weight loss reduces serum total cholesterol, triglycerides, and ldl cholesterol levels in obese women," *The American Journal of Chinese Medicine*, vol. 33, no. 4, pp. 525–533, 2005.

[33] S. J. Wang, H. Z. Xu, and H. L. Xiao, "Effect of high-frequency electroacupuncture on lipid metabolism in obesity rats," *Zhen Ci Yan Jiu*, vol. 33, no. 3, pp. 154–158, 2008.

[34] Z. Liu, F. Sun, J. Li et al., "Prophylactic and therapeutic effects of acupuncture on simple obesity complicated by cardiovascular diseases," *Journal of Traditional Chinese Medicine*, vol. 12, no. 1, pp. 21–29, 1992.

[35] M. T. Cabyoglu, N. Ergene, and U. Tan, "The mechanism of acupuncture and clinical applications," *International Journal of Neuroscience*, vol. 116, no. 2, pp. 115–125, 2006.

[36] K. J. Tracey, "The inflammatory reflex," *Nature*, vol. 420, no. 6917, pp. 853–859, 2002.

[37] J. S. Yudkin, C. D. A. Stehouwer, J. J. Emeis, and S. W. Coppack, "C-reactive protein in healthy subjects: associations with obesity, insulin resistance, and endothelial dysfunction: a potential role for cytokines originating from adipose tissue?" *Arteriosclerosis, Thrombosis, and Vascular Biology*, vol. 19, no. 4, pp. 972–978, 1999.

[38] S. D. A. Zanette, I. G. Born, J. C. T. Brenol, and R. M. Xavier, "A pilot study of acupuncture as adjunctive treatment of rheumatoid arthritis," *Clinical Rheumatology*, vol. 27, no. 5, pp. 627–635, 2008.

[39] L. Casimiro, L. Barnsley, L. Brosseau et al., "Acupuncture and electroacupuncture for the treatment of rheumatoid arthritis," *Cochrane Database of Systematic Reviews*, no. 4, Article ID CD003788, 2005.

[40] R. Wang, C. Jiang, Z. Lei, and K. Yin, "The role of different therapeutic courses in treating 47 cases of rheumatoid arthritis with acupuncture," *Journal of Traditional Chinese Medicine*, vol. 27, no. 2, pp. 103–105, 2007.

9

Bioimpedance Vector Pattern in Taiwanese and Polish College Students Detected by Bioelectric Impedance Vector Analysis: Preliminary Observations

Teresa Malecka-Massalska,[1] Agata Smolen,[2] Elzbieta Madro,[3] and Wojciech Surtel[4]

[1] *Physiology Department, Medical University of Lublin, Radziwiłłowska 11 Street, 20-080 Lublin, Poland*
[2] *Department of Mathematics and Biostatistics, Medical University of Lublin, Jaczewskiego 4 Street, 20-090 Lubin, Poland*
[3] *Institute of Hematology and Transfusiology, Indiry Gandhi 14 Street, 02-776 Warsaw, Poland*
[4] *Department of Electronics, University of Technology, Nadbystrzycka 38a Street, 20-618 Lublin, Poland*

Correspondence should be addressed to Teresa Malecka-Massalska, tmalecka@gmail.com

Academic Editor: Biagio R. Di Iorio

Background and Objectives. The study was conducted to evaluate soft tissue hydration and mass through pattern analysis of vector plots as height, normalized resistance, and reactance measurements by bioelectric impedance vector analysis in Taiwanese and Polish college students. *Methods.* Whole-body measurements were made with ImpediMed bioimpedance analysis SFB7 BioImp v1.55 (Pinkenba Qld 4008, Australia) in 16 Taiwanese and Polish men and 16 Taiwanese and Polish women. *Results.* Mean vectors of Taiwanese men and women groups versus the Polish men and women groups were characterized by almost the same normalized resistance component with reactance component (separate 95% confidence limits, $P < 0.05$) indicating that there were no differences of soft tissue hydration and mass. *Interpretation and Conclusion.* The evaluation of soft tissue hydration and mass through pattern analysis of vector plots as height, normalized resistance, and reactance measurements by bioelectric impedance vector analysis in Taiwanese and Polish college students did not differ between these two diverse ethnic groups. Further observational research investigating these properties in larger groups would be welcomed to elucidate and/or confirm these findings.

1. Introduction

There are many methods for nutritional status assessment. One of them is bioimpedance analysis (BIA) and the assessment of direct bioimpedance measures (resistance (R), reactance (X_c), and phase angle (PA)). The use of these raw data has gained popularity in nutrition assessment and monitoring of nutrition status in patients [1]. BIA is based on the principle that a fixed, low-voltage, high-frequency alternating current introduced into the human body is conducted almost completely through the fluid compartment of the fat-free mass [2]. BIA evaluates the body components, resistance (R) and reactance (X_c), by recording a voltage drop in applied current [3]. Resistance is the restriction to the flow of an electric current, primarily related to the amount of water present in the tissues. Reactance is the resistive effect produced by the tissue interfaces and cell membranes [3]. Part of the electrical current is stored by the cell membranes, which acts as capacitors, creating resistive force. It is this reactance that causes the current to lag behind the voltage ultimately creating a phase shift, which is quantified geometrically as the angular transformation of the ratio of reactance to resistance, or PA [4].

BIVA technique is a promising tool, using the pure data obtained by BIA evaluation, for the screening and monitoring of nutrition and hydration status. BIVA has the potential to be used as a routine method at the bedside for assessment and management of body fluids [5]. Bioelectrical impedance vector analysis allows noninvasive evaluation of soft tissue hydration and mass through pattern analysis of vector plots as height, normalized resistance, and reactance measurements [6]. BIVA has been used to allow detection, monitoring, and control of hydration and nutrition status using vector displacement for the feedback on treatment among patients with Alzheimer's disease [7], in stable and nonstable heart failure patients [8], in critically ill and cardiorenal patients [9], in haemodialysis patients [10], in peritoneal dialysis patients [11], and in cancer patients [12].

In healthy populations, BIVA method has been used in modeling the human body shape [13] and monitoring the variation of the hydrate status in healthy term newborns [14].

In particular, raw BIA measurements measured at 50 kHz, because of its reproducibility quality, has been used to determine the differences in soft tissue hydration and mass [6–14].

The aim of our observational study was to perform bioelectrical impedance analysis to investigate whether the position on the R-X_c plane of impedance vectors from Taiwanese men and women differed from Polish men and women.

2. Materials and Methods

2.1. Study Design. This observational study investigated whether the position on the R-X_c plane of impedance vectors from Taiwanese men and women differed from Polish men and women.

2.2. Study Populations. Between October 2009 and May 2010, BIA examinations of tissue electrical properties were conducted in sixty-four college students. Thirty-two healthy Taiwanese students were examined: 16 men and 16 women aged between 18 and 40 years old. Thirty-two healthy Polish students were also examined: 16 men and 16 women aged between 20 and 26 years old.

Baseline nutritional assessment was performed by Subjective Global Assessment (SGA). Subjective Global Assessment has been widely used to assess nutritional needs and monitor nutrition therapy in the hospitalized population. It is a simple, safe, and inexpensive test to administer. BIA was performed by a medical doctor using ImpediMed bioimpedance analysis SFB7 BioImp v1.55 (Pinkenba Qld 4008, Australia). Due to previously published research indicating that exercise influences BIA measurements, in particular phase angle, we controlled for this variable in our study. BIA was performed, after a 10-minute rest period. All patients were positioned supine on a bed, with their legs apart and their arms not touching their torso. All evaluations were conducted on the patients' right side by using the 4 surface standard electrode (tetra polar) techniques on the hand and foot. R and X_c were measured directly in ohms at 5, 50, 100, and 200 kHz. R and X_c values were measured three times in each patient, and the mean values were used. PA was obtained from the arc-tangent ratio $X_c : R$. To transform the result from radians to degrees, the result that was obtained was multiplied by $180°/\pi$. For further analysis, values of R, X_c, and PA measured at 50 kHz were taken. Fat mass (kg), as a difference between fat-free mass and weight and fat-free mass (kg) derived from total body water divided by the hydration constant were automatically received on the ImpediMed bioimpedance analysis SFB7 BioImp v1.55 equipment.

2.3. Bioimpedance. BIA was performed by a medical doctor using ImpediMed bioimpedance analysis SFB7 BioImp v1.55 (Pinkenba Qld 4008, Australia). BIA was performed, after a 10-minute rest period, while the patients were lying supine on a bed, with their legs apart and their arms not touching their torso. All evaluations were conducted on the patients' right side by using the 4 surface standard electrode (tetra polar) technique on the hand and foot. R and X_c were measured directly in ohms at 5, 50, 100, 200 kHz. R and X_c values were measured three times in each patient, and the mean values were used. PA was obtained from the arc-tangent ratio $X_c : R$. To transform the result from radians to degrees, the result that was obtained was multiplied by $180°/\pi$.

2.4. Bioelectrical Impedance Vector Analysis. According to the RX_c graph method [15], measurements of R and X_c were standardized by the H subjects (i.e., R/H and X_c/H) and expressed in ohms per meter. By using the bivariate normal distribution of R/H and X_c/H, we calculated the bivariate 95% confidence limits for mean impedance vectors of cancer patients and healthy subjects (i.e., the limit containing the magnitude and the phase angle of the mean vectors with 95% probability). Separate 95% confidence limits indicate a statistically significant difference between mean vector positions on the R-X_c plane, that is, in their R/H, X_c/H, or both components or in their magnitude, phase angle, or both ($P < 0.05$, which is equivalent to a significant Hotelling t^2 test) [15].

2.5. Statistical Methods. Our results are expressed as mean ± SD. The Shapiro-Wilk (S-W) test was used to assess the distribution conformity of examined parameters with a normal distribution; the Fisher (F) test was used to assess variance homogeneity. For group comparisons of metric data, we used the Mann-Whitney U test. A P value < 0.05 was considered statistically significant. The statistical analysis for this study was performed using the computer software STATISTICA v.8.0 (StatSoft, Poland). BIVA was done with BIVA software (version 2002).

3. Results

As previously stated, many research studies refer to great reproducibility of direct bioimpedance measurements (R, X, PA) at 50 kHz. Due to the logic of this reasoning, our RX_c graph method refers to 50 kHz.

Taiwanese and Polish college male and female student's characteristics with average values of protocol variables are reported in Tables 1, 2, 3, and 4.

4. Discussion

Phase angle analysis has become a valuable tool to assess health. Even though the biological meaning of PA is not

Table 1: Baseline characteristics of the Taiwanese and Polish college male students[1].

Characteristic	Value (Taiwanese men)	Value (Polish men)	P
Age (y)	25.81 ± 5.5	21.13 ± 1.54	**0.0001**
BMI kg/m^2	23.06 ± 2.59	23.09 ± 2.81	0.9
Height (cm)	171.5 ± 7.32	179.13 ± 6.18	0.95
Weight (kg)	68.13 ± 10.81	74.34 ± 11.80	0.92
R at 50 kHz (ohm)	582.44 ± 59.32	584.38±68.42	0.19
R/H (ohm/m)	340 ± 34.86	327.34±43.88	0.15
X_c at 50 kHz (ohm)	63.38 ± 4.88	62.9 ± 7.51	0.71
X_c/H (ohm/m)	37.03 ± 3.36	35.22 ± 5.03	0.35
Phase angle at 50 kHz (°)	6.23 ± 0.43	6.16 ± 0.5	0.85

[1] $n = 16$; ±SD; range in parentheses (all such values).

Table 2: Electrical tissue properties characteristics of the Taiwanese and Polish college male students[1].

Characteristic	Value (Taiwanese college male students)	Value (Polish college male students)
Resistance at 5 kHz (ohm)	673.8 ± 63.08	676.21 ± 75.41
Reactance at 5 kHz (ohm)	34.24 ± 3.54	34.26 ± 3.81
Phase angle at 5 kHz (°)	2.93 ± 0.3	2.93 ± 0.34
Resistance at 100 kHz (ohm)	552.08 ± 57.33	554.32 ± 65.55
Reactance at 100 kHz (ohm)	52.96 ± 4.95	52.71 ± 6.10
Phase angle at 100 kHz (°)	5.51 ± 0.46	5.45 ± 0.46
Resistance at 200 kHz (ohm)	526.88 ± 56.78	528.76 ± 62.88
Reactance at 200 kHz (ohm)	47.2 ± 5.67	45.61 ± 5.7
Phase angle at 200 kHz (°)	5.13 ± 0.53	4.93 ± 0.31

[1] $n = 16$; ±SD; range in parentheses (all such values).

Table 3: Baseline characteristics of the Taiwanese and Polish college female students[1].

Characteristic	Value (Taiwanese men)	Value (Polish men)	P
Age (y)	25.81 ± 5.5	21.13 ± 1.54	**0.000001**
BMI kg/m^2	23.06 ± 2.59	23.09 ± 2.81	0.4
Height (cm)	171.5 ± 7.32	179.13 ± 6.18	0.5
Weight (kg)	68.13 ± 10.81	74.34 ± 11.80	0.26
R at 50 kHz (ohm)	582.44 ± 59.32	584.38±68.42	0.59
R/H (ohm/m)	340 ± 34.86	327.34±43.88	0.47
X_c at 50 kHz (ohm)	63.38 ± 4.88	62.9 ± 7.51	0.72
X_c/H (ohm/m)	37.03 ± 3.36	35.22 ± 5.03	0.84
Phase angle at 50 kHz (°)	6.23 ± 0.43	6.16 ± 0.5	0.47

well understood, what is known about PA has awakened new possibilities for its used. It reflects body cell mass and is one of the best markers of cell membrane function because it is related to the ratio between extracellular water and intracellular water. Variations in phase angle values have been reported between women and men, healthy and diseased patients, and in young and older people. Variations in PA have also been noted among individuals at fixed frequency. The observed variations could be due to differences in the capacitive behavior of this group' tissues, associated variability in cell size, membrane permeability, or intracellular composition or associated with differences in the distribution of body fluids among individuals, which may affect the amount of shunting of the current through the interstitial spaces [16].

Table 4: Electrical tissue properties characteristics of the Taiwanese and Polish college female students[1].

Characteristic	Value (Taiwanese college female students)	Value (Polish college female students)
Resistance at 5 kHz (ohm)	799.24 ± 49.79	787.25 ± 46.78
Reactance at 5 kHz (ohm)	34.26 ± 12.16	32.11 ± 3.16
Phase angle at 5 kHz (°)	2.48 ± 0.98	2.34 ± 0.25
Resistance at 100 kHz (ohm)	681.91 ± 54.14	669.28 ± 42.93
Reactance at 100 kHz (ohm)	55.19 ± 9.03	56.5 ± 4.63
Phase angle at 100 kHz (°)	4.68 ± 0.9	4.84 ± 0.38
Resistance at 200 kHz (ohm)	654.64 ± 53.95	642.11 ± 42.74
Reactance at 200 kHz (ohm)	52.88 ± 6.04	49.23 ± 5.98
Phase angle at 200 kHz (°)	4.65 ± 0.68	4.39 ± 0.4

[1] $n = 16$; ±SD; range in parentheses (all such values).

In healthy populations, there can be considerable differences between phase angle reference values, and these values vary by population. Kyle et al. [17] found that in the Swiss population, PA values were lower (10.5% in men and 7.7% in women) in comparison to the American study sample. Barbosa-Silva et al. [18] also observed similar variations in PA values between gender and age groups. To our knowledge, the lowest values of PA reference values have been found in the German population, in a study by Dittmar [19]. Thus far, there are no phase angle reference values available for healthy Polish and Taiwanese populations. In light of history, there are some shared cultural between the German and Polish populations. German population reference values are probably most closely related to the Polish population.

BIVA allows noninvasive evaluation of soft tissue hydration [6]. In our study, we observed no significant difference vector distribution in either Taiwanese and Polish women or Taiwanese and Polish men by sex and age. The vector displacement of Taiwanese and Polish healthy subjects was characterized by a similar X_c component and similar R component [Figures 1 and 2].

Further research is needed to investigate direct bioimpedance measures (resistance, reactance and PA value) on a larger group of Polish and Taiwanese subjects to confirm the similarity of tissue electrical properties for subjects in the age range of our study. This information would also be valuable also in establishing PA reference values for the Polish and Taiwanese populations.

We could consider age to be a factor in our results since the Taiwanese group of students was overall slightly older than the Polish group. However, previous research mentions age as a factor for lower PA due to the influence of exercise or rather, lack of exercise. Since it is shown that as people age, they exercise less [19]. Perhaps because both groups are

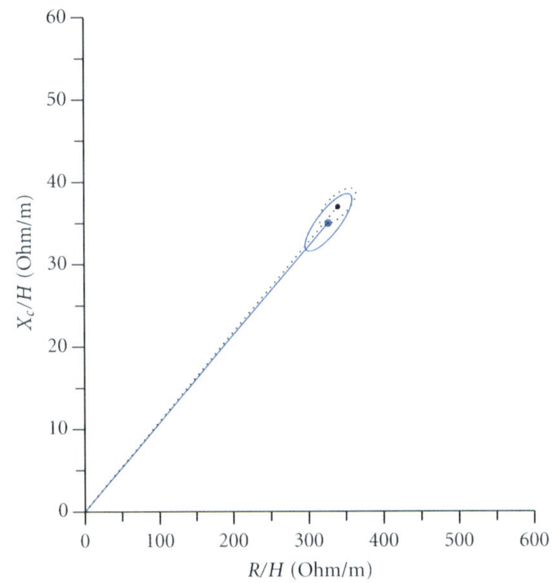

FIGURE 1: Mean vectors of 95% confidence limits in Taiwanese (black dotted line) and Polish (solid blue line) college men.

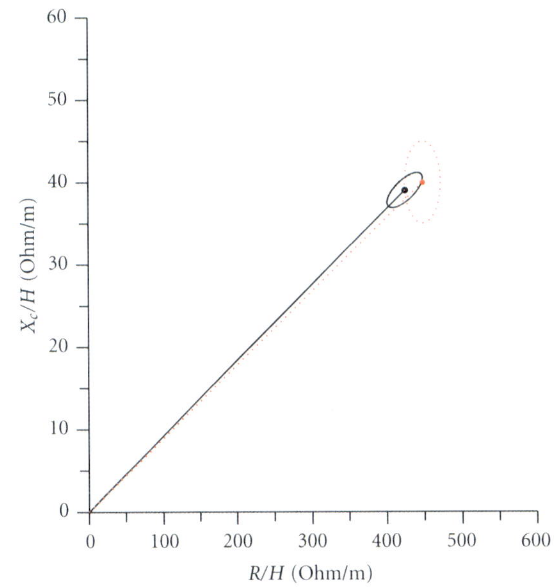

FIGURE 2: Mean vectors of 95% confidence limits in Taiwanese (red dotted line) and Polish (solid black line) college women.

college students, the activity of college life balanced out any age-related influences.

We cannot understand why we did not observe, as reported by other researchers, statistically significant differences between our student populations. It seems unlikely that these two diverse ethnic groups' results would have such similar PA, resistance, and reactance values.

5. Conclusion

In conclusion, our study did not indicate any statistically significant differences in electrical tissue properties, expressed by resistance, reactance, and phase angle between Taiwanese and Polish college students. Mean vectors of Taiwanese men and women groups versus the Polish men and women groups were characterized by almost the same normalized resistance component with reactance component. We observed no statistically significant differences either at different frequencies, among women, men, and/or overall. Further observational research investigating these properties in larger groups would be welcomed to elucidate and/or confirm these findings.

Authors' Contributions

T. Malecka-Massalska was the main author of the paper and participated in concept, design, data collection, data analysis, data interpretation, and writing. A. Smolen and W. Surtel assisted with the statistical analysis and data interpretation. E. Madro participated in data collection, data analysis, and data interpretation.

Conflict of Interests

The authors declare that they have no conflict of interests.

Acknowledgment

The authors wish to thank Professor Antonio Piccoli, University of Padua, Italy, for kindly providing the BIVA Software 2002.

References

[1] A. Bosy-Westphal, S. Danielzik, R. P. Dörhöfer, W. Later, S. Wiese, and M. J. Müller, "Phase angle from bioelectrical impedance analysis: population reference values by age, sex, and body mass index," *Journal of Parenteral and Enteral Nutrition*, vol. 30, no. 4, pp. 309–316, 2006.

[2] J. P. F. H. A. Simons, A. M. W. J. Schols, K. R. Westerterp, G. P. M. Ten Velde, and E. F. M. Wouters, "The use of bioelectrical impedance analysis to predict total body water in patients with cancer cachexia," *American Journal of Clinical Nutrition*, vol. 61, no. 4, pp. 741–745, 1995.

[3] B. J. Zarowitz and A. M. Pilla, "Bioelectrical impedance in clinical practice," *DICP, Annals of Pharmacotherapy*, vol. 23, no. 7-8, pp. 548–555, 1989.

[4] M. C. G. Barbosa-Silva and A. J. D. Barros, "Bioelectrical impedance analysis in clinical practice: a new perspective on its use beyond body composition equations," *Current Opinion in Clinical Nutrition and Metabolic Care*, vol. 8, no. 3, pp. 311–317, 2005.

[5] A. Piccoli, "Bioelectric impedance measurement for fluid status assessment," *Contributions to Nephrology*, vol. 164, pp. 143–152, 2010.

[6] S. Toso, A. Piccoli, M. Gusella et al., "Bioimpedance vector pattern in cancer patients without disease versus locally advanced or disseminated disease," *Nutrition*, vol. 19, no. 6, pp. 510–514, 2003.

[7] R. Buffa, R. M. Mereu, P. F. Putzu, G. Floris, and E. Marini, "Bioelectrical impedance vector analysis detects low body cell mass and dehydration in patients with Alzheimer's disease," *Journal of Nutrition, Health and Aging*, vol. 14, no. 10, pp. 823–827, 2010.

[8] P. Gastelurrutia, L. Nescolarde, J. Rosell-Ferrer, M. Domingo, N. Ribas, and A. Bayes-Genis, "Bioelectrical impedance vector analysis (BIVA) in stable and non-stable heart failure patients: a pilot study," *International Journal of Cardiology*, vol. 146, no. 2, pp. 262–264, 2010.

[9] W. F. Peacock, "Use of bioimpedance vector analysis in critically ill and cardiorenal patients," *Contributions to Nephrology*, vol. 165, pp. 226–235, 2010.

[10] L. Nescolarde, A. Piccoli, A. Román et al., "Bioelectrical impedance vector analysis in haemodialysis patients: relation between oedema and mortality," *Physiological Measurement*, vol. 25, no. 5, pp. 1271–1280, 2004.

[11] A. Piccoli, "Bioelectric impedance vector distribution in peritoneal dialysis patients with different hydration status," *Kidney International*, vol. 65, no. 3, pp. 1050–1063, 2004.

[12] S. Toso, A. Piccoli, M. Gusella et al., "Altered tissue electric properties in lung cancer patients as detected by bioelectric impedance vector analysis," *Nutrition*, vol. 16, no. 2, pp. 120–124, 2000.

[13] C. H. Kim, J. H. Park, H. Kim, S. Chung, and S. H. Park, "Modeling the human body shape in Bioimpedance Vector Measurements," in *Proceedings of the 32nd Annual International Conference of the IEEE Engineering in Medicine and Biology Society (EMBC '10)*, pp. 3872–3874, September 2010.

[14] A. V. B. Margutti, J. P. Monteiro, and J. S. Camelo Jr., "Reference distribution of the bioelectrical impedance vector in healthy term newborns," *British Journal of Nutrition*, vol. 104, no. 10, pp. 1508–1513, 2010.

[15] A. Piccoli, B. Rossi, L. Pillon, and G. Bucciante, "A new method for monitoring body fluid variation by bioimpedance analysis: the RXc graph," *Kidney International*, vol. 46, no. 2, pp. 534–539, 1994.

[16] J. J. Ackmann and M. A. Seitz, "Methods of complex impedance measurements in biologic tissue," *Critical Reviews in Biomedical Engineering*, vol. 11, no. 4, pp. 281–311, 1984.

[17] U. G. Kyle, L. Genton, D. O. Slosman, and C. Pichard, "Fat-free and fat mass percentiles in 5225 healthy subjects aged 15 to 98 years," *Nutrition*, vol. 17, no. 7-8, pp. 534–541, 2001.

[18] M. C. G. Barbosa-Silva, A. J. D. Barros, J. Wang, S. B. Heymsfield, and R. N. Pierson, "Bioelectrical impedance analysis: population reference values for phase angle by age and sex," *American Journal of Clinical Nutrition*, vol. 82, no. 1, pp. 49–52, 2005.

[19] M. Dittmar, "Reliability and variability of bioimpedance measures in normal adults: effects of age, gender and body mass index," *American Journal of Physical Anthropology*, vol. 122, no. 4, pp. 361–370, 2003.

10

The Antioxidant Status and Concentrations of Coenzyme Q10 and Vitamin E in Metabolic Syndrome

Chi-Hua Yen,[1,2,3] Nae-Cherng Yang,[4,5] Bor-Jen Lee,[6] Jui-Yuan Lin,[4] Simon Hsia,[7] and Ping-Ting Lin[4,5]

[1] *Department of Family and Community Medicine, Chung Shan Medical University Hospital, Taichung 40201, Taiwan*
[2] *School of Medicine, Chung Shan Medical University, Taichung 40201, Taiwan*
[3] *Center for Education and Research on Geriatrics and Gerontology, Chung Shan Medical University, Taichung 40201, Taiwan*
[4] *School of Nutrition, Chung Shan Medical University, Taichung 40201, Taiwan*
[5] *Department of Nutrition, Chung Shan Medical University Hospital, Taichung 40201, Taiwan*
[6] *The Intensive Care Unit, Taichung Veterans General Hospital, Taichung 40705, Taiwan*
[7] *Department of Nutrition and Institute of Biomedical Nutrition, Hungkuang University, Taichung 43346, Taiwan*

Correspondence should be addressed to Ping-Ting Lin; apt810@csmu.edu.tw

Academic Editors: A. Chicco and A. Turrini

The purpose of this study was to investigate the levels of coenzyme Q10 and vitamin E and the antioxidant status in subjects with metabolic syndrome (MS). Subjects with MS ($n = 72$) were included according to the criteria for MS. The non-MS group ($n = 105$) was comprised of healthy individuals with normal blood biochemical values. The plasma coenzyme Q10, vitamin E concentrations, lipid profiles, and antioxidant enzymes levels (catalase, superoxide dismutase, and glutathione peroxidase) were measured. The subjects with MS had significantly higher concentrations of plasma coenzyme Q10 and vitamin E than those in the non-MS group, but these differences were not significant after being normalized for triglyceride level. The levels of antioxidant enzymes were significantly lower in the MS group than in the non-MS group. The subjects with the higher antioxidant enzymes activities had significant reductions in the risk of MS ($P < 0.01$) after being adjusted for coenzyme Q10 and vitamin E. In conclusion, the subjects with MS might be under higher oxidative stress resulting in low levels of antioxidant enzyme activities. A higher level of antioxidant enzymes activities was significantly associated with a reduction in the risk of MS independent of the levels of coenzyme Q10 and vitamin E.

1. Introduction

Metabolic syndrome (MS) represents a cluster of physiological and anthropometric abnormalities [1] and is recognized as a significant risk factor for cardiovascular disease and type II diabetes [2]. The Third National Health and Nutrition Examination Survey (1988–1994) reported that more than 20% of the adult population in the USA suffered from MS [3, 4]. A recent report from the Elderly Nutrition and Health Survey in Taiwan (NAHSIT) conducted during 1999-2000 noted that 26% of men and 47% of women suffered from MS [5]. The health and dietary transition in Taiwan is beginning to have some similarities with western nations. The NAHSIT (2005–2008) observed that dietary habits in Taiwan were changing, particularly in regard to intake of cakes, sweets, and sugary drinks. The energy intake in young people has increased because of the popularity of fast food chains, and combined with an increasingly sedentary lifestyle, this may have led to the increase in obesity and associated metabolic diseases [6]. The markers of MS, including insulin resistance, type II diabetes, hypertension, dyslipidemia, and visceral obesity, may increase oxidative stress [7–9] and reduce antioxidant defenses [10–12]. Increases in oxidative stress contribute to impaired vascular function, inflammation, thrombosis, and atherosclerosis and ultimately give rise to vascular disease [13].

Coenzyme Q10 and vitamin E are lipid-soluble vitamins known for their excellent antioxidant qualities. The Third

National Health and Nutrition Examination Survey indicated that adults with MS have suboptimal concentrations of antioxidants [14]. However, the French SU.VI.MAX (Supplementation en Vitamines et Minéraux AntioXydants) trials followed subjects without MS for 7.5 years and showed that there was no beneficial effect of antioxidant supplementation (such as vitamin E) on the incidence of MS [15]. Coenzyme Q10 (also called ubiquinone) is a lipid-soluble benzoquinone containing 10 isoprenyl units in its side chain. Coenzyme Q10 is a key component of the mitochondrial respiratory chain and is required for adenosine triphosphate (ATP) synthesis [16, 17]. Coenzyme Q10 is an intracellular antioxidant that protects low-density lipoprotein cholesterol (LDL-C) from free radical-induced oxidative damage [18, 19]. It has demonstrated potential cardioprotective properties and reduces the risk of coronary artery disease [20]; however, few studies have examined the concentration of coenzyme Q10 in patients with MS. In the present study, we hypothesize that subjects with MS might be under higher oxidative stress, which influences their antioxidant status. Therefore, the purpose of this study was to investigate the antioxidant status and the levels of coenzyme Q10 and vitamin E in the subjects with MS.

2. Materials and Methods

2.1. Subjects. This study was a cross-sectional study. We expected the differences in the mean levels of plasma coenzyme Q10 between the MS and non-MS groups to be 0.2 ± 0.3 μmol/L based on the Miles et al. study [21]. The desired power was set at 0.8 to detect a true effect, alpha was set at 0.05 ($\alpha = 0.05$), and a minimum sample size of 50 participants was required for each group. Subjects with MS ($n = 72$) were recruited from the Department of Family and Community Medicine of Chung Shan Medical University Hospital in Taiwan. The inclusion criteria for the MS group were based on the definition published by the Taiwan Bureau of Health Promotion, Department of Health (2007). The subjects were diagnosed with MS if they had 3 of the following 5 characteristics: (1) abdominal obesity (waist circumference ≥90 cm in men and ≥80 cm in women), (2) impaired fasting glucose (≥5.6 mmol/L), (3) hypertriglyceridemia (≥1.7 mmol/L), (4) low high-density lipoprotein cholesterol (HDL-C < 1.0 mmol/L in men and <1.3 mmol/L in women), and (5) increased blood pressure (systolic blood pressure ≥130 mmHg and diastolic blood pressure ≥85 mmHg). The diagnostic criteria for MS of Taiwan are according to the National Cholesterol Education Program Adult Treatment Panel III (ATP III, 2001), International Diabetes Federation (IDF, 2005), and the American Heart Association/National Heart, Lung, and Blood Institute (AHA/NHLBI, 2005) criteria [1, 22, 23]. Therefore, the diagnostic criteria for MS of Taiwan are similar to these international criteria. The subjects who were using antidiabetic, antihypertensive, or lipid-lowering medications were considered to have elevated fasting blood glucose, elevated blood pressures, and dyslipidemia, respectively. The concentration of coenzyme Q10 might be affected by statin therapy [24]; therefore, the subjects with MS who were receiving statin therapy were excluded. The subjects in the non-MS group ($n = 105$) were recruited from the physical examination unit of the hospital. The inclusion criteria for the non-MS group were based on the subjects' medical records from the previous month. The subjects were included in the non-MS group if they did not have a diagnosis of any of the following diseases or conditions: gastrointestinal disorder, hypertension, hyperlipidemia, liver disease, renal disease, diabetes, or other metabolic diseases. The subjects also had to exhibit normal blood biochemical values, including all of the following characteristics: fasting glucose <5.6 mmol/L, blood urea nitrogen <7.9 mmol/L, creatinine <123.8 μmol/L, alkaline phosphate <190 U/L, glutamic oxaloacetic transaminase <35 U/L, and glutamic pyruvate transaminase <45 U/L. The subjects in both MS and non-MS groups who were taking antioxidant vitamin supplements (including coenzyme Q10 and vitamin E supplementation) were excluded from the study. This study was approved by the Institutional Review Board of Chung Shan Medical Hospital in Taiwan, and the written informed consent was obtained from each subject.

The age, blood pressures, and smoking habits of each subject were recorded. The blood pressure was measured by a sphygmomanometer with repeated measurements for concordance in each subject after resting for at least 5 min. The body weight, height, and waist and hip circumferences of each subject were measured by a trained examiner of the same gender as the study subjects, and the body mass index (kg/m^2) and the waist to hip ratio were then calculated. The subjects were instructed to complete a 24 h dietary recall of the day before blood sample collection. The nutrient composition was calculated with Nutritionist Professional software (E-Kitchen Business Corp., Taiwan); the nutrient database was based on the Taiwan food composition table (Food and Drug Administration, Department of Health, Taiwan; http://www.doh.gov.tw/FoodAnalysis/ingredients.htm).

2.2. Blood Collection and Biochemical Measurement. Fasting venous blood samples (15 mL) were obtained to estimate the levels of fasting glucose, blood lipid profiles, antioxidant enzymes activities, coenzyme Q10, vitamin E, and inflammatory markers. The researchers advised that all subjects fast for 10–12 h before blood collection and avoid exercise for 24 h before blood collection. Blood specimens were collected in vacutainer tubes with and without EDTA as an anticoagulant as necessary. Serum and plasma were prepared and frozen (−80°C) for storage until analysis. Blood lipid parameters (i.e., total cholesterol (TC), triglyceride (TG), LDL-C, and HDL-C) concentrations were measured using an automated biochemical analyzer (Hitachi-7180E, Tokyo, Japan).

Plasma coenzyme Q10 and vitamin E were measured by high-performance liquid chromatography (HPLC) and detected by a UV detector at 275 nm and 292 nm, respectively [25, 26]. Red blood cells (RBCs) were diluted with 25x sodium phosphate buffer for SOD (superoxide dismutase) and GPx (glutathione peroxidase) measurements and 250x sodium phosphate buffer for CAT (catalase) measurement. The methods for measuring CAT, SOD, and GPx in RBCs have previously been described [27–29]; measurements were

TABLE 1: Characteristics of subjects.

	MS (n = 72)	Non-MS (n = 105)
Male/female (n)	43/29	52/53
Age (y)	53.3 ± 11.6[1]	52.0 ± 8.1
Systolic blood pressure (mmHg)	141.9 ± 11.8*	118.8 ± 16.8
Diastolic blood pressure (mmHg)	88.5 ± 10.3*	77.7 ± 9.8
Waist circumference (cm)	96.0 ± 12.4*	80.6 ± 13.6
Fasting glucose (mmol/L)	7.5 ± 2.6*	5.2 ± 1.1
TC (mmol/L)	4.9 ± 1.0	5.1 ± 0.9
TG (mmol/L)	1.9 ± 0.9*	1.3 ± 0.6
LDL-C (mmol/L)	3.2 ± 0.9*	2.9 ± 0.7
HDL-C (mmol/L)	1.2 ± 0.3*	1.4 ± 0.4
TC/HDL-C	4.4 ± 1.2*	3.9 ± 1.2
Dietary intake		
Energy (Kcal/d)	2002.8 ± 529.9	1905.0 ± 694.4
Protein (g/d)	67.7 ± 20.8	76.3 ± 36.9
Percentage of total calories	(13.6%)	(16.0%)
Fat (g/d)	74.7 ± 27.3*	60.5 ± 32.3
Percentage of total calories	(33.4%)	(28.6%)
Carbohydrate (g/d)	264.1 ± 76.3	265.8 ± 104.1
Percentage of total calories	(53.0%)	(55.8%)
Polyunsaturated fatty acid (g/d)	26.9 ± 13.2*	21.2 ± 12.3
Percentage of total calories	(12.1%)	(10.0%)
Monounsaturated fatty acid (g/d)	22.6 ± 11.0*	18.8 ± 12.6
Percentage of total calories	(10.2%)	(8.9%)
Saturated fatty acid (g/d)	20.4 ± 10.3*	17.2 ± 11.5
Percentage of total calories	(9.2%)	(8.1%)
Vitamin E (mg α-T.E./d)	6.6 ± 3.4*	5.5 ± 3.4
Vitamin E/fat (mg α-T.E./g)	0.1 ± 0.0	0.1 ± 0.1

[1]Mean ± SD. *Values were significantly different between case and control groups.
HDL-C: high-density lipoprotein-cholesterol; LDL-C: low density lipoprotein-cholesterol; TC: total cholesterol; TG: triglyceride.

acquired with a spectrophotometer at 240 nm, 325 nm, and 340 nm, respectively. The RBC protein content was determined based on the Biuret reaction of the BCA kit (Thermo, Rockford, IL, USA). The antioxidant enzymes levels were expressed as units/mg protein. All analyses were performed in duplicate and repeated measurements of the same sample varied by less than 10%.

2.3. Statistical Analyses. The data were analyzed using SigmaPlot software (version 12.0, Systat, San Jose, California, USA). The normal distribution of variables was evaluated using the Shapiro-Wilk test. The differences in demographic and hematological measurement data between the MS and non-MS groups were analyzed using Student's t-test or the Mann-Whitney rank sum test. For categorical response variables, differences between the two groups were assessed using the Chi-square test or Fisher's exact test. Adjusted odds ratios with 95% confidence intervals (CI) for MS were calculated from the logistic regression models base on the fifth level (50th percentile) of antioxidant enzymes activities. The data are expressed as the means ± the standard deviations (SD). The results were considered statistically significant at $P < 0.05$.

TABLE 2: The odds ratios of metabolic syndrome based on the antioxidant enzymes activities.

	Odds ratio (95% CI)	P value
CAT < 22.5 U/mg protein	1.00	—
CAT ≥ 22.5 U/mg protein		
Model 1[1]	0.45 (0.24–0.84)	0.01
Model 2[2]	0.29 (0.11–0.75)	0.01
SOD < 42.2 U/mg protein	1.00	—
SOD ≥ 42.2 U/mg protein		
Model 1	0.25 (0.13–0.47)	<0.01
Model 2	0.29 (0.11–0.75)	0.01
GPx < 34.1 U/mg protein	1.00	—
GPx ≥ 34.1 U/mg protein		
Model 1	0.03 (0.01–0.08)	<0.01
Model 2	0.06 (0.02–0.19)	<0.01

[1]None adjusted.
[2]Adjusted for age, gender, waist circumferences, triglyceride, coenzyme Q10, and vitamin E.
CAT: catalase activity; CI: confidence interval; GPx: glutathione peroxidase; SOD: superoxide dismutase.

3. Results

Table 1 shows the demographic data and health characteristics of the subjects. The subjects with MS had significantly higher values of systolic blood pressure, diastolic blood pressure, waist circumference, fasting glucose, TG, LDL-C, and TC/HDL-C and lower HDL-C values than those in the non-MS group. With respect to dietary intake, the subjects with MS had higher fat ($P < 0.01$), saturated fatty acid (P = 0.03), and unsaturated fatty acid (P = 0.01), and vitamin E (P = 0.02) intakes than those in the non-MS group. However, the vitamin E intake was not significantly different between the two groups after normalization by fat intake.

The levels of plasma coenzyme Q10, vitamin E, and antioxidant enzymes are shown in Figures 1 and 2. The subjects with MS had significantly higher plasma coenzyme Q10 and vitamin E concentrations ($P < 0.01$). After normalization to TG, the ratio of coenzyme Q10 to TG (P = 0.91) and the ratio of vitamin E to TG (P = 0.15) were not significantly different between the MS and non-MS groups. With respect to the antioxidant enzymes activities, the subjects with MS had lower CAT (P = 0.02), SOD ($P < 0.01$), and GPx activities ($P < 0.01$) than those in the non-MS group.

Furthermore, we calculated the odds ratio of MS base on the antioxidant enzymes activities (Table 2). The subjects with higher antioxidant enzymes activities had significant reductions in the risk of MS, even after being adjusted for the potential confounders of MS and the levels of coenzyme Q10 and vitamin E.

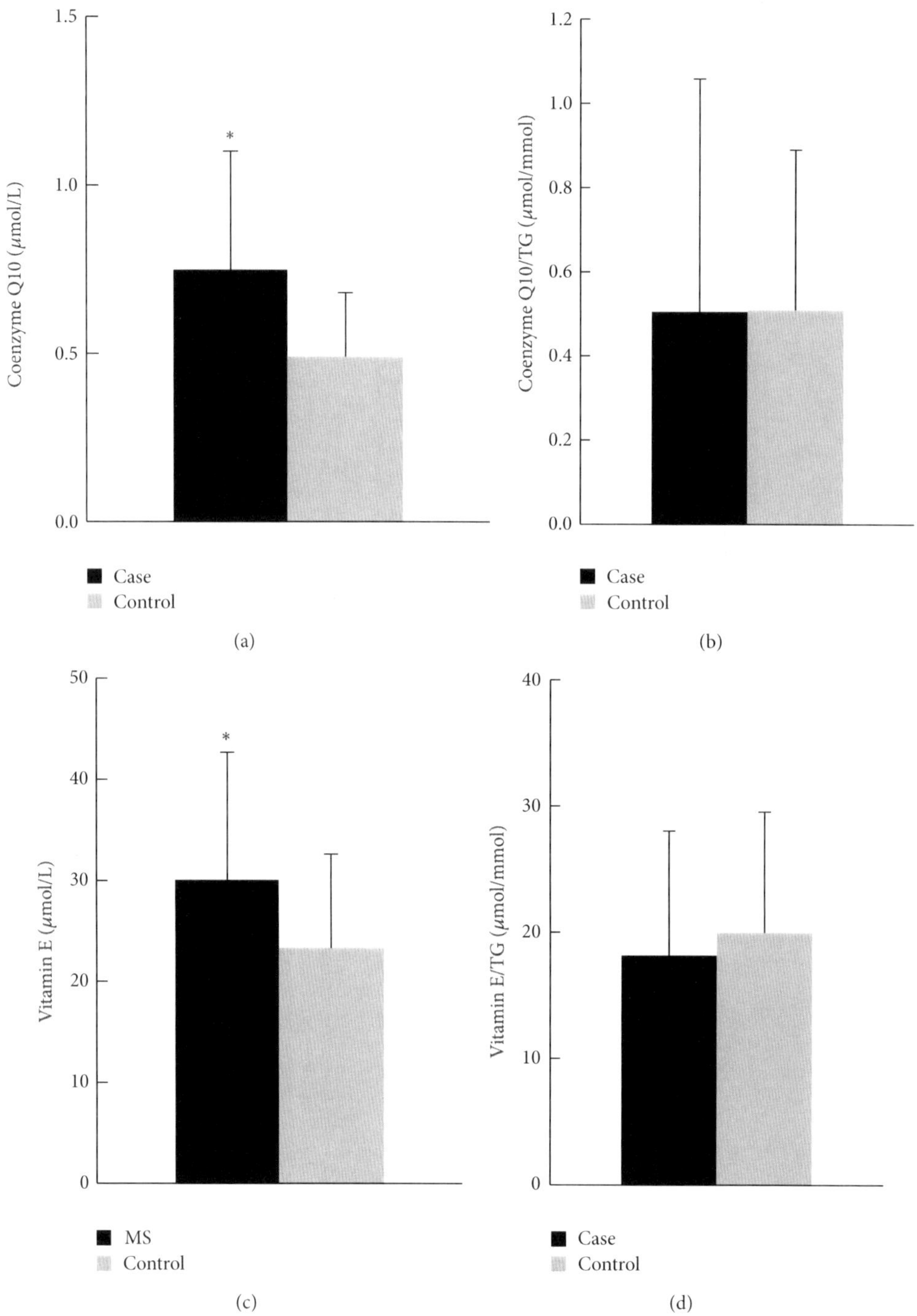

FIGURE 1: The levels of plasma coenzyme Q10 and vitamin E. *Values were significantly different between case and control groups; $P < 0.01$. TG: triglyceride.

4. Discussion and Conclusion

The present study showed a statistically significant difference in the antioxidant status and levels of coenzyme Q10 and vitamin E in the subjects with MS. The subjects with MS had significantly higher levels of plasma coenzyme Q10 and vitamin E than those in the non-MS group, but these differences were not statistically significant after normalization to TG. A previous study was conducted by Miles et al. [21], who found that the coenzyme Q10 level was significantly higher in subjects with MS and proposed that an increase in the level of coenzyme Q10 might be a result of the natural antioxidant defense to certain features of MS. The Third National Health and Nutrition Examination Survey [14] also noted that subjects with MS had a significantly higher level of vitamin E compared with non-MS subjects ($P < 0.01$).

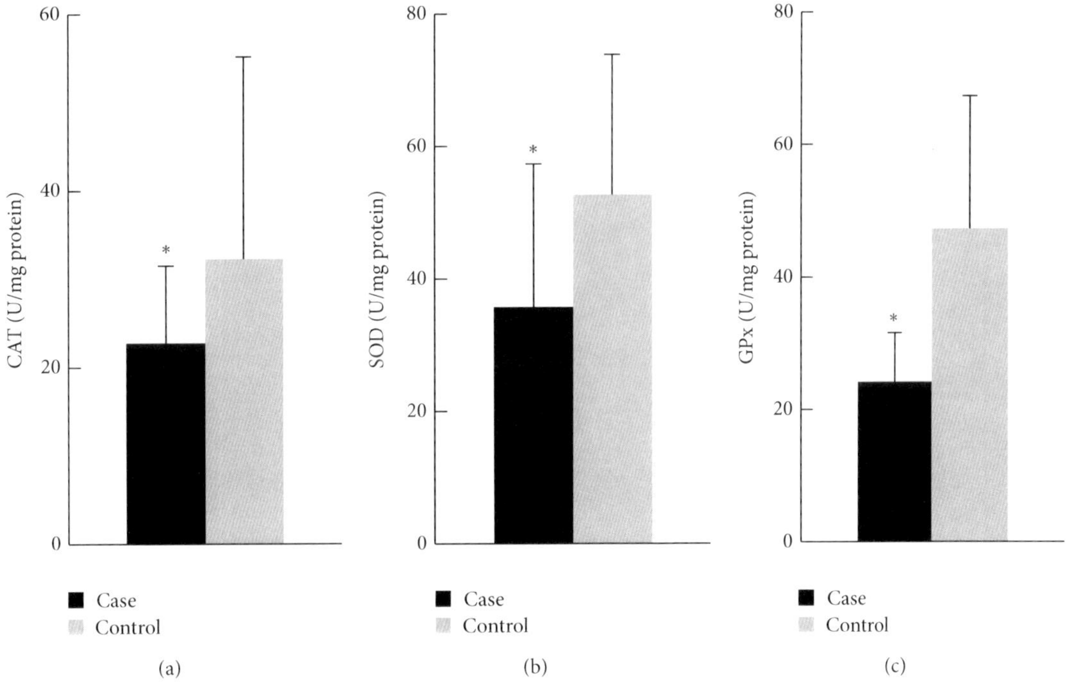

Figure 2: The levels of antioxidant enzymes. *Values were significantly different between case and control groups; $P < 0.05$. CAT: catalase activity; GPx: glutathione peroxidase; SOD: superoxide dismutase.

The concentrations of coenzyme Q10 and vitamin E were closely correlated with lipid profiles. The subjects with MS had a higher level of TG, which may carry the greatest risk of atherogenicity [23], and the levels of antioxidant vitamins (such as coenzyme Q10 and vitamin E) may be increased in triglyceride-rich lipoprotein to provide the lipoprotein lipid with highly efficient antioxidant protection [30].

A recent report from NAHSIT (2005–2008) found that the frequency of vegetable and fruit consumption was low in the Taiwanese population [31]. The dietary results showed that the subjects with MS had significantly higher fat, saturated fatty acid, unsaturated fatty acid, and vitamin E intakes, but the vitamin E intake was not significantly different between the two groups after normalization by fat intake (Table 1). Vegetable oil is a major dietary source of vitamin E, and the Taiwanese commonly used vegetable oil (especially soybean oil) in their cooking method (such as stir frying) [6]. In the present study, we did not assess coenzyme Q10 intake, but there was a significant correlation between the level of plasma coenzyme Q10 and fat intake ($r = 0.17$, $P = 0.04$). Meat, fish, nuts, and some oils are the richest nutritional sources of coenzyme Q10 [32]. As a result, a higher fat intake might be an another reason why we observed the higher levels of coenzyme Q10 and vitamin E in the subjects with MS, and the concentrations were not significantly different after adjusted for the lipid.

Oxidative stress is thought to play an important role in the development of MS [8]. In the present study, we assessed the activities of the major antioxidant enzymes that are directly involved in the neutralization of reactive oxygen species (ROS). The subjects with MS had significantly lower CAT, SOD, and GPx activities (Figure 2), and the subjects with higher antioxidant enzymes activities were significantly associated with a reduction in the risk of MS independent of the levels of coenzyme Q10 and vitamin E (Table 2). Strictly speaking, MS is a type of metabolic disorder rather than a disease. Subjects with MS might be under higher oxidative stress; antioxidant enzymes are the first line of defense against ROS and may decrease to adjust for higher levels of oxidative stress [12]. In addition, MS subjects in general were typically abdominally obese. Obesity is also an oxidative burden that may lead to the reduction of antioxidant enzymes activities [33].

There are some limitations of the present study. First, this study was cross-sectional; therefore, no causal relationship could be defined. Larger prospective studies are required to establish the relationship between antioxidant status in subjects with MS. Second, we did not assess coenzyme Q10 intake because of insufficient data in the nutrients databank. Further developments in analytical chemistry (HPLC) are needed to provide the better information about the coenzyme Q10 content in various foods. Third, we preformed the 24 h dietary recall to evaluate the nutrients intake in this study; however, the MS does not derive from a short-term shock. Further study is needed to clarify the differences of usual dietary intake between MS and non-MS subjects by long-term dietary assessment.

In conclusion, the subjects suffering from MS might be under higher oxidative stress, resulting in low levels of antioxidant enzyme activities. A higher level of antioxidant enzymes activities was significantly associated with a reduction in the risk of MS independent of the levels of coenzyme Q10 and vitamin E.

Acknowledgments

This study was supported by a grant from the National Science Council (NSC 99-2320-B-040-011), Taiwan. The authors would like to express their sincere appreciation to the subjects for their participation. They thank the nurses at the Chung Shan Medical University Hospital for providing expert assistance in blood sample collection and data analysis.

References

[1] J. I. Cleeman, "Executive summary of the third report of the National Cholesterol Education Program (NCEP) expert panel on detection, evaluation, and treatment of high blood cholesterol in adults (adult treatment panel III)," *Journal of the American Medical Association*, vol. 285, no. 19, pp. 2486–2497, 2001.

[2] E. Ferrannini, S. M. Haffner, B. D. Mitchell, and M. P. Stern, "Hyperinsulinaemia: the key feature of cardiovascular and metabolic syndrome," *Diabetologia*, vol. 34, no. 6, pp. 416–422, 1991.

[3] E. S. Ford and W. H. Giles, "A comparison of the prevalence of the metabolic syndrome using two proposed definitions," *Diabetes Care*, vol. 26, no. 3, pp. 575–581, 2003.

[4] Y.-W. Park, S. Zhu, L. Palaniappan, S. Heshka, M. R. Carnethon, and S. B. Heymsfield, "The metabolic syndrome: prevalence and associated risk factor findings in the US population from the Third National Health and Nutrition Examination Survey, 1988–1994," *Archives of Internal Medicine*, vol. 163, no. 4, pp. 427–436, 2003.

[5] L. T. Lee, Y. C. Chang, K. C. Huang, W. H. Pan, and C. Y. Chen, "The prevalence survey of metabolic syndrome of the elderly in Taiwan," *Taiwan Geriatrics & Gerontology*, vol. 1, no. 1, pp. 9–17, 2005.

[6] W.-H. Pan, H.-J. Wu, C.-J. Yeh et al., "Diet and health trends in Taiwan: comparison of two nutrition and health surveys from 1993–1996 and 2005–2008," *Asia Pacific Journal of Clinical Nutrition*, vol. 20, no. 2, pp. 238–250, 2011.

[7] A. Ceriello, A. Quatraro, and D. Giugliano, "Diabetes mellitus and hypertension: the possible role of hyperglycaemia through oxidative stress," *Diabetologia*, vol. 36, no. 3, pp. 265–266, 1993.

[8] D. Giugliano, A. Ceriello, and G. Paolisso, "Diabetes mellitus, hypertension, and cardiovascular disease: which role for oxidative stress?" *Metabolism*, vol. 44, no. 3, pp. 363–368, 1995.

[9] I. C. West, "Radicals and oxidative stress in diabetes," *Diabetic Medicine*, vol. 17, no. 3, pp. 171–180, 2000.

[10] C. Antoniades, D. Tousoulis, C. Tentolouris, P. Toutouzas, and C. Stefanadis, "Oxidative stress, antioxidant vitamins, and atherosclerosis. From basic research to clinical practice," *Herz*, vol. 28, no. 7, pp. 628–638, 2003.

[11] R. Stocker and J. F. Keaney Jr., "Role of oxidative modifications in atherosclerosis," *Physiological Reviews*, vol. 84, no. 4, pp. 1381–1478, 2004.

[12] S. Penckofer, D. Schwertz, and K. Florczak, "Oxidative stress and cardiovascular disease in type 2 diabetes: the role of antioxidants and pro-oxidants," *The Journal of Cardiovascular Nursing*, vol. 16, no. 2, pp. 68–85, 2002.

[13] D. Giugliano, "Dietary antioxidants for cardiovascular prevention," *Nutrition, Metabolism and Cardiovascular Diseases*, vol. 10, no. 1, pp. 38–44, 2000.

[14] E. S. Ford, A. H. Mokdad, W. H. Giles, and D. W. Brown, "The metabolic syndrome and antioxidant concentrations: findings from the Third National Health and Nutrition Examination Survey," *Diabetes*, vol. 52, no. 9, pp. 2346–2352, 2003.

[15] S. Czernichow, A.-C. Vergnaud, P. Galan et al., "Effects of long-term antioxidant supplementation and association of serum antioxidant concentrations with risk of metabolic syndrome in adults," *American Journal of Clinical Nutrition*, vol. 90, no. 2, pp. 329–335, 2009.

[16] L. Ernster and G. Dallner, "Biochemical, physiological and medical aspects of ubiquinone function," *Biochimica et Biophysica Acta*, vol. 1271, no. 1, pp. 195–204, 1995.

[17] H. N. Bhagavan and R. K. Chopra, "Coenzyme Q10: absorption, tissue uptake, metabolism and pharmacokinetics," *Free Radical Research*, vol. 40, no. 5, pp. 445–453, 2006.

[18] R. Alleva, M. Tomasetti, M. Battino, G. Curatola, G. P. Littarru, and K. Folkers, "The roles of coenzyme Q10 and vitamin E on the peroxidation of human low density lipoprotein subfractions," *Proceedings of the National Academy of Sciences of the United States of America*, vol. 92, no. 20, pp. 9388–9391, 1995.

[19] U. Singh, S. Devaraj, and I. Jialal, "Coenzyme Q10 supplementation and heart failure," *Nutrition Reviews*, vol. 65, no. 6, pp. 286–293, 2007.

[20] B. J. Lee, Y. C. Lin, Y. C. Huang, Y. W. Ko, S. Hsia, and P. T. Lin, "The relationship between coenzyme Q10, oxidative stress, and antioxidant enzymes activities and coronary artery disease," *The Scientific Word Journal*, vol. 2012, Article ID 792756, 8 pages, 2012.

[21] M. V. Miles, P. S. Horn, J. A. Morrison, P. H. Tang, T. DeGrauw, and A. J. Pesce, "Plasma coenzyme Q10 reference intervals, but not redox status, are affected by gender and race in self-reported healthy adults," *Clinica Chimica Acta*, vol. 332, no. 1-2, pp. 123–132, 2003.

[22] K. G. M. M. Alberti and P. Zimmet, "The metabolic syndrome—a new worldwide definition," *The Lancet*, vol. 366, no. 9491, pp. 1059–1062, 2005.

[23] S. M. Grundy, J. I. Cleeman, S. R. Daniels et al., "Diagnosis and management of the metabolic syndrome: an American Heart Association/National Heart, Lung, and Blood Institute scientific statement," *Circulation*, vol. 112, no. 17, pp. 2735–2752, 2005.

[24] H. Mabuchi, T. Higashikata, M. Kawashiri et al., "Reduction of serum ubiquinol-10 and ubiquinone-10 levels by atorvastatin in hypercholesterolemic patients," *Journal of Atherosclerosis and Thrombosis*, vol. 12, no. 2, pp. 111–119, 2005.

[25] G. P. Littarru, F. Mosca, D. Fattorini, and S. Bompadre, "Method to assay coenzyme Q10 in blood plasma or blood serum," United State Patent 7303921, 2007.

[26] L. J. Hatam and H. J. Kayden, "A high-performance liquid chromatographic method for the determination of tocopherol in plasma and cellular elements of the blood," *Journal of Lipid Research*, vol. 20, no. 5, pp. 639–645, 1979.

[27] D. E. Paglia and W. N. Valentine, "Studies on the quantitative and qualitative characterization of erythrocyte glutathione peroxidase," *The Journal of Laboratory and Clinical Medicine*, vol. 70, no. 1, pp. 158–169, 1967.

[28] S. Marklund and G. Marklund, "Involvement of the superoxide anion radical in the autoxidation of pyrogallol and a convenient assay for superoxide dismutase," *European Journal of Biochemistry*, vol. 47, no. 3, pp. 469–474, 1974.

[29] H. Aebi, "Catalase in vitro," *Methods in Enzymology*, vol. 105, no. C, pp. 121–126, 1984.

[30] D. Mohr and R. Stocker, "Radical-mediated oxidation of isolated human very-low-density lipoprotein," *Arteriosclerosis and Thrombosis*, vol. 14, no. 7, pp. 1186–1192, 1994.

[31] K.-J. Chen, W.-H. Pan, Y.-C. Lin, and B.-F. Lin, "Trends in folate status in the Taiwanese population aged 19 years and older from the Nutrition and Health Survey in Taiwan 1993–1996 to 2005–2008," *Asia Pacific Journal of Clinical Nutrition*, vol. 20, no. 2, pp. 275–282, 2011.

[32] I. Pravst, K. Žmitek, and J. Žmitek, "Coenzyme Q10 contents in foods and fortification strategies," *Critical Reviews in Food Science and Nutrition*, vol. 50, no. 4, pp. 269–280, 2010.

[33] N. Karaouzene, H. Merzouk, M. Aribi et al., "Effects of the association of aging and obesity on lipids, lipoproteins and oxidative stress biomarkers: a comparison of older with young men," *Nutrition, Metabolism and Cardiovascular Diseases*, vol. 21, no. 10, pp. 792–799, 2011.

11

Consumption of Chinese Tea-Flavor Liquor Improves Circulating Insulin Levels without Affecting Hepatic Lipid Metabolism-Related Gene Expression in Sprague-Dawley Rats

Ju-Sheng Zheng,[1,2] Yuan-Qing Fu,[1,2] Qi Chen,[1,2] Tao Huang,[1,2] Jing Yang,[1,2] and Duo Li[1,2]

[1] *Department of Food Science and Nutrition, Zhejiang University, 866 Yuhangtang Road, Hangzhou 310058, China*
[2] *APCNS Centre of Nutrition and Food Safety, 866 Yuhangtang Road, Hangzhou 315200, China*

Correspondence should be addressed to Duo Li; duoli@zju.edu.cn

Academic Editors: A. Chicco, Y.-C. Huang, and P. Pérez-Martínez

Objective. To examine the effect of two Chinese liquors with quite different nonalcoholic components on insulin sensitivity, tissue polyunsaturated fatty acids (PUFA), and hepatic lipid metabolism in SD rats. *Methods*. Thirty-three SD rats were randomized into four groups and maintained in each treatment for 10 weeks: Chinese tea-flavor liquor (TFL, $n = 9$), traditional Chinese liquor (TCL, $n = 8$), ethanol control (EC, $n = 8$), and water control (WC, $n = 8$). *Results*. TFL significantly decreased plasma insulin ($P = 0.009$) and marginally decreased Homeostatic Model Assessment-Insulin Resistance (HOMA-IR) ($P = 0.05$), compared with WC. Hepatic total and n-6 PUFA compositions were significantly decreased in TFL, TCL, and EC groups compared with WC group ($P < 0.05$). TFL significantly increased kidney n-6 PUFA ($P = 0.05$) and total PUFA ($P = 0.039$), compared with EC group. EC group showed significant higher gene expressions of acetyl-CoA carboxylase and steroid response element-binding protein (1c and 2), while there were no significant differences of these gene expressions in TFL or TCL group compared with WC. *Conclusions*. TFL has a beneficial effect on metabolic disorder in relation to improved circulating insulin levels without affecting hepatic lipid metabolism-related gene expressions in rats.

1. Introduction

Moderate alcohol consumption (1-2 drinks per day) has been reported to be associated with improved insulin sensitivity [1, 2] and lower risk of cardiovascular disease (CVD) in humans [3, 4]. Red wine is supposed to exert an evident protective effect on cardiovascular system, and nonalcoholic components, such as polyphenols in the red wine, might play a significant role in its protection effects [5–7]. In addition, alcohol could decrease tissue polyunsaturated fatty acids (PUFA) including C20:4n-6 and C22:6n-3 in animal studies [8–11], while this decrease could be attenuated or even reversed by red wine consumption, which might be attributed to the effects of nonalcoholic components [9, 10]. Chinese liquor contains abundant nonalcoholic components [12] and is consumed widely around China. However, to our knowledge, few studies have examined the effects of Chinese liquors on insulin sensitivity and tissue fatty acid compositions in rodent model.

Hepatic lipids metabolism is mainly controlled by two transcription factors, the peroxisome proliferator-activated receptor-α (PPAR-α) and the steroid response element-binding protein (SREBP). PPAR-α is a receptor for free fatty acids (FFA) and could activate genes involved in transport, oxidation, and export of FFA, while SREBP (SREBP-1c, SREBP-2) is a sensor for cholesterol level and could activate genes involved in synthesis of cholesterol and FFA [13]. In addition, adenosine monophosphate-dependent protein kinase (AMPK) is another key regulator of metabolism, which could drive fatty acid oxidation and export through activation of PPAR-α and suppression of SREBP and acetyl-CoA carboxylase (ACC) (Figure 1). Chronic ethanol treatment of cells or animals could activate SREBP and AMPK and inhibit PPAR-α, contributing to the potential alcoholic fatty liver [13, 14]. However, whether Chinese liquor would affect the expression of these critical genes in lipid metabolism in the same way as pure ethanol is unclear.

Tea-flavor liquor (TFL) and traditional Chinese liquor (TCL) are two Chinese liquors with abundant but quite different nonalcoholic components. Our previous randomized trial indicates that one-month consumption of both TFL and TCL significantly decreases serum glucose concentrations in healthy young humans [15]. However, whether the effect of these two Chinese liquors on glucose or insulin sensitivity differs from that of pure ethanol is less clear. Therefore, the present study was conducted to test whether daily consumption of TFL and TCL, compared with ethanol control and water control, could affect insulin sensitivity and fatty acid compositions in different tissues of SD rats. In addition, the effect of TFL and TCL treatments on rat hepatic lipid metabolism-related gene expression was examined.

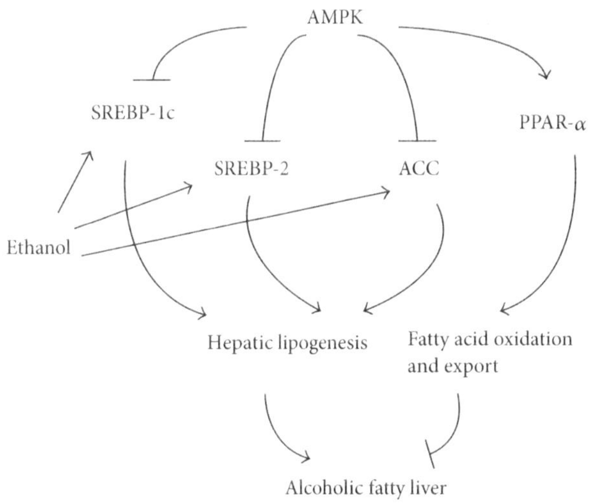

FIGURE 1: Effect of ethanol treatment on the AMPK-related lipid metabolism pathway. SREBP: steroid response element-binding protein; AMPK: adenosine monophosphate-dependent protein kinase; PPAR-α: peroxisome proliferator-activated receptor alpha; ACC: acetyl-CoA carboxylase.

2. Methods and Materials

2.1. Study Animals and Study Design. Thirty-three male SD rats, three to four months old (518 ± 33.9 g), were purchased from Zhejiang Laboratory Animal Center (Hangzhou, China). The rats were housed in a room under a 12 h light/12 h dark cycle at 22°C. The rats were allowed for acclimatization for three weeks before they were randomized into four groups: a TFL group ($n = 9$), a TCL group ($n = 8$), an ethanol control (EC, $n = 8$) group, and a water control (WC, $n = 8$) group. TFL, TCL, and EC groups received standard rat chow diet together with drinking water containing 3% ethanol in the form of TFL, TCL, and ethanol. WC group received plain water in addition to the standard rat diet. Drinking water, liquors, and rat chow diet were all provided ad lib. The rats were weighed every week, and the amounts of water, liquor and chow diet the rats consumed were measured every day. 10 weeks later, after an overnight fast, all the rats were decapitated and blood was collected in tubes containing ethylenediaminetetra-acetic acid. Plasma was separated from cells by spinning at 2000 rpm for 15 min at 4°C and stored at −20°C if not immediately analyzed. Liver and kidney were removed rapidly, frozen in liquid nitrogen, and stored at −70°C for further analysis. The study protocol was approved by the Ethics Committee of Department of Food Science of Nutrition, Zhejiang University.

2.2. Determination of Liquor Composition. TFL and TCL (both 45% (v/v) alcohol) were provided by Guizhou Meijiao Co., Ltd., Guizhou, China. Total acid and ester of the liquors were analyzed by the method issued by the Chinese National Standardization Committee (GB/T 10345-2007). The total polyphenols in the liquors were determined by a colorimetric method using the Folin-Ciocalteu Phenol reagent with gallic acid as equivalent [16]. Briefly, 0.5 mL of supernatant was placed in a 25 mL test tube and mixed with 5 mL Folin-Ciocalteu Phenol reagent. Then 4 mL of Na_2CO_3 solution (75 g/L) was added to the tube, and the solution was allowed to stand for 2 hours at room temperature. Absorbance of the blue color complex was measured under 675 nm. Volatile nonalcoholic compounds of the liquors were detected using gas chromatographic together with flame ionization detection. A DB-FFAP capillary column (30 m × 0.25 mm id, 0.25 μm film thickness, J&W, USA) was used. The oven temperature was initially set at 50°C for 6 minutes, then increased to 240°C at 4°C/min, and held for 5 minutes, and nitrogen was used as carrier gas. Butyl acetate was used as the internal standard.

2.3. Determination of Plasma Parameters. Total cholesterol (TC), triacylglycerol (TG), high-density lipoprotein cholesterol (HDL-C), low-density lipoprotein cholesterol (LDL-C), alanine aminotransferase (ALT), aspartate aminotransferase (AST), alkaline phosphatase (ALP), creatinine, uric acid, urea nitrogen, and glucose were analyzed on HITACHI 7020 chemistry analyzer using colorimetric test supplied by Diasys Diagnostic Systems (Shanghai) Co., Ltd. Plasma apolipoprotein A1 (apoA1), apolipoprotein B (apoB), and tumor necrosis factor-α (TNF-α); insulin, interleukin-6 (IL-6), and adiponectin were detected using ELISA (R&D Systems). Homeostatic Model Assessment-Insulin Resistance (HOMA-IR) was calculated as (fasting plasma insulin (in mU/L) × fasting plasma glucose (in mmol/L))/22.5.

2.4. Determination of Plasma, Kidney, and Liver Total Fatty Acid Compositions. The total lipid contents of plasma, kidney, and liver were extracted with solvents, and the fatty acid methyl esters were prepared and separated by gas-liquid chromatography as described previously [17].

2.5. Determination of Lipid Metabolism-Related mRNA Expressions. Total RNA from liver was extracted with Trizol reagent, and reverse transcription was performed in a total volume of 20 μL. After denaturing at 95°C for 5 min, the RT products were preceded for real-time RT PCR using SYBR Green RT-PCR kit (TaKaRa Biotechnology (Dalian) Co.,

Table 1: Primers used in the polymerase chain reaction.

Gene	Primers
Srebf2	F: 5′-CGCTCCACAGACCAGGATCA-3′
	R: 5′-TGTCACGAGGCTTTGCACTTG-3′
Srebf1	F: 5′-GGAGCCATGGATTGCACATT-3′
	R: 5′-AGGAAGGCTTCCAGAGAGGA-3′
Ppara	F: 5′-GACAAGGCCTCAGGATACCACTATG-3′
	R: 5′-TTGCAGCTTCGATCACACTTGTC-3′
Prkaa1	F: 5′-GGCTCGCCCAATTATGCTG-3′
	R: 5′-AGAGTTGGCACGTGGTCATCA-3′
Acaca	F: 5′-CAATCCTCGGCACATGGAGA-3′
	R: 5′-GCTCAGCCAAGCGGATGTAGA-3′
β-actin	F: 5′-GGAGATTACTGCCCTGGCTCCTA-3′
	R: 5′-GACTCATCGTACTCCTGCTTGCTG-3′

Srebf1: sterol regulatory element binding transcription factor 1; *Srebf2*: sterol regulatory element binding transcription factor 2; *Ppara*: peroxisome proliferator-activated receptor alpha; *Acaca*: acetyl-coenzyme A carboxylase alpha; *Prkaa1*: protein kinase, AMP-activated, alpha 1 catalytic subunit.

Ltd., China) using Bio-Rad's ICycler IQ Fluorescent Quantity RCR Detecting System. Primers used were listed in Table 1.

Comparative C_T method was used to quantitate gene expression. The amount of target, normalized to a housekeeping gene (β-actin) and relative to the control group (water control), was given by the formula $2^{-\Delta\Delta C_T}$ [18].

2.6. Statistical Analyses. Data analyses were performed using SPSS 16.0 (SPSS Inc., Chicago, IL, USA). One-way analysis of variance and Tukey's post hoc test were used for statistical analyses. $P < 0.05$ was considered as statistically significant. All the data were expressed as mean ± SD.

3. Results

3.1. Analyses of Chinese Liquor. Total organic acid was 0.22 g/L and 0.83 g/L for TFL and TCL, respectively, and total ester was 1.58 g/L and 2.64 g/L for TFL and TCL. Ethyl lactate (0.76 g/L). Ethyl hexanoate (0.70 g/L) and isoamylol (0.27 g/L) were the most abundant volatile compounds in TFL, while ethyl hexanoate (1.20 g/L), ethyl lactate (0.71 g/L), and acetic acid (0.63 g/L) in TCL. Total polyphenol was 2.45 mg/L in TFL and 1.88 mg/L in TCL.

3.2. Food Consumption, Body Weight Gain, and Plasma Parameters of SD Rats. No significant difference for body weight gain was observed among the four groups, although food consumption in WC group was significantly higher than that of the other three groups (Table 2).

As is shown in Table 3, LDL-C in TFL group was significantly higher than in TCL group ($P = 0.04$), while apoB in TFL group was significantly higher than in EC group ($P = 0.004$). However, there was no significant difference for blood lipids in TFL and TCL groups, compared with WC group. Plasma creatinine was higher in TFL ($P = 0.02$) and TCL ($P = 0.049$) groups than in WC group. ALP in EC group was significantly lower than in WC group ($P = 0.048$).

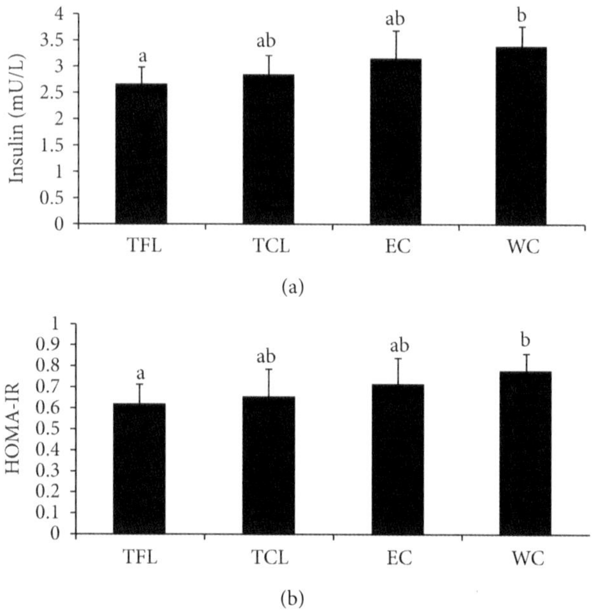

Figure 2: TFL and TCL consumption and plasma insulin and HOMA-IR levels. (a) Effect of TFL and TCL consumption on plasma insulin; (b) Effect of TFL and TCL consumption on HOMA-IR. TFL: tea-flavor liquor; TCL: traditional Chinese liquor; EC: ethanol control; WC: water control.

3.3. Plasma Insulin, Glucose, and HOMA-IR. TFL consumption significantly decreased fasting plasma insulin compared with WC ($P = 0.009$), while TCL nonsignificantly decreased insulin compared with WC ($P = 0.077$) (Figure 2(a)). There was no significant difference for plasma glucose among the four groups. TFL consumption marginally decreased HOMA-IR compared with WC ($P = 0.05$) (Figure 2(b)).

3.4. Fatty Acid Composition of Plasma, Kidney, and Liver. For plasma total fatty acid compositions (Table 4), TCL group showed lower total SFA composition than WC group ($P = 0.015$), while total MUFA composition in TFL group was lower compared with EC group ($P = 0.031$). N-6 PUFA ($P = 0.05$) and total PUFA ($P = 0.039$) contents of kidney were significantly higher in TFL group than in EC group (Table 5). TFL ($P = 0.006$) and EC ($P = 0.014$) groups showed significant increases in hepatic total SFA composition compared with WC group, and TFL group also had a higher liver MUFA composition than WC group ($P = 0.041$). N-6 PUFA, C20:5n-3 + C22:6n-3, n-3 PUFA, and total PUFA contents of liver were all lower in TFL, TCL, and EC groups than in WC group; total and n-6 PUFA compositions were significantly lower in TFL, TCL, and EC groups compared with WC group ($P < 0.05$) (Table 6).

3.5. Lipid Metabolism-Related Gene mRNA Expression. No significant change was observed for AMPK (encoded by gene *Prkaa1*) and PPAR-α (encoded by gene *Ppara*) mRNA expression in TFL, TCL, and EC groups, compared with WC group. However compared with WC group, EC group showed significantly higher mRNA expression of ACC (encoded by

TABLE 2: Body weight change and ethanol and food intake of SD rats.

	TFL ($n = 9$)	TCL ($n = 8$)	EC ($n = 8$)	WC ($n = 8$)
Body weight change (kg)	92.3 ± 38.1	116.4 ± 57.5	103.3 ± 50.4	105.5 ± 51.6
Ethanol consumption (g/d/kg body weight)	2.5 ± 0.5	2.4 ± 0.6	2.7 ± 0.5	0
Food consumption (g/d/kg body weight)	39.8 ± 4.4^a	40.7 ± 5.8^a	39.3 ± 6.3^a	47.2 ± 6.6^b

TFL: tea-flavor liquor; TCL: traditional Chinese liquor; EC: ethanol control; WC: water control; Different letters represent statistically significant difference ($P < 0.05$) between the two groups (e.g., a versus b, b versus c). No significant difference was observed if two groups contain the same letters (e.g., ab versus b, a versus ab).

TABLE 3: Plasma lipids and other parameters after consumption of TFL and TCL.

	TFL ($n = 9$)	TCL ($n = 8$)	EC ($n = 8$)	WC ($n = 8$)
HDL-C (mmol/L)	1.14 ± 0.18	1.08 ± 0.18	1.12 ± 0.18	1.01 ± 0.13
LDL-C (mmol/L)	0.26 ± 0.07^a	0.18 ± 0.04^b	0.19 ± 0.04^{ab}	0.19 ± 0.09^{ab}
TC (mmol/L)	2.07 ± 0.26	1.99 ± 0.30	2.04 ± 0.27	1.89 ± 0.20
LDL/HDL	0.23 ± 0.07	0.17 ± 0.04	0.17 ± 0.03	0.18 ± 0.07
TC/HDL	1.83 ± 0.12	1.85 ± 0.05	1.82 ± 0.07	1.86 ± 0.08
TG (mmol/L)	0.70 ± 0.17	0.74 ± 0.29	0.78 ± 0.18	0.79 ± 0.17
Glucose (mmol/L)	5.40 ± 0.49	5.20 ± 0.62	5.17 ± 0.66	5.26 ± 0.58
ApoA1 (mg/L)	4.48 ± 0.52	4.36 ± 0.61	4.30 ± 0.49	4.52 ± 0.55
ApoB (μg/L)	79.02 ± 5.83^a	74.67 ± 6.16^{ab}	67.69 ± 5.89^b	73.07 ± 6.80^{ab}
Adiponectin (μg/L)	17.51 ± 1.43	16.82 ± 1.37	16.12 ± 1.41	16.87 ± 1.09
IL-6 (ng/L)	21.72 ± 2.25	20.06 ± 1.20	19.94 ± 1.48	20.23 ± 1.98
TNF-α (ng/L)	45.60 ± 6.82	44.49 ± 3.99	46.67 ± 4.43	43.49 ± 5.29
Uric acid (μmol/L)	21.36 ± 4.55	21.48 ± 3.19	19.66 ± 3.61	21.34 ± 3.93
Urea nitrogen (mmol/L)	4.18 ± 0.45	4.29 ± 0.88	3.97 ± 0.61	4.43 ± 0.60
Creatinine (μmol/L)	56.66 ± 2.84^a	56.21 ± 4.23^a	52.98 ± 2.99^{ab}	51.74 ± 2.90^b
ALT (U/L)	50.22 ± 8.15	53.00 ± 11.65	48.25 ± 7.48	57.12 ± 5.44
AST (U/L)	157.0 ± 31.28	178.75 ± 60.34	169.88 ± 46.53	199.12 ± 70.07
ALP (U/L)	7.33 ± 4.21^{ab}	6.88 ± 2.42^{ab}	5.25 ± 1.17^a	9.38 ± 3.16^b

TFL: tea-flavor liquor; TCL: traditional Chinese liquor; EC: ethanol control; WC: water control; HDL-C: high-density lipoprotein cholesterol; LDL-C: low-density lipoprotein cholesterol; TC: total cholesterol; TG: triacylglycerol; ApoA1: apolipoprotein A1; ApoB: apolipoprotein B; IL-6: interleukin-6; TNF-α: tumor necrosis factor-α; ALT: alanine aminotransferase; AST: aspartate aminotransferase; ALP: alkaline phosphatase; Different letters represent statistically significant difference ($P < 0.05$) between the two groups (e.g., a versus b, b versus c). No significant difference was observed if two groups contain the same letters (e.g., ab versus b, a versus ab).

gene *Acaca*) ($P = 0.007$), SREBP-1c (encoded by gene *Srebf1*) ($P < 0.001$), and SREBP-2 (encoded by gene *Srebf2*) ($P = 0.048$) (Figures 1 and 3), while there was no significant difference in TFL or TCL group for all these gene expressions compared with WC group.

4. Discussion

Neither TFL nor TCL exerted any significant effect on plasma lipids compared with WC. TFL consumption might have a beneficial effect on metabolic disorder in relation to decreased plasma insulin and improved insulin sensitivity. Both TFL and TCL consumption decreased hepatic total and n-6 PUFA compositions compared with WC, while TFL consumption increased total and n-6 PUFA compositions of kidney compared with EC. In addition, compared with WC group, EC group showed significant higher gene expressions of ACC, SREBP-1c, and SREBP-2, which would lead to hepatic fat accumulation, while there was no significant difference of these gene expressions in TFL or TCL group compared with WC.

The protective effects of moderate alcohol consumption against coronary heart disease appeared to be mediated in large part by alcohol-induced increases in HDL-C [19, 20]. However, alcohol consumption in this study did not increase HDL-C level and this might be due to the low ethanol content in drinking liquor and the relatively short alcohol consumption duration in the present study.

Moderate alcohol consumption (1-2 drinks per day) was reported to improve insulin sensitivity in both men and women [2, 21, 22]. Davies et al. [21] concluded that consumption of 30 g/d of alcohol had beneficial effects on insulin and

TABLE 4: Plasma total fatty acid profiles after consumption of TFL and TCL.

	TFL ($n = 9$)	TCL ($n = 8$)	EC ($n = 8$)	WC ($n = 8$)
14:0	0.44 ± 0.13	0.46 ± 0.11	0.53 ± 0.17	0.50 ± 0.10
15:0	0.33 ± 0.09	0.38 ± 0.09	0.36 ± 0.11	0.36 ± 0.06
16:0	17.30 ± 0.88	16.20 ± 0.99	16.92 ± 1.41	17.83 ± 0.99
18:0	8.27 ± 0.53	7.95 ± 0.62	7.94 ± 0.94	8.57 ± 0.86
20:0	0.41 ± 0.19	0.37 ± 0.06	0.39 ± 0.18	0.28 ± 0.07
SFA	26.76 ± 0.10^{ab}	25.37 ± 1.28^{a}	26.03 ± 1.26^{ab}	27.54 ± 1.14^{b}
16:1n7	1.26 ± 0.54	1.02 ± 0.35	1.00 ± 0.13	1.31 ± 0.22
18:1n9	8.19 ± 0.98^{a}	8.37 ± 1.53^{a}	12.43 ± 4.23^{b}	9.01 ± 0.88^{a}
18:1n7	1.85 ± 0.30	1.83 ± 0.13	1.82 ± 0.30	1.79 ± 0.17
20:1n9	0.27 ± 0.09^{a}	0.56 ± 0.33^{b}	0.25 ± 0.18^{a}	0.29 ± 0.13^{ab}
MUFA	11.57 ± 1.60^{a}	11.78 ± 1.78^{ab}	15.50 ± 4.41^{b}	12.40 ± 1.09^{ab}
18:2n6	19.93 ± 2.42	19.86 ± 1.39	20.26 ± 3.63	20.25 ± 1.73
18:3n6	0.94 ± 0.53	1.10 ± 0.59	0.79 ± 0.19	0.63 ± 0.17
20:2n6	0.25 ± 0.07	0.23 ± 0.03	0.22 ± 0.05	0.22 ± 0.01
20:3n6	0.71 ± 0.24	0.67 ± 0.21	0.53 ± 0.08	0.67 ± 0.12
20:4n6	30.00 ± 4.03	29.86 ± 2.34	26.61 ± 7.40	28.88 ± 1.73
22:4n6	0.28 ± 0.04^{ab}	0.25 ± 0.05^{a}	0.34 ± 0.07^{b}	0.28 ± 0.04^{ab}
N-6 PUFA	52.11 ± 2.05	51.98 ± 1.47	48.74 ± 5.01	50.94 ± 1.61
18:3n3	1.01 ± 0.35	1.07 ± 0.33	0.86 ± 0.29	1.11 ± 0.20
20:3n3	0.12 ± 0.04	0.13 ± 0.03	0.12 ± 0.07	0.10 ± 0.03
20:5n3	1.80 ± 0.41	2.23 ± 0.62	1.65 ± 0.35	1.69 ± 0.40
22:5n3	0.86 ± 0.17	0.90 ± 0.27	0.92 ± 0.18	0.86 ± 0.11
22:6n3	5.09 ± 0.50	5.28 ± 1.13	4.54 ± 1.03	4.49 ± 0.51
DHA + EPA	6.89 ± 0.72	7.52 ± 1.62	6.20 ± 1.09	6.18 ± 0.60
N-3 PUFA	8.89 ± 1.01	9.61 ± 2.14	8.10 ± 1.46	8.25 ± 0.76
Total PUFA	60.99 ± 1.98	61.59 ± 1.68	56.84 ± 5.97	59.20 ± 1.78
N-3/N-6 PUFA	0.17 ± 0.02	0.19 ± 0.04	0.17 ± 0.03	0.16 ± 0.02

TFL: tea-flavor liquor; TCL: traditional Chinese liquor; EC: ethanol control; WC: water control; SFA: saturated fatty acid; PUFA: polyunsaturated fatty acid; DHA: docosahexaenoic acid; EPA: eicosapentaenoic acid; Different letters represent statistically significant difference ($P < 0.05$) between the two groups (e.g., a versus b, b versus c). No significant difference was observed if two groups contain the same letters (e.g., ab versus b, a versus ab).

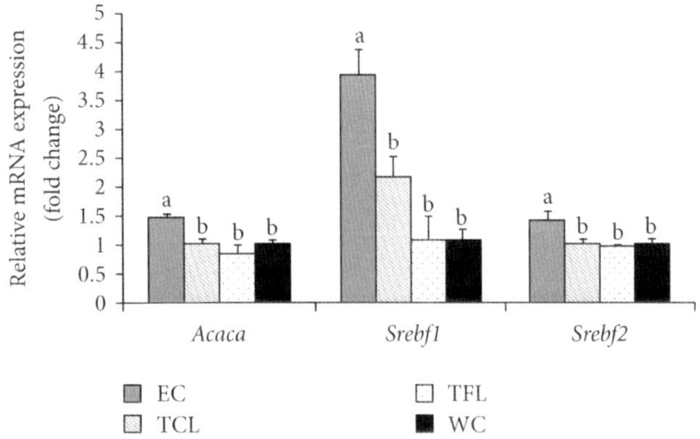

FIGURE 3: Relative mRNA expressions of key lipid metabolism-related genes. *Acaca*: acetyl-coenzyme A carboxylase alpha; *Srebf1*: sterol regulatory element binding transcription factor 1; *Srebf2*: sterol regulatory element binding transcription factor 2; TFL: tea-flavor liquor; TCL: traditional Chinese liquor; EC: ethanol control; WC: water control.

insulin sensitivity in nondiabetic postmenopausal women. Joosten et al. [2] also reported that moderate alcohol consumption for 6 weeks could improve insulin sensitivity in 36 postmenopausal women. In addition, alcohol consumption could promote insulin sensitivity in mice consuming both low-fat and high-fat diets [23]. In the present study, insulin and HOMA-IR in TFL group, but not TCL or EC group, were significantly lower than in WC group. Low and short-term ethanol consumption may contribute to the nonsignificant effects of TCL and EC on insulin sensitivity. However, nonalcoholic components of TFL might also contribute to the improved insulin sensitivity which was not observed in the other groups. Green tea was reported to improve insulin sensitivity [24, 25]; for TFL, nonalcoholic components derived from green tea, one of the fermentation materials, might partially contribute to the improved insulin sensitivity, and the total polyphenols concentration was also higher in TFL than TCL. However, nonalcoholic components taking effect were still to be determined.

Table 5: Kidney total fatty acid profiles after consumption of TFL and TCL.

	TFL ($n = 9$)	TCL ($n = 8$)	EC ($n = 8$)	WC ($n = 8$)
14:0	0.48 ± 0.14^{a}	0.63 ± 0.18^{ab}	0.72 ± 0.25^{ab}	0.78 ± 0.15^{b}
15:0	0.23 ± 0.03	0.22 ± 0.04	0.20 ± 0.04	0.21 ± 0.03
16:0	19.11 ± 1.01^{a}	19.43 ± 0.93^{ab}	20.82 ± 1.64^{b}	20.76 ± 1.04^{bc}
18:0	11.89 ± 1.88	10.30 ± 3.00	9.77 ± 3.74	8.98 ± 2.19
20:0	0.21 ± 0.15	0.10 ± 0.06	0.11 ± 0.04	0.11 ± 0.08
SFA	31.92 ± 2.03	30.68 ± 2.47	31.62 ± 2.08	30.85 ± 2.03
16:1n7	1.72 ± 0.73	1.99 ± 0.59	3.14 ± 1.79	2.70 ± 0.76
18:1n9	11.63 ± 3.46	13.92 ± 4.57	9.77 ± 3.74	8.98 ± 2.19
18:1n7	2.56 ± 0.21	2.55 ± 0.10	2.72 ± 0.65	2.65 ± 0.17
20:1n9	0.14 ± 0.10	0.13 ± 0.06	0.11 ± 0.04	0.12 ± 0.04
MUFA	16.04 ± 4.28	18.59 ± 5.06	22.03 ± 7.76	21.74 ± 4.32
18:2n6	21.10 ± 3.21	24.06 ± 6.53	22.03 ± 4.28	25.26 ± 5.27
18:3n6	0.27 ± 0.10	0.26 ± 0.08	0.23 ± 0.08	0.21 ± 0.08
20:2n6	0.28 ± 0.06	0.26 ± 0.05	0.24 ± 0.10	0.28 ± 0.11
20:3n6	0.79 ± 0.21	0.62 ± 0.24	0.59 ± 0.25	0.51 ± 0.19
20:4n6	22.70 ± 4.50	18.54 ± 7.77	17.26 ± 8.34	15.37 ± 5.77
22:4n6	0.37 ± 0.06	0.30 ± 0.10	0.28 ± 0.12	0.29 ± 0.08
N-6 PUFA	45.52 ± 2.48^{a}	44.04 ± 2.77^{ab}	40.63 ± 5.86^{b}	41.88 ± 2.54^{ab}
18:3n3	0.76 ± 0.36	1.26 ± 0.68	1.24 ± 0.59	1.42 ± 0.45
20:3n3	0.18 ± 0.06^{a}	0.13 ± 0.07^{ab}	0.13 ± 0.08^{ab}	0.09 ± 0.04^{b}
20:5n3	0.68 ± 0.19	0.63 ± 0.24	0.52 ± 0.16	0.51 ± 0.26
22:5n3	0.63 ± 0.14	0.63 ± 0.29	0.56 ± 0.15	0.54 ± 0.18
22:6n3	2.84 ± 0.62	2.64 ± 1.01	2.20 ± 0.59	2.00 ± 0.75
DHA + EPA	3.53 ± 0.79	3.28 ± 1.23	2.71 ± 0.74	2.51 ± 1.00
N-3 PUFA	5.09 ± 0.61	5.29 ± 1.22	4.63 ± 0.50	4.56 ± 0.88
Total PUFA	50.62 ± 2.90^{a}	49.34 ± 2.55^{ab}	45.26 ± 5.89^{b}	46.44 ± 3.23^{ab}
N-3/N-6 PUFA	0.11 ± 0.01	0.12 ± 0.03	0.12 ± 0.02	0.11 ± 0.02

TFL: tea-flavor liquor; TCL: traditional Chinese liquor; EC: ethanol control; WC: water control; SFA: saturated fatty acid; PUFA: polyunsaturated fatty acid; DHA: docosahexaenoic acid; EPA: eicosapentaenoic acid; Different letters represent statistically significant difference ($P < 0.05$) between the two groups (e.g., a versus b, b versus c). No significant difference was observed if two groups contain the same letters (e.g., ab versus b, a versus ab).

Although the alcohol consumption of SD rats in the present study was relatively low (from 2.4 to 2.7 g/d/kg body weight), it was demonstrated that chronic periods of moderate alcohol consumption (from 1.2 to 2.6 g/d/kg body weight) were sufficient to decrease PUFA contents of liver [11, 26, 27]. The results of present study were consistent with previous studies [11, 26, 27], and compositions of total n-3 PUFA, n-6 PUFA, and C20:5n-3 + C22:6n-3 decreased in alcohol group compared with WC group. However, the effect of alcohol on plasma and kidney fatty acids was less evident compared with changes of hepatic fatty acid composition, while TFL could even significantly increase kidney n-6 PUFA and total PUFA content compared with EC. It might be due to that ethanol is mainly metabolized in the liver and ethanol metabolism is capable of generating reactive oxygen species (ROS), which mainly react with PUFA in the liver [11, 28]. In contrast, red wine was reported to preserve kidney long-chain PUFA and nonalcoholic components were reported to contribute to the result [9, 10]. This was consistent with our present findings. TFL could also preserve n-6 and total PUFA contents compared with EC in kidney. And it can be postulated that nonalcoholic components in TFL might partly contribute to the PUFA preservation effect; however, the mechanisms were largely unknown.

Another topic of concern was the fish-like effect of moderate alcohol drinking recently suggested by some researchers [29–31]. Guiraud et al. [30] demonstrated that ethanol drinking would result in a significant increase in plasma docosahexaenoic acid in rats. But the authors did not show changes of fatty acids in liver. As the ethanol intake in that study was much higher than our present study, the PUFA depletion in the liver would be even stronger than the present study. So the fish-like effect of alcohol should be explained with caution as the effect of ethanol on hepatic fatty acid was very sensitive.

Ethanol was reported to increase hepatic lipogenesis by activating SREBP-1 and ACC [32]. Our results were consistent with previous findings that SREBP-1c and ACC mRNA

Table 6: Hepatic total fatty acid profiles after consumption of TFL and TCL.

	TFL ($n = 9$)	TCL ($n = 8$)	EC ($n = 8$)	WC ($n = 8$)
14:0	0.77 ± 0.19^{a}	0.59 ± 0.07^{ab}	0.77 ± 0.21^{a}	0.42 ± 0.07^{b}
15:0	0.22 ± 0.06	0.21 ± 0.03	0.26 ± 0.06	0.21 ± 0.02
16:0	25.73 ± 3.12^{a}	23.16 ± 1.18^{ab}	26.45 ± 3.54^{a}	21.84 ± 1.47^{b}
18:0	12.92 ± 2.55	11.55 ± 1.79	11.99 ± 2.43	11.51 ± 2.93
20:0	0.07 ± 0.04	0.05 ± 0.01	0.09 ± 0.03	0.04 ± 0.02
SFA	39.71 ± 2.42^{a}	35.56 ± 2.45^{ab}	39.54 ± 4.39^{a}	34.00 ± 3.69^{b}
16:1n7	1.22 ± 0.30	1.31 ± 0.52	1.26 ± 0.33	1.00 ± 0.47
18:1n9	12.52 ± 2.87	12.31 ± 2.89	10.34 ± 1.90	9.28 ± 2.27
18:1n7	2.61 ± 0.34	2.73 ± 0.34	2.71 ± 0.44	2.25 ± 0.28
20:1n9	0.21 ± 0.04^{a}	0.18 ± 0.04^{ab}	0.19 ± 0.06^{a}	0.12 ± 0.03^{b}
MUFA	16.56 ± 2.79^{a}	16.53 ± 3.50^{ab}	14.50 ± 2.15^{ab}	12.66 ± 2.71^{b}
18:2n6	18.62 ± 3.35	20.41 ± 2.87	18.37 ± 3.97	21.85 ± 4.19
18:3n6	0.07 ± 0.03	0.09 ± 0.02	0.09 ± 0.04	0.10 ± 0.04
20:2n6	0.39 ± 0.13	0.40 ± 0.06	0.34 ± 0.04	0.41 ± 0.08
20:3n6	0.63 ± 0.15^{ab}	0.70 ± 0.16^{ab}	0.58 ± 0.12^{a}	0.80 ± 0.16^{b}
20:4n6	15.71 ± 3.33	15.63 ± 2.07	17.19 ± 2.29	18.49 ± 3.88
22:4n6	0.31 ± 0.12	0.41 ± 0.12	0.40 ± 0.12	0.49 ± 0.15
N-6 PUFA	35.70 ± 2.07^{a}	37.61 ± 3.50^{a}	36.94 ± 2.61^{a}	42.12 ± 2.48^{b}
18:3n3	0.69 ± 0.33	0.76 ± 0.15	0.73 ± 0.23	0.88 ± 0.34
20:3n3	0.10 ± 0.04	0.09 ± 0.04	0.10 ± 0.04	0.10 ± 0.02
20:5n3	0.62 ± 0.31^{ab}	0.83 ± 0.29^{ab}	0.56 ± 0.12^{a}	0.98 ± 0.32^{b}
22:5n3	1.18 ± 0.32^{a}	1.47 ± 0.37^{ab}	1.32 ± 0.24^{ab}	1.88 ± 0.60^{b}
22:6n3	5.34 ± 0.92^{a}	6.35 ± 0.74^{bc}	6.07 ± 0.76^{ab}	7.22 ± 0.47^{c}
DHA + EPA	5.96 ± 0.97^{a}	7.17 ± 0.99^{bc}	6.63 ± 0.72^{ab}	8.20 ± 0.76^{c}
N-3 PUFA	7.92 ± 1.21^{a}	9.48 ± 1.29^{ab}	8.72 ± 0.60^{a}	11.05 ± 1.59^{b}
Total PUFA	43.61 ± 2.91^{a}	47.09 ± 2.86^{a}	45.66 ± 2.85^{a}	53.17 ± 3.23^{b}
N-3/N-6 PUFA	0.22 ± 0.03	0.26 ± 0.06	0.24 ± 0.02	0.26 ± 0.04

TFL: tea-flavor liquor; TCL: traditional Chinese liquor; EC: ethanol control; WC: water control; SFA: saturated fatty acid; PUFA: polyunsaturated fatty acid; DHA: docosahexaenoic acid; EPA: eicosapentaenoic acid; Different letters represent statistically significant difference ($P < 0.05$) between the two groups (e.g., a versus b, b versus c). No significant difference was observed if two groups contain the same letters (e.g., ab versus b, a versus ab).

expression were significantly increased in EC group. SREBP-2 is also very important in regulating genes involved in cholesterol metabolism (e.g., HMG-CoA synthase, HMG-CoA reducase) [33]. EC group showed significantly higher SREBP-2 mRNA expressions, which may indicate minor disruption of cholesterol metabolism. However TFL and TCL groups in the present study did not cause any significant change for all these mentioned gene expressions, which might attenuate the impacts of ethanol on lipid metabolism. Given that the ethanol contents in TFL, TCL, and EC groups were the same, nonalcoholic components in TFL and TCL may contribute to the results. The detailed functional nonalcoholic components in the liquors were yet to be determined. However these results should be explained with caution, as the lipid metabolism between humans and rodents is different, and results from rodent model could not be fully extrapolated to humans.

In conclusion, hepatic total and n-6 PUFA compositions were decreased in all the alcoholic groups, while in kidney, TFL may preserve total and n-6 PUFA compositions. TFL has a beneficial effect for metabolic disorder in relation to improved circulating insulin levels without affecting hepatic lipid metabolism-related gene expressions in rats. Nonalcoholic components may contribute to these results.

Abbreviations

- ALT: Alanine aminotransferase
- AST: Aspartate aminotransferase
- ALP: Alkaline phosphatase
- ApoA1: Apolipoprotein A1
- ApoB: Apolipoprotein B
- AMPK: Adenosine monophosphate-dependent protein kinase
- ACAC-α: Acetyl-coenzyme A carboxylase alpha
- EC: Ethanol control
- TCL: Traditional Chinese liquor
- HDL-C: High-density lipoprotein cholesterol
- IL-6: Interleukin-6
- LDL-C: Low-density lipoprotein cholesterol
- PUFA: Polyunsaturated fatty acid
- PRKA-α1: Protein kinase, AMP-activated, alpha 1 catalytic subunit
- PPAR-α: Peroxisome proliferator-activated receptor alpha
- SREBF-1c: Sterol regulatory element binding transcription factor 1c
- SREBF-2: Sterol regulatory element binding transcription factor 2

TFL: Tea-flavor liquor
TC: Total cholesterol
TG: Triacylglycerol
TNF-α: Tumor necrosis factor-α
WC: Water control.

Conflict of Interests

The authors declared that there is no conflict of interests.

Acknowledgments

The authors would like to thank Guizhou Meijiao Co., Ltd., China, for providing the two liquors. The project was funded by the National Natural Science Foundation of China (NSFC, no. 30972464), the National Basic Research Program of China (973 Program: 2011CB504002), and Zhejiang University (no. H20091920).

References

[1] S. Kiechl, J. Willeit, W. Poewe et al., "Insulin sensitivity and regular alcohol consumption: large, prospective, cross sectional population study (Bruneck study)," *British Medical Journal*, vol. 313, no. 7064, pp. 1040–1044, 1996.

[2] M. M. Joosten, J. W. J. Beulens, S. Kersten, and H. F. J. Hendriks, "Moderate alcohol consumption increases insulin sensitivity and ADIPOQ expression in postmenopausal women: a randomised, crossover trial," *Diabetologia*, vol. 51, no. 8, pp. 1375–1381, 2008.

[3] R. A. Kloner and S. H. Rezkalla, "To drink or not to drink? That is the question," *Circulation*, vol. 116, no. 11, pp. 1306–1317, 2007.

[4] L. L. J. Koppes, J. M. Dekker, H. F. J. Hendriks, L. M. Bouter, and R. J. Heine, "Meta-analysis of the relationship between alcohol consumption and coronary heart disease and mortality in type 2 diabetic patients," *Diabetologia*, vol. 49, no. 4, pp. 648–652, 2006.

[5] E. Sacanella, M. Vázquez-Agell, M. P. Mena et al., "Down-regulation of adhesion molecules and other inflammatory biomarkers after moderate wine consumption in healthy women: a randomized trial," *American Journal of Clinical Nutrition*, vol. 86, no. 5, pp. 1463–1469, 2007.

[6] M. Naissides, J. C. L. Mamo, A. P. James, and S. Pal, "The effect of chronic consumption of red wine on cardiovascular disease risk factors in postmenopausal women," *Atherosclerosis*, vol. 185, no. 2, pp. 438–445, 2006.

[7] R. Estruch, E. Sacanella, E. Badia et al., "Different effects of red wine and gin consumption on inflammatory biomarkers of atherosclerosis: a prospective randomized crossover trial: effects of wine on inflammatory markers," *Atherosclerosis*, vol. 175, no. 1, pp. 117–123, 2004.

[8] J. Villanueva, C. J. Chandler, N. Shimasaki et al., "Effects of ethanol feeding on liver, kidney and jejunal membranes of micropigs," *Hepatology*, vol. 19, no. 5, pp. 1229–1240, 1994.

[9] J. Araya, R. Rodrigo, M. Orellana, and V. García, "Effects of red wine consumption on kidney FA composition," *Lipids*, vol. 38, no. 3, pp. 275–279, 2003.

[10] J. Araya, R. Rodrigo, M. Orellana, and G. Rivera, "Red wine raises plasma HDL and preserves long-chain polyunsaturated fatty acids in rat kidney and erythrocytes," *British Journal of Nutrition*, vol. 86, no. 2, pp. 189–195, 2001.

[11] R. J. Pawlosky, B. M. Flynn, and N. Salem, "The effects of low dietary levels of polyunsaturates on alcohol-induced liver disease in rhesus monkeys," *Hepatology*, vol. 26, no. 6, pp. 1386–1392, 1997.

[12] W. Fan and M. C. Qian, "Characterization of aroma compounds of Chinese "Wuliangye" and "Jiannanchun" liquors by aroma extract dilution analysis," *Journal of Agricultural and Food Chemistry*, vol. 54, no. 7, pp. 2695–2704, 2006.

[13] M. Sozio and D. W. Crabb, "Alcohol and lipid metabolism," *American Journal of Physiology*, vol. 295, no. 1, pp. E10–E16, 2008.

[14] Y. Li, S. Xu, M. M. Mihaylova et al., "AMPK phosphorylates and inhibits SREBP activity to attenuate hepatic steatosis and atherosclerosis in diet-induced insulin-resistant mice," *Cell Metabolism*, vol. 13, no. 4, pp. 376–388, 2011.

[15] J.-S. Zheng, J. Yang, T. Huang, X.-J. Hu, M. Luo, and D. Li, "Effects of Chinese liquors on cardiovascular disease risk factors in healthy young humans," *The Scientific World Journal*, vol. 2012, Article ID 372143, 9 pages, 2012.

[16] V. L. Singleton and J. A. Rossi Jr., "Colorimetry of total phenolics with phosphomolybdic-phosphotungstic acid reagents," *American Journal of Enology and Viticulture*, vol. 16, pp. 144–158, 1965.

[17] D. Li, A. Sinclair, A. Wilson et al., "Effect of dietary α-linolenic acid on thrombotic risk factors in vegetarian men," *American Journal of Clinical Nutrition*, vol. 69, no. 5, pp. 872–882, 1999.

[18] C. A. Heid, J. Stevens, K. J. Livak, and P. M. Williams, "Real time quantitative PCR," *Genome Research*, vol. 6, no. 10, pp. 986–994, 1996.

[19] J. M. Gaziano, J. E. Buring, J. L. Breslow et al., "Moderate alcohol intake, increased levels of high-density lipoprotein and its subfractions, and decreased risk of myocardial infarction," *New England Journal of Medicine*, vol. 329, no. 25, pp. 1829–1834, 1993.

[20] E. B. Rimm, E. L. Giovannucci, W. C. Willett et al., "Prospective study of alcohol consumption and risk of coronary disease in men," *The Lancet*, vol. 338, no. 8765, pp. 464–468, 1991.

[21] M. J. Davies, D. J. Baer, J. T. Judd, E. D. Brown, W. S. Campbell, and P. R. Taylor, "Effects of moderate alcohol intake on fasting insulin and glucose concentrations and insulin sensitivity in postmenopausal women: a randomized controlled trial," *Journal of the American Medical Association*, vol. 287, no. 19, pp. 2559–2562, 2002.

[22] A. Sierksma, H. Patel, N. Ouchi et al., "Effect of moderate alcohol consumption on adiponectin, tumor necrosis factor-alpha, and insulin sensitivity," *Diabetes Care*, vol. 27, no. 1, pp. 184–189, 2004.

[23] J. Hong, R. R. Smith, A. E. Harvey, and N. P. Núñez, "Alcohol consumption promotes insulin sensitivity without affecting body fat levels," *International Journal of Obesity*, vol. 33, no. 2, pp. 197–203, 2009.

[24] L. Y. Wu, C. C. Juan, L. T. Ho, Y. P. Hsu, and L. S. Hwang, "Effect of green tea supplementation on insulin sensitivity in Sprague-Dawley rats," *Journal of Agricultural and Food Chemistry*, vol. 52, no. 3, pp. 643–648, 2004.

[25] L. Y. Wu, C. C. Juan, L. S. Hwang, Y. P. Hsu, P. H. Ho, and L. T. Ho, "Green tea supplementation ameliorates insulin resistance and increases glucose transporter IV content in a fructose-fed rat model," *European Journal of Nutrition*, vol. 43, no. 2, pp. 116–124, 2004.

[26] R. J. Pawlosky and N. Salem Jr., "Alcohol consumption in rhesus monkeys depletes tissues of polyunsaturated fatty acids and

alters essential fatty acid metabolism," *Alcoholism*, vol. 23, no. 2, pp. 311–317, 1999.

[27] R. J. Pawlosky and N. Salem Jr., "Ethanol exposure causes a decrease in docosahexaenoic acid and an increase in docosapentaenoic acid in feline brains and retinas," *American Journal of Clinical Nutrition*, vol. 61, no. 6, pp. 1284–1289, 1995.

[28] E. A. Meagher, O. P. Barry, A. Burke et al., "Alcohol-induced generation of lipid peroxidation products in humans," *Journal of Clinical Investigation*, vol. 104, no. 6, pp. 805–813, 1999.

[29] M. de Lorgeril, P. Salen, J. L. Martin, F. Boucher, and J. de Leiris, "Interactions of wine drinking with omega-3 fatty acids in patients with coronary heart disease: a fish-like effect of moderate wine drinking," *American Heart Journal*, vol. 155, no. 1, pp. 175–181, 2008.

[30] A. Guiraud, M. de Lorgeril, S. Zeghichi et al., "Interactions of ethanol drinking with n-3 fatty acids in rats: potential consequences for the cardiovascular system," *British Journal of Nutrition*, vol. 100, no. 6, pp. 1237–1244, 2008.

[31] R. Di Giuseppe, M. De Lorgeril, P. Salen et al., "Alcohol consumption and n-3 polyunsaturated fatty acids in healthy men and women from 3 European populations," *American Journal of Clinical Nutrition*, vol. 89, no. 1, pp. 354–362, 2009.

[32] M. You, M. Matsumoto, C. M. Pacold, W. K. Cho, and D. W. Crabb, "The role of AMP-activated protein kinase in the action of ethanol in the liver," *Gastroenterology*, vol. 127, no. 6, pp. 1798–1808, 2004.

[33] I. Shimomura, H. Shimano, J. D. Horton, J. L. Goldstein, and M. S. Brown, "Differential expression of exons 1a and 1c in mRNAs for sterol regulatory element binding protein-1 in human and mouse organs and cultured cells," *Journal of Clinical Investigation*, vol. 99, no. 5, pp. 838–845, 1997.

12

Radioprotective Effect of Alk(en)yl Thiosulfates Derived from Allium Vegetables against DNA Damage Caused by X-Ray Irradiation in Cultured Cells: Antiradiation Potential of Onions and Garlic

Hye-Sook Chang,[1] Daiji Endoh,[2] Yushi Ishida,[2] Hiroyuki Takahashi,[3] Shuji Ozawa,[4] Masanobu Hayashi,[2] Akira Yabuki,[1] and Osamu Yamato[1]

[1] *Laboratory of Clinical Pathology, Department of Veterinary Medicine, Kagoshima University, 1-21-24 Kohrimoto, Kagoshima 890-0065, Japan*
[2] *Department of Veterinary Radiology, School of Veterinary Medicine, Rakuno Gakuen University, 582 Midorimachi, Bunkyodai, Hokkaido 069-8501, Ebetsu, Japan*
[3] *Information Systems Department, Industrial Research Institute, Hokkaido Research Organization, Kita-19 Nishi-11, Hokkaido 060-0819, Sapporo, Japan*
[4] *Laboratory of Natural Products Chemistry, Department of Sustainable Agriculture, Rakuno Gakuen University, 582 Midorimachi, Bunkyodai, Hokkaido 069-8501, Ebetsu, Japan*

Correspondence should be addressed to Osamu Yamato, osam@vet.kagoshima-u.ac.jp

Academic Editors: Y.-C. Huang and B. Venn

To evaluate a radioprotective effect of sodium *n*-propyl thiosulfate (NPTS) and sodium 2-propenyl thiosulfate (2PTS) derived from onions and garlic, respectively, rat hepatoma H4IIE cells and mouse lymphoma L5178Y cells were preincubated with each of these compounds for 48 hours at 37°C before receiving 10 Gy of X-ray irradiation. Cell damage caused by the irradiation was quantified as comet tail moment, which represents the degree of DNA damage. X-ray-induced DNA damage was significantly decreased in both H4IIE and L5178Y cells by micromolar concentrations of NPTS and 2PTS compared with the control without the compounds. The protective effect was more potent with 2PTS than NPTS. Onions and garlic have antiradiation potential.

1. Introduction

Radiation exposure, either accidentally or during radiotherapy and radio imaging, has deterministic or stochastic effects on living systems. The development of effective and nontoxic radioprotective agents is therefore of considerable interest, and a large number of chemical and biological agents have been screened over the past decade [1, 2]. As yet, however, there is not a single agent available which meets all the prerequisites of an ideal radio protector, that is, produces no cumulative or irreversible toxicity, offers effective long-term protection, possesses a shelf life of 2–5 years, and can be easily administered [1].

Garlic extract and its chemical constituents such as allicin, alliin, and diallyl sulfide have inhibitory effects on chemical mutagenesis and carcinogenesis [3–5]. Furthermore, experiments *in vitro* using *Salmonella* tester strains and Chinese hamster ovary cells showed that garlic exerts an antimutagenic effect against gammaradiation possibly through the scavenging of free radicals [4]. Other researchers also demonstrated a radioprotective effect of garlic against tissue damage in liver and lung, reducing the radiation-induced mortality in albino rats [6]. Based on these observations, some constituents in Allium vegetables such as onions and garlic are expected to be radioprotective.

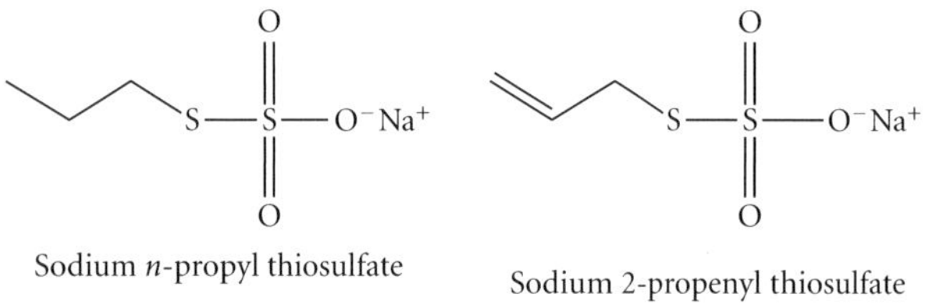

FIGURE 1: Structure of sodium *n*-propyl thiosulfate (NPTS) and sodium 2-propenyl thiosulfate (2PTS).

Two alk(en)yl thiosulfates (Figure 1), sodium *n*-propyl thiosulfate (NPTS) and sodium 2-propenyl thiosulfate (2PTS), isolated from onions (*Allium cepa*) and garlic (*A. sativum*), respectively, were originally identified as causative agents of onion- and garlic-induced hemolytic anemia in dogs [7–10]. To date, however, NPTS and 2PTS have been shown to have a number of beneficial properties for humans, that is, an inhibitory effect on tumor cell growth [11–13], an immune-enhancing effect on polymorphonuclear leukocytes [14], an antiaggregatory effect on platelets [14, 15], and an inductive effect on phase II detoxification enzymes [16]. In contrast, there has not been any report of anemia associated with the consumption of onions or garlic in humans.

In view of the usefulness of these Allium vegetables and the multifunction of these alk(en)nyl thiosulfates for human health, the present study was undertaken to evaluate a possible radioprotective effect of NPTS and 2PTS against X-ray-induced DNA damage in cultured mammalian cells. In addition, the radioprotective effect of these compounds was compared with that of lignan, recently reported to have a radioprotective effect in cultured cells [17] and in mice [18].

2. Materials and Methods

All experiments in the present study were carried out in laboratories specific for radiation experiments in the Rakuno Gakuen University under the supervision of a radiology specialist (D. Endoh, one of the authors).

2.1. Chemicals and Reagents. NPTS and 2PTS were synthesized and purified according to a method described previously [7, 10]. Lignan-containing flaxseed extract was prepared as reported previously [19]. Normal melting-point agarose (NMA) was obtained from the Nacalai Tesque (Kyoto, Japan) and low melting-point agarose (LMA) from Funakoshi (Tokyo, Japan).

2.2. Cell Culture and Treatments. The rat hepatoma H4IIE cell line was purchased from the Dainippon Sumitomo Pharma (Osaka, Japan). H4IIE cells were grown in Dulbecco's modified eagle's medium supplemented with 10% fetal bovine serum, 100 U/mL penicillin, and 100 μg/mL streptomycin. The mouse lymphoma L5178Y cell line was provided by the Riken Bio Resource Center (Tsukuba, Japan). L5178Y cells were grown in RPMI 1640 medium supplemented with 10% heat-inactivated horse serum, 100 U/mL penicillin, and 100 μg/mL streptomycin. NPTS and 2PTS were dissolved in culture medium and adjusted to the concentrations required for the experiments. Lignan-containing flaxseed extract was diluted with culture medium and adjusted to the required concentration. The cells were seeded at an initial density of 7×10^5 cells into a 25 cm^2 flask, preincubated for 24 hours at 37°C, and then exposed to final concentrations (1–50 μM) of NPTS, 2PTS, or 2.5 mg/mL of lignan-containing flaxseed extract for 48 hours at 37°C. Control cells were exposed to nothing.

2.3. Comet Assay. The comet assay was carried out according to procedures reported previously [20, 21], with some modifications. A microscope slide was precoated in 1% NMA and allowed to dry at room temperature. The cell suspension was mixed with an equal volume of 2% LMA at 37°C. Sixty microliter of the LMA cell suspension was rapidly pipetted over an NMA precoated slide and covered with a coverslip as the cells were spread homogeneously. After solidification of the LMA cell suspension for 15 min at 4°C, the coverslip was gently removed. On the solidified LMA cell suspension, 100 μL of cell-free LMA was layered, covered with a coverslip, and then allowed to solidify for 20 min at 4°C. After removal of the coverslip, the slide for irradiation experiments was exposed to a 10 Gy dose of X-rays. Following completion of the irradiation, the slide was immediately immersed into alkaline lysis solution containing 1 M NaCl, 0.03 M NaOH, and 0.1% sodium sarcosinate for 30 min at 4°C, being protected from light. Next the slide was placed in electrophoresis solution (pH 13) containing 0.3 M NaOH and 2 mM EDTA, and electrophoresis was conducted for 25 min at 25 V and 400 mA. After the electrophoresis, the slide was neutralized in neutralization buffer (pH 7.4) containing 154 mM NaCl, 1 mM $CaCl_2$, 0.5 mM $MgCl_2$, and 100 mM Tris, for 20 min, and stained with PicoGreen (Invitrogen, Eugene, OR, USA) diluted to 200-fold in the neutralization buffer, and photographed using an inspection device (Bioplorer FJ-VKH-01; Koyo Sangyo, Tokyo, Japan; Panasonic Ecology Systems, Kasugai-shi, Japan). Image analysis of the photograph was performed using originally developed software (Hokkaido Industrial Research Institute, Sapporo, Japan) on cells selected randomly by the software (Japanese Patent no. 4355832). The extent of DNA damage was quantified as the tail moment of 50–100 individual cells per treatment.

2.4. X-Ray Irradiation. The cells were irradiated to a dose of 10 Gy using an X-ray generator (Model MBR-1520R, Hitachi, Tokyo, Japan) operated at 150 kVp and 20 mA with 0.5 mm Cu and 0.5 mm Al filtration. The source-to-surface distance was 30 cm, and the dose rate was approximately 1.12 Gy/min.

2.5. Statistical Analyses. All data are presented as the mean ± standard deviation of the tail moment in 50–100 cells selected randomly by the software for image analysis. For comparisons between groups, data were analyzed by a one-way factorial analysis of variance with post hoc tests (Tukey's method). Differences were considered significant at $P < 0.05$.

3. Results

The results of the comet assay using H4IIE cells are shown in Figure 2. NPTS and 2PTS did not change comet tail moment in H4IIE cells without irradiation (Figure 2(a)). In control cells without any compound, tail moment was increased 3.0-fold by irradiation (Figure 2(b)) compared with that in control cells without irradiation shown in Figure 2(a). Tail moment was significantly reduced by 26% by treatment with lignan, compared with control cells with irradiation (Figure 2(b)). In cells treated with NPTS, tail moment was decreased dose-dependently and by a maximum of 25% at 50 μM. The values at 5–50 μM NPTS were significantly lower than those in the control. In 2PTS, the values at all concentrations were significantly lower than those in the control, but the change was not dose dependent: the lowest (by 39%) was at 5 μM and the highest (by 19%) at 50 μM. In comparisons between NPTS and 2PTS, tail moment was significantly lower in 2PTS than that in the latter at 1–10 μM, but significantly higher at 50 μM.

The results in the comet assay using L5178Y cells are shown in Figure 3. Even in nonirradiation experiments, tail moment was significantly reduced at 10 and 50 μM NPTS and at all concentrations of 2PTS (Figure 3(a)). The value was significantly lower in 2PTS than in NPTS at all concentrations. In irradiation experiments (Figure 3(b)), the results were similar to those in H4IIE cells shown in Figure 2(b). In control cells, tail moment was increased 3.3-fold by irradiation (Figure 3(b)). Tail moment was significantly reduced by 35% by treatment with lignan. Both NPTS and 2PTS reduced tail moment, but the changes were not dose dependent. In NPTS, tail moment was significantly decreased at 1–10 μM and the lowest value (by 17%) was at 5 μM. In 2PTS, tail moment was significantly decreased at all concentrations and the lowest value (by 48%) was at 10 μM. Tail moment was significantly lower in 2PTS than that in NPTS at all concentrations.

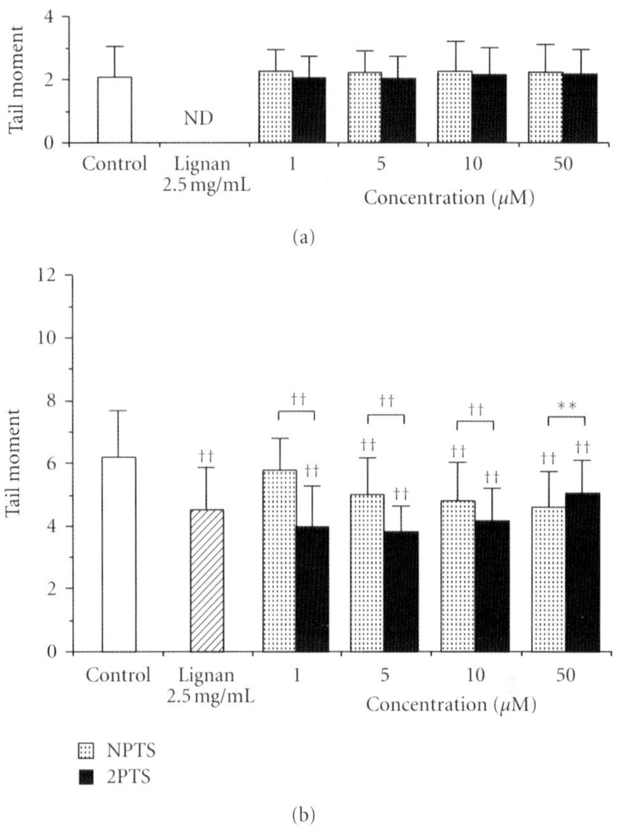

FIGURE 2: The effect of alk(en)yl thiosulfates on X-ray-induced DNA damage in rat hepatoma H4IIE cells. Cells were pretreated with different concentrations (1–50 μM) of sodium *n*-propyl thiosulfate (NPTS), sodium 2-propenyl thiosulfate (2PTS), or 2.5 mg/mL lignan-containing flaxseed extract for 48 hours at 37°C before X-ray irradiation (10 Gy). Control cells (white column) were not exposed to any compound. The experiments were divided into nonirradiated (a) and X-ray-irradiated (b) groups. The assessment of DNA damage was carried out on 50–100 individual cells per treatment using a comet assay. Data were analyzed by a one-way factorial analysis of variance with post hoc tests (Tukey's method). $^{**}P < 0.01$ and $^{\dagger\dagger}P < 0.001$ versus control or between groups. ND: not determined.

4. Discussion

In the present study, we investigated a radioprotective effect of two alk(en)yl thiosulfates and lignan against DNA damage caused by X-ray irradiation in 2 kinds of cultured mammalian cells. Based on the results, it was demonstrated that a 48-hour culture with NPTS and 2PTS reduced the degree of DNA damage caused by subsequent irradiation in both cell lines, like lignan, an effect of which had been reported previously [17, 18]. The radioprotective effect of NPTS and 2PTS is consistent with findings from studies *in vitro*, which demonstrated an antimutagenic effect of garlic against gammaradiation in *Salmonella* and Chinese hamster ovary cells [4].

Since free radicals play an important role in irradiation-induced damage, the underlying radioprotective mechanism of a majority of radioprotective compounds has been linked, either directly or indirectly, to their antioxidative capabilities by scavenging free radicals responsible for DNA damage [22]. Garlic oil is rich in sulfhydryl compounds that are capable of protecting against tissue-damaging effects of irradiation [6]. The mechanism of the protective effect by sulfhydryl compounds is considered to be free radical extinction. Diallyl trisulfide, a principal constituent of garlic oil, significantly induced the production of glutathione peroxidase, one of the most important antioxidative enzymes in living systems [23]. Other researchers investigated effects of onions on red cell antioxidants such as superoxide dismutase, catalase, glucose-6-phosphate, and reduced glutathione (GSH) by feeding onion soup to dogs [24]. In this experiment, there was a transient decrease in the antioxidants, but values then began to increase progressively toward a peak, before returning to normal. In our previous experiment *in vivo* using NPTS, the concentration of erythrocyte GSH was significantly increased

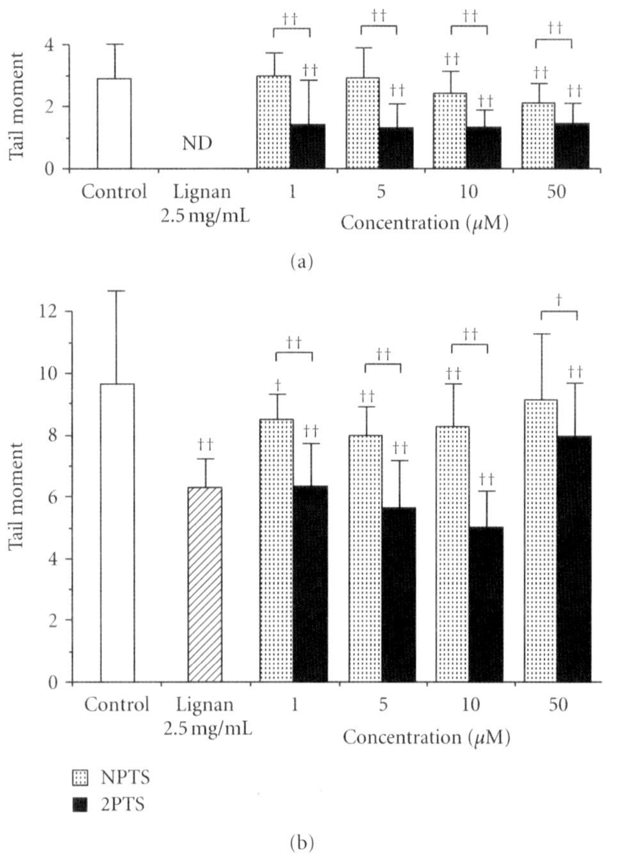

Figure 3: The effect of alk(en)yl thiosulfates on X-ray-induced DNA damage in mouse lymphoma L5178Y cells. Cells were pretreated with different concentrations (1–50 μM) of sodium *n*-propyl thiosulfate (NPTS), sodium 2-propenyl thiosulfate (2PTS), or 2.5 mg/mL lignan-containing flaxseed extract for 48 hours at 37°C before the X-ray irradiation (10 Gy). Control cells (white column) were not exposed to any compound. The experiments were divided into nonirradiated (a) and X-ray-irradiated (b) groups. The assessment of DNA damage was carried out on 50–100 individual cells per treatment using a comet assay. Data were analyzed by a one-way factorial analysis of variance with post hoc tests (Tukey's method). $^{\dagger}P < 0.005$ and $^{\dagger\dagger}P < 0.001$ versus control or between groups. ND: not determined.

after the oral administration of NPTS to dogs although NPTS acts as an oxidant-inducing hemolytic anemia in dogs [8]. These observations suggest that the body's antioxidation system could be stimulated by pre-exposure to certain worthwhile oxidants, which enhances endogenous protective mechanisms against oxidative stress. There is considerable evidence that Allium vegetables prevent cancer in humans [25–28]. The radioprotective effect of NPTS and 2PTS may be one of the mechanisms of cancer prevention.

In the present study, significantly effective radioprotection was not always obtained dose dependently. The radioprotective effect at relatively high concentrations of alk(en)yl thiosulfates seemed to become weaker rather than stronger. In H4IIE cells, 2PTS showed higher levels of DNA damage at 10 and 50 μM than at 1 and 5 μM (Figure 2(b)). Likewise, in L5178Y cells, both NPTS and 2PTS showed higher levels of DNA damage at 50 μM than those at the other lower concentrations (Figure 3(b)). Therefore, it is thought that overexposure to alk(en)yl thiosulfates could result in excessive oxidative stress rather than the level of stress appropriate for stimulating the body's antioxidation system. In other words, NPTS and 2PTS exert an antioxidative effect by stimulating the antioxidation system at low concentrations, but as their concentrations increase, their natural characteristics as oxidants become evident and the radioprotective effect might be offset. In fact, NPTS and 2PTS have an antitumor effect through the induction of apoptosis initiated by oxidative stress at relatively high concentrations (>50 μM) [11].

Computed tomography (CT) is one of the largest contributors to man-made irradiation doses in medical populations, and its use continues to grow rapidly all over the world. The principal concern regarding irradiation exposure is that the subject may develop malignancies. Many studies have shown that organ doses associated with routine diagnostic CT scans are similar to the low-dose range of irradiation received by atomic-bomb survivors, and the US Food and Drug Administration estimates that a CT examination with an effective dose of 10 mSv may be associated with an increased chance of developing fatal cancer for approximately one in 2000 patients [29]. In addition, there is a risk of radioactive pollutants being released into the environment by serious accidents at nuclear power plants, as happened at Fukushima in 2011 and Chernobyl in 1986.

We believe that the daily intake of Allium vegetables such as onions and garlic containing alk(en)yl thiosulfates and other effective compounds could be beneficial to decrease toxic effects of irradiation.

Acknowledgments

This study was supported financially by grants (nos. 17658135, O. Yamato, and 20-08445, H.-S. Chang) from the Ministry of Education, Culture, Sports, Science and Technology of Japan and the Japan Society for Promotion of Science.

References

[1] R. Arora, D. Gupta, R. Chawla et al., "Radioprotection by plant products: present status and future prospects," *Phytotherapy Research*, vol. 19, no. 1, pp. 1–22, 2005.

[2] S. Amer, K. J. Na, M. Motobu et al., "Radioprotective effect of sugar cane extract in chickens," *Phytotherapy Research*, vol. 19, no. 6, pp. 496–500, 2005.

[3] V. L. Sparnins, G. Barany, and L. W. Wattenberg, "Effects of organosulfur compounds from garlic and onions on benzo[*a*]pyrene-induced neoplasia and glutathione s-transferase activity in the mouse," *Carcinogenesis*, vol. 9, no. 1, pp. 131–134, 1988.

[4] S. Knasmuller, R. de Martin, G. Domjan, and A. Szakmary, "Studies on the antimutagenic activities of garlic extract," *Environmental and Molecular Mutagenesis*, vol. 13, no. 4, pp. 357–365, 1989.

[5] J. Liu, R. I. Lin, and J. A. Milner, "Inhibition of 7,12-dimethylbenz[*a*]anthracene-induced mammary tumors and

DNA adducts by garlic powder," *Carcinogenesis*, vol. 13, no. 10, pp. 1847–1851, 1992.

[6] S. K. Jaiswal and A. Bordia, "Radio-protective effect of garlic Allium sativum Linn. in albino rats," *Indian Journal of Medical Sciences*, vol. 50, no. 7, pp. 231–233, 1996.

[7] O. Yamato, T. Yoshihara, A. Ichihara, and Y. Maede, "Novel Heinz body hemolysis factors in onion (*Allium cepa*)," *Bioscience, Biotechnology and Biochemistry*, vol. 58, no. 1, pp. 221–222, 1994.

[8] O. Yamato, M. Hayashi, M. Yamasaki, and Y. Maede, "Induction of onion-induced haemolytic anaemia in dogs with sodium n-propylthiosulphate," *Veterinary Record*, vol. 142, no. 9, pp. 216–219, 1998.

[9] O. Yamato, M. Hayashi, E. Kasai, M. Tajima, M. Yamasaki, and Y. Maede, "Reduced glutathione accelerates the oxidative damage produced by sodium *n*-propylthiosulfate, one of the causative agents of onion-induced hemolytic anemia in dogs," *Biochimica et Biophysica Acta*, vol. 1427, no. 2, pp. 175–182, 1999.

[10] O. Yamato, Y. Sugiyama, H. Matsuura et al., "Isolation and identification of sodium 2-propenyl thiosulfate from boiled garlic (*Allium sativum*) that oxidizes canine erythrocytes," *Bioscience, Biotechnology and Biochemistry*, vol. 67, no. 7, pp. 1594–1596, 2003.

[11] H. S. Chang, O. Yamato, M. Yamasaki, M. Ko, and Y. Maede, "Growth inhibitory effect of alk(en)yl thiosulfates derived from onion and garlic in human immortalized and tumor cell lines," *Cancer Letters*, vol. 223, no. 1, pp. 47–55, 2005.

[12] R. Sabelli, E. Iorio, A. de Martino et al., "Rhodanese-thioredoxin system and allyl sulfur compounds: implications in apoptosis induction," *FEBS Journal*, vol. 275, no. 15, pp. 3884–3899, 2008.

[13] R. Nepravishta, R. Sabelli, E. Iorio, L. Micheli, M. Paci, and S. Melino, "Oxidative species and S-glutathionyl conjugates in the apoptosis induction by allyl thiosulfate," *FEBS Journal*, vol. 279, no. 1, pp. 154–167, 2012.

[14] H. S. Chang, O. Yamato, Y. Sakai, M. Yamasaki, and Y. Maede, "Acceleration of superoxide generation in polymorphonuclear leukocytes and inhibition of platelet aggregation by alk(en)yl thiosulfates derived from onion and garlic in dogs and humans," *Prostaglandins Leukotrienes and Essential Fatty Acids*, vol. 70, no. 1, pp. 77–83, 2004.

[15] H. S. Chang, O. Yamato, M. Yamasaki, and Y. Maede, "Modulatory influence of sodium 2-propenyl thiosulfate from garlic on cyclooxygenase activity in canine platelets: possible mechanism for the anti-aggregatory effect," *Prostaglandins Leukotrienes and Essential Fatty Acids*, vol. 72, no. 5, pp. 351–355, 2005.

[16] H. S. Chang, M. Ko, M. Ishizuka et al., "Sodium 2-propenyl thiosulfate derived from garlic induces phase II detoxification enzymes in rat hepatoma H4IIE cells," *Nutrition Research*, vol. 30, no. 6, pp. 435–440, 2010.

[17] R. Checker, S. Chatterjee, D. Sharma et al., "Immunomodulatory and radioprotective effects of lignans derived from fresh nutmeg mace (*Myristica fragrans*) in mammalian splenocytes," *International Immunopharmacology*, vol. 8, no. 5, pp. 661–669, 2008.

[18] A. L. Bhatia, A. Sharma, S. Patni, and A. L. Sharma, "Prophylactic effect of flaxseed oil against radiation-induced hepatotoxicity in mice," *Phytotherapy Research*, vol. 21, no. 9, pp. 852–859, 2007.

[19] D. Endoh, T. Okui, S. Ozawa et al., "Protective effect of a lignan-containing flaxseed extract against CCl_4-induced hepatic injury," *Journal of Veterinary Medical Science*, vol. 64, no. 9, pp. 761–765, 2002.

[20] N. P. Singh, M. T. McCoy, R. R. Tice, and E. L. Schneider, "A simple technique for quantitation of low levels of DNA damage in individual cells," *Experimental Cell Research*, vol. 175, no. 1, pp. 184–191, 1988.

[21] P. J. McCarthy, S. F. Sweetman, P. G. McKenna, and V. J. McKelvey-Martin, "Evaluation of manual and image analysis quantification of DNA damage in the alkaline comet assay," *Mutagenesis*, vol. 12, no. 4, pp. 209–214, 1997.

[22] T. K. Lee, R. M. Johnke, R. R. Allison, K. F. O'Brien, and L. J. Dobbs Jr., "Radioprotective potential of ginseng," *Mutagenesis*, vol. 20, no. 4, pp. 237–243, 2005.

[23] T. Fukao, T. Hosono, S. Misawa, T. Seki, and T. Ariga, "The effects of allyl sulfides on the induction of phase II detoxification enzymes and liver injury by carbon tetrachloride," *Food and Chemical Toxicology*, vol. 42, no. 5, pp. 743–749, 2004.

[24] E. Ogawa, T. Shinoki, F. Akahori, and T. Masaoka, "Effect of onion ingestion on anti-oxidizing agents in dog erythrocytes," *Nippon Juigaku Zasshi*, vol. 48, no. 4, pp. 685–691, 1986.

[25] E. Dorant, P. A. van den Brandt, R. A. Goldbohm, and F. Sturmans, "Consumption of onions and a reduced risk of stomach carcinoma," *Gastroenterology*, vol. 110, no. 1, pp. 12–20, 1996.

[26] F. Bianchini and H. Vainio, "Allium vegetables and organosulfur compounds: do they help prevent cancer?" *Environmental Health Perspectives*, vol. 109, no. 9, pp. 893–902, 2001.

[27] A. T. Fleischauer and L. Arab, "Garlic and cancer: a critical review of the epidemiologic literature," *Journal of Nutrition*, vol. 131, no. 3, pp. 1032S–1040S, 2001.

[28] A. W. Hsing, A. P. Chokkalingam, Y. T. Gao et al., "Allium vegetables and risk of prostate cancer: a population-based study," *Journal of the National Cancer Institute*, vol. 94, no. 21, pp. 1648–1651, 2002.

[29] R. C. Semelka, D. M. Armao, J. Elias Jr., and W. Huda, "Imaging strategies to reduce the risk of radiation in CT studies, including selective substitution with MRI," *Journal of Magnetic Resonance Imaging*, vol. 25, no. 5, pp. 900–909, 2007.

13

Chemical Composition and Fatty Acid Content of Some Spices and Herbs under Saudi Arabia Conditions

Fahad Mohammed Al-Jasass[1] and Mohammed Saud Al-Jasser[2]

[1] *General Directorate of Research Grants, King Abdulaziz City for Science and Technology, P.O. Box 6086, Riyadh 11442, Saudi Arabia*
[2] *Department of Food Science and Nutrition, College of Food and Agricultural Sciences, King Saud University, P.O. Box 2460, Riyadh 11451, Saudi Arabia*

Correspondence should be addressed to Fahad Mohammed Al-Jasass, aljasass@kacst.edu.sa

Academic Editors: H.-W. Chang, L.-Y. Chuang, and S. Yasmin

Some Saudi herbs and spices were analyzed. The results indicated that mustard, black cumin, and cress seeds contain high amount of fat 38.45%, 31.95% and 23.19%, respectively, as compared to clove (16.63%), black pepper (5.34%) and fenugreek (4.51%) seeds. Cress, mustard, black cumin and black pepper contain higher protein contents ranging from 26.61 to 25.45%, as compared to fenugreek (12.91%) and clove (6.9%). Crude fiber and ash content ranged from 6.36 to 23.6% and from 3.57 to 7.1%, respectively. All seeds contain high levels of potassium (ranging from 383 to 823 mg/100g), followed by calcium (ranging from 75 to 270 mg/100g), Magnesium (ranged from 42 to 102 mg/100g) and iron (ranged from 20.5 to 65 mg/100g). However, zinc, manganese and copper were found at low levels. The major fatty acids in cress and mustard were linolenic acid (48.43%) and erucic acid (29.81%), respectively. The lenoleic acid was the major fatty acid in black cumin, fenugreek, black pepper and clove oils being 68.07%, 34.85%, 33.03% and 44.73%, respectively. Total unsaturated fatty acids were 83.24, 95.62, 86.46, 92.99, 81.34 and 87.82% for cress, mustard, black cumin, fenugreek, black pepper and clove, respectively. The differences in the results obtained are due to environmental factors, production areas, cultivars used to produce seeds and also due to the different methods used to prepare these local spices.

1. Introduction

Some seeds are grown primarily for their use as condiments or for herbal medicine such as fenugreek (*Trigonella foenum-gracecum* L.), cress (*Lepidium sativum* L.), mustard (*Sinapis alba* L.), black cumin (*Nigella sativa* L.), black pepper (*Piper nigrum* L.), and clove (*Dianthus* sp.). Fenugreek is an annual crop belonging to the Fabaceae family. This crop is native to an area extending from Iran to northern India, but is now widely cultivated in China, north and east Africa, Ukraine, and Greece [1]. In parts of Asia, the young plants are used as pot herbs and the seeds as a spice or as herbal medicine [2]. Medically, fenugreek is reported to have antidiabetic, antifertility, anticancer, antimicrobial, and antiparasitic, and hypocholesterolaemic effects [3]. Seeds contain 26% mucilage, 22% protein comprising of globulin, histidine, and albumin with a good amount of phosphorus, sulphur, and also lecithin, it contains also 50% of soluble and insoluble fiber found essential for good health [4]. Fenugreek oil contains ω-3, ω-6, and ω-9 fatty acids along with many saponins, alkaloids, and sterols that serve as a source of proestrogens and inhibit intestinal cholesterol absorption [5]. Kochhar et al. [6] reported that fenugreek seeds contain 11.8% moisture, 25.8% crude protein, 6.53% oil, 3.26% ash, and 6.28% crude fiber and 58.13% total carbohydrates on dry basis. However, El-Nasri and El-Tinay [7] found that protein content of fenugreek was found to be 28.4%, crude fiber content was 9.3%, and crude fat was 7.1%. The fatty acid profile was dominated by unsaturated acids, namely, oleic, linoleic, and linolenic acids accounting for 16.3%, 50% and 24.4%, respectively of the total fatty acids. However, El-Sebaiy and El-Mahdy [8] reported that the fatty acids $C_{18:2}$ and $C_{18:3}$ were the most abundant fatty acids in the lipids of the fenugreek seeds. Thus fenugreek seeds may serve to be a beneficial health food if consumed regularly.

Cress is known as garden cress or garden cress pepper weed, and it is a fast growing annual herb. It belongs to the Brassicaceae family that is native to Egypt and west Asia but is widely cultivated in temperate climates throughout the world for various culinary and medicinal uses [9]. It was also reported cress seeds contain 22.5% protein, 27.5% fat, 30% dietary fiber, and 1193 mg/100 g potassium. Hence, it was assumed that these seeds can be used as a functional food. Moreover, Moser et al. [10] found that the oil content of dried cress seeds was 22.7% and the primary fatty acids found in cress oil were oleic (30.6%) and linolenic acids (29.3%). Cress oil contained high concentrations of γ-(1422 ppm) and (356 ppm) tocopherols. However, Gokavi et al. [9] reported that the primary fatty acids found in cress oil were oleic ($C_{18:1}$; 30.6%), linolenic ($C_{18:3}$; 29.3%), palmitic ($C_{16:0}$; 9.4%), linoleic ($C_{18:2}$; 7.6%), erucic ($C_{22:1}$; 3.0%), stearic ($C_{18:0}$; 2.8%), and arachidic ($C_{20:0}$; 2.3%) acids among the minor fatty acids found in cress oil.

Mustard is a herb belonging to the Brassicaceae family and the dry seeds are the only part used. It stimulates digestion and salivary secretion [11]. Mustard seeds have an advantageous chemical composition such as its protein content and fairly well-balanced amino acid composition, rich in dietary fiber and natural antioxidants. In addition to its nutritional value, mustard seed flour offers rather unique functional properties; therefore, it could be taken into consideration as potential component of many food products [12]. White mustard has been used effectively for food and medical applications, one of the limiting factors for human use of mustard products is the spicy flavor produced by myrosinase enzyme activities. Mustard seeds have high-energy content, having 28–32% oil with relatively high protein content (28–36%). The amino acid composition of mustard protein is well balanced; it is rich in essential amino acids. Mustard seeds until now have been used mainly for condiment production, however, this advantageous chemical composition and its relatively low price offer wide possibilities for utilization of this valuable seed, for example, in human foods as additive and to feed animals. Mustard oil has a special fatty acid composition, it contains about 20–28% oleic acid, 10–12% linoleic, 9.0–9.5% linolenic acid, and 30–40% erucic acid, which is indigestible for human and animal organisms. The high erucic acid content of mustard seed could be reduced by breeding, some low erucic acid content genotypes are in cultivation in several countries. Mustard oil is rich in tocopherols, as a consequence of their antioxidant characteristic, they act as a preservative against rancidity [10].

Black cumin is a herb belonging to the Ranunculaceae family and it is widely distributed in countries bordering the Mediterranean Sea, middle Europe, and western Asia [13]. The seeds of N. sativa have been known also as black cumin or black caraway in English and corek out in Turkish, and used as spice and culinary purposes [14]. Black cumin contains 30 to 40% oil and 20 to 30% protein, 3.7–4.7% ash and 25–40% total carbohydrates with antioxidants lignans such as saponin, melantin [15]. Fatty acid compositions of black cumin were $C_{14:0}$ (12.97–13.23%), $C_{16:0}$ (9.47–13.34%), $C_{18:1}$ (15.17–24.15%), and $C_{18:2}$ (54.32–70.81%) as reported by Cheikh-Rouhou et al. [13] and Tulukcu [16]. On the other hand, black cumin oil is considered as one among the newer sources of edible oils. Linoleic acid, undoubtedly one of the most important polyunsaturated fatty acids in human food because of its prevention of distinct heart vascular diseases is present in all the seed oils [17]. It was revealed that the oleic and linoleic acids are the most abundant monounsaturated and polyunsaturated fatty acids in all samples, respectively. The total MUFA composition of the studied species is assigned between 15.17 and 24.15%.

Pepper is a flowering vine belonging to the Piperaceae family and is the most widely used of all condiments. The components contributing to its value are the alkaloids, of which piperine is the most important, for pregnancy, and the volatile (essential) oil for odor and flavor as well as for massage [18]. Black pepper contains (11–14%) protein, (47–53%) fiber, and (10–13.5%) starch [19]. The content of piperine, volatile oil, starch, and fiber can vary markedly in different pepper varieties and is indicative of the quality of black pepper [20]. Black pepper contains about 5–9% of the alkaloids piperine and piperettine and about 1.2–5% of volatile oil [21]. Essential oil is a small portion of a plant material, which consists mainly of terpenes, sequiterpenes, and their derivatives that are responsible for the characteristic aroma, and imparts the identifying flavor and odor most closely associated with the plant itself [22].

Clove is the dried unopened flower bunds of *D. caryophyllus* L. that belong to the Caryophyllaceae family. The dried bulbs resemble a round-headed nail, are dark reddish-brown in color, have a strong aromatic odor and a hot pungent taste. Cloves are now cultivated in many parts of the tropics, particularly Tanzania, Madagascar, Malaysia, India, Srilanka, Jamaica, and French Guiana [23]. Oil of cloves has some antiseptic qualities and is recommended by some dentists as a flavoring aid. Milind and Deepa [24] revealed that clove seeds contains 5.98% protein, 20% total fat, 61.21% carbohydrates, 34.2 fibers, and 5.88% ash. However, it contains also high levels of potassium (1102 mg/100 g) and magnesium (268 mg/100 g). Milind and Deepa [24] also found total saturated fatty acids (5.38%), total monounsaturated fatty acids (1.47%), and total polyunsaturated acids (7.09%).

Although numerous studies on the effects of cultural practices on spices were conducted, changes in their chemical compositions are still far from being finalized specially in Saudi Arabia. Hence, the aim of this study was to investigate the chemical composition, mineral content, and fatty acid profiles of some locally produced spicesand herbs obtained from markets in Saudi Arabia.

2. Material and Methods

2.1. Materials. Fenugreek, cress, mustard, black cumin, black pepper, and clove were *grown in Saudi Arabia.*

2.2. Chemical Composition. Moisture, crude protein, crude fat, crude fiber, and ash were determined according to the AOAC [25] in 2 g, 2 g, 5 g, 2 g, and 5 g sample of each spice.

Table 1: Chemical composition (%) of cress, mustard, black cumin, fenugreek, black pepper, and clove seeds*.

Analysis	Cress	Mustard	Black cumin	Fenugreek	Black pepper	Clove
Moisture	2.88 ± 0.1	4.36 ± 0.1	2.55 ± 0.2	7.71 ± 0.2	4.68 ± 0.3	7.74 ± 0.2
Crude fat	23.19 ± 0.2	38.45 ± 0.5	31.95 ± 0.3	4.51 ± 0.2	5.34 ± 0.6	16.63 ± 0.3
Crude protein	24.19 ± 0.5	25.39 ± 0.3	20.61 ± 0.3	12.91 ± 0.4	25.45 ± 0.4	6.9 ± 0.4
Crude fiber	11.9 ± 0.4	6.36 ± 0.1	10.37 ± 0.1	13.14 ± 0.3	23.6 ± 0.3	11.47 ± 0.5
Ash	7.1 ± 0.1	4.25 ± 0.1	4.51 ± 0.1	4.23 ± 0.05	3.57 ± 0.1	5.96 ± 0.1
Total carbohydrate**	30.74 ± 1.2	21.19 ± 0.9	30.0 ± 1.2	57.5 ± 2.2	37.36 ± 1.4	51.3 ± 2.7

*Means ($n = 3$) ± SD.
**Calculated by difference.

Table 2: Mineral content (mg/100g) of cress, mustard black cumin, fenugreek, black pepper, and clove seeds*.

Mineral	Cress	Mustard	Black cumin	Fenugreek	Black pepper	Clove
K	663 ± 20.0	383.0 ± 10.0	823.0 ± 30.0	603.0 ± 15.0	663 ± 25.0	650.0 ± 30.0
Mg	102.0 ± 10.0	100.0 ± 8.0	80.0 ± 10.0	42.0 ± 5.0	52.0 ± 8.0	97.0 ± 10.0
Ca	105.0 ± 10.0	159.0 ± 15.0	160.0 ± 10.0	75.0 ± 9.0	195.0 ± 15.0	270.0 ± 20
Zn	3.7 + 0.3	3.4 + 0.3	2.5 ± 0.2	2.4 ± 0.2	0.9 ± 0.1	0.7 + 0.1
Mn	1.1 ± 0.1	1.8 ± 0.2	1.5 ± 0.1	0.9 ± 0.1	3.5 ± 0.2	43.8 ± 1.5
Cu	4.8 ± 0.2	0.7 ± 0.1	0.9 ± 0.1	0.9 ± 0.1	1.3 ± 0.1	0.8 ± 0.1
Fe	21.0 ± 1.1	25.5 ± 1.5	65.0 ± 2.5	25.8 ± 1.2	20.5 ± 0.5	36.0 ± 0.8

*Means ($n = 3$) ± SD.

Potassium, magnesium, calcium, zinc, manganese, copper, and iron were extracted with acids from 5 g samples according to McGrath and Cubliffe [26] and their concentrations were detected using a PE model 2380 atomic absorption spectrophotometer.

2.3. Fatty Acids Analysis. Oil samples extracted from 5 g seed samples were methylated with 14% boron trifluoride (BF_3, BDH-Company) in methanol [27]. Analysis of the fatty acids was carried out with a GLC-Varian 6000 gas chromatograph with Flame Ionization Detector (FID), 2 m length, 0.32 cm internal diameter stainless steel column, packed with 15% OV-275, chrome P/AW/80-100 mesh stationary phase which operated at 180°C, injection temperature 230°C, detector temperature 250°C with carrier-gas (Helium) at a flow rate of 25 mL/min, hydrogen flow 30 mL/min, and air flow 300 mL/min. Identification of the fatty acid methyl esters was carried out by comparison of their retention times with that of the standards (Polyscience Corporation, Kit number 61 CX) and the quantities were calculated from the area obtained by the LKB 2200 recorded integrator.

3. Statistical Analyses

The factorial experiment in the completely randomized design was done with three replicates. Then all data were statistically analyzed using analysis of variance.

4. Results and Discussion

Chemical composition of spices is given in Table 1. The results indicated that mustard, black cumin, and cress seeds had higher fat content of (38.45%), (31.95%), and (23.19%), respectively, as compared to clove (16.63%), black pepper (5.34%), and fenugreek (4.51%) seeds. It could be noticed that cress, mustard, black cumin, and black pepper had higher protein content that ranged from 20.61% to 25.45%, as compared to fenugreek (12.91%) and clove (6.9%). Crude fiber and ash contents ranged from 6.36 to 23.6% and from 3.57 to 7.1%, respectively. Table 1 shows the obtained results. Kochhar et al. [6] and El Nasri and El Tinay [7] reported that fat, protein, and fiber content of fenugreek seeds ranged from 6.53% to 7.1%, 24.4% to 25.8%, and 6.28% to 9.3%, respectively. On the other hand, Ildikó et al. [12] found that mustard seeds contain 28–32% fat and 28–36% proteins. Gokavi et al. [9], mentioned that cress seeds contain fat, protein and fiber of 27.5, 22.5, and 30%, respectively. It has also been reported that black cumin had 30–40% fat, 20–30% protein, 3.7–4.7% ash, while the protein and fat contents of black pepper ranged from 11–14 and 47–53%, respectively, as reported by Jayashree et al. [19]. Moreover, clove contains 20% fat, 5.98% protein, 34.2% fiber, and 5.88% ash [10].

The low percentage of moisture in cress and black cumin as compared to the others may increase the shelf life of these spices during packaging and storage. They also limit fungal and contamination effects. Data presented in Table 2 shows the mineral contents of the different seeds under investigation. It could be noticed that all seeds contains higher levels of potassium (ranged from 383 to 823 mg/100 g) followed by calcium (ranged from 75 to 270 mg/100 g), magnesium (ranged from 42 to 102 mg/100 g), and iron (ranged from 20.5 to 65 mg/100 g). However, zinc, manganese, and copper metals were found at lower levels. These results differed mainly in the amount of potassium, magnesium,

TABLE 3: Fatty acid (%) extracted from cress, mustard, black cumin, fenugreek, black pepper, and clove seeds*.

Fatty acid	Cress	Mustard	Black cumin	Fenugreek	Black pepper	Clove
$C_{14:0}$	1.55	—	1.0	1.38	—	1.29
$C_{16:0}$	5.86	3.2	10.5	3.85	3.15	6.21
$C_{16:1}$	2.02	—	—	8.29	11.91	20.96
$C_{18:0}$	6.56	1.18	2.04	1.78	—	—
$C_{18:1}$ (Cis)	15.35	18.32	16.23	8.29	16.17	13.0
$C_{18:1}$ (Trans)	4.05	—	—	10.76	9.89	6.20
$C_{18:2}$	11.79	23.57	68.07	34.85	33.03	44.73
$C_{18:3}$	48.43	23.92	2.16	30.8	10.34	2.93
$C_{20:0}$	2.79	—	—	—	15.51	4.68
$C_{20:2}$	1.60	—	—	—	—	—
$C_{22:1}$	—	29.81	—	—	—	—
TSF	16.76	4.38	13.54	7.01	18.66	12.18
TUSF	83.24	95.62	86.46	92.99	81.34	87.82

calcium and iron, as compared to previous results obtained by Nergiz and Otles [28], for black cumin and fenugreek seeds (El-Mahdy, and El-Sebaiy [29]). However, Gokavi et al. [9] found that cress seeds contain 1193 mg/100 g potassium. While, clove seeds contain high levels of potassium (1102 mg/100 g) and magnesium (268 mg/100 g) as reported by Milind and Deepa [24]. The differences in the results obtained and that reported in previous studies may be due to environmental factors that prevail in production areas, cultivars used to produce seeds and also due to the different methods used to prepare these local spices.

Fatty acids composition of cress, mustard, black cumin, fenugreek, black pepper, and clove seed oils are presented in Table 3. The major fatty acids in cress and mustard were lenolenic acid (48.43%) and erucic acid (29.81%), respectively. While, linoleic acid was the major fatty acid in black cumin, fenugreek, black pepper, and clove oils being 68.07%, 34.85%, 33.03%, and 44.73%, respectively. Total unsaturated fatty acids were 83.24, 95.62, 86.46, 92.99, 81.34, and 87.82% for cress, mustard, black cumin, fenugreek, black pepper, and clove, respectively. These results are in good agreement with most of the previous studies. Moser et al., [10] reported that oleic (30.60%) and linolenic (29.3%) acids were the major fatty acids in cress seed oil. However, erucic acid (30–40%) was the major fatty acid in mustard oil according to Ali and McKay [11] and Ildikó et al. [12]. Nergiz and Otles [28], Tulukcu [16], and Sultan et al. [30] demonstrated that the predominant fatty acid in black cumin, fenugreek, black pepper and clove seed oils was linoleic acid.

From the results of this study, it could be concluded that the spices and herbs under investigation contain appreciable amounts of nutrients which may serve as beneficial health sources if consumed regularly specially cress and fenugreek and can be used as food supplements for edible oils, besides its uses as a condiments in home. Spices and herbs are used at relatively low levels in foods, these data indicate that spices may provide a meaningful level of protein, fat, and minerals when consumed in a variety of foods. Also, these results were obtained with relatively different results of others and this requires further studies on the impact of soil and weather conditions on the composition of these crops.

Acknowledgments

The authors would like to thank King Abdulaziz City for Science and Technology and King Saud University for their support of this work and allowing them to use their equipment and laboratories.

References

[1] G. A. Petropoulos, *Fenugreek—The Genus Trigonella*, Taylor & Francis, London, UK, 2002.

[2] J. B. Lust, *The Herb Book*, Bantam, New York, NY, USA, 1986.

[3] M. Al-Habori and A. Raman, "Pharmacological Properties," in *Fenugreek—The Genus Trigonella*, G. A. Petropoulos, Ed., vol. 10, pp. 163–182, Taylor & Francis, London, UK, 1st edition, 2002.

[4] C. Gopalan, B. V. Ramshastri, and S. C. Balasubramanian, *Nutritive Value of Indian Foods*, National Institute of Nutrition, India, 1989, Revised and updated by B. S. Narsinga Rao, Y. G. Deoshale, K . C, Pant Hyderabad.

[5] L. Heller, "Fenugreek. A noteworthy hypoglycemic, Pacific College of oriental medicine," 2001, http://www.ormed.Edu/newsletters/fenugreek.html.

[6] A. Kochhar, M. Nagi, and R. Sachdeva, "Proximate composition available carbohydrates, dietary fiber and anti-nutritional factors of selected traditional medicinal plants," *Journal of Human Ecology*, vol. 19, pp. 195–199, 2006.

[7] N. A. El Nasri and A. H. El Tinay, "Functional properties of fenugreek (*Trigonella foenum graecum*) protein concentrate," *Food Chemistry*, vol. 103, no. 2, pp. 582–589, 2007.

[8] L. A. El-Sebaiy and A. R. El-Mahdy, "Lipid changes during germination of fenugreek seeds (*Trigonella foenum graecum*)," *Food Chemistry*, vol. 10, no. 4, pp. 309–319, 1983.

[9] S. S. Gokavi, N. G. Malleshi, and M. Guo, "Chemical composition of garden cress (*Lepidium sativum*) seeds and its fractions and use of bran as a functional ingredient," *Plant Foods for Human Nutrition*, vol. 59, no. 3, pp. 105–111, 2004.

[10] B. R. Moser, S. N. Shah, J. K. Winkler-Moser, S. F. Vaughn, and R. L. Evangelista, "Composition and physical properties

of cress (*Lepidium sativum* L.) and field pennycress (*Thlaspi arvense* L.) oils," *Industrial Crops and Products*, vol. 30, no. 2, pp. 199–205, 2009.

[11] A. Ali and J. E. McKay, "The chemical and physical characteristics and fatty acid composition of seed oils extracted from cruciferous species cultivated in Pakistan," *Food Chemistry*, vol. 8, no. 3, pp. 225–231, 1982.

[12] S.-G. Ildikó, K. A. Klára, T.-M. Marianna, B. Ágnes, M.-B. Zsuzsanna, and C. Bálint, "The effect of radio frequency heat treatment on nutritional and colloid-chemical properties of different white mustard (*Sinapis alba* L.) varieties," *Innovative Food Science and Emerging Technologies*, vol. 7, no. 1-2, pp. 74–79, 2006.

[13] S. Cheikh-Rouhou, S. Besbes, B. Hentati, C. Blecker, C. Deroanne, and H. Attia, "*Nigella sativa* L.: chemical composition and physicochemical characteristics of lipid fraction," *Food Chemistry*, vol. 101, no. 2, pp. 673–681, 2007.

[14] G. Kokdil, A. Dlcim, B. Ozbilgin, and C. Uygun, "Morphology and stem anatomy of some species of genus *Nigella* L. in Turkey," *Journal of Faculty of Pharmacy of Ankara*, vol. 35, no. 1, pp. 19–41, 2006.

[15] M. B. Atta, "Some characteristics of nigella (*Nigella sativa* L.) seed cultivated in Egypt and its lipid profile," *Food Chemistry*, vol. 83, no. 1, pp. 63–68, 2003.

[16] E. Tulukcu, "A comparative study on fatty acid composition of black cumin obtained from different regions of Turkey, Iran and Syria," *African Journal of Agricultural Research*, vol. 6, no. 4, pp. 892–895, 2011.

[17] I. A. Ajayi, R. A. Oderinde, D. O. Kajogbola, and J. I. Uponi, "Oil content and fatty acid composition of some underutilized legumes from Nigeria," *Food Chemistry*, vol. 99, no. 1, pp. 115–120, 2006.

[18] J. R. Piggot and Z. Othman, "Effect of irradiation on volatile oils of black pepper," *Food Chemistry*, vol. 46, no. 2, pp. 115–119, 1993.

[19] E. Jayashree, J. T. Zachariah, and P. Gobinath, "Physicochemical properties of black pepper from selected varieties in relation to market grades," *Journal of Food Science and Technology*, vol. 46, no. 3, pp. 263–265, 2009.

[20] V. S. Govindarajan, "Pepper chemistry, technology, and quality evaluation," *CRC Critical Reviews in Food Science and Nutrition*, vol. 9, no. 2, pp. 115–225, 1977.

[21] S. Tewtrakul, K. Hase, S. Kadota, T. Namba, K. Komatsu, and K. Tanaka, "Fruit oil composition of *Piper chaba* Hunt., *P. longum* L. and *P. nigrum* L.," *Journal of Essential Oil Research*, vol. 12, no. 5, pp. 603–608, 2000.

[22] A. C. Kimoro, M. Hasan, and H. Singh, "Extraction Of sarawak black pepper essential oil using supercritical carbon dioxide," *Arabian Journal for Science and Engineering*, vol. 35, no. 2, pp. 7–16, 2010.

[23] K. T. Farrell, *Spices, Condiments and Seasonings*, AVI, Westport, Conn, USA, 1985.

[24] P. Milind and K. Deepa, "Clove: a champion spice," *International Journal of Research in Ayurveda and Pharmacy*, vol. 2, no. 1, pp. 47–54, 2011.

[25] Association of Official Analytical Chemists, *Official Methods of Analysis*, Washington, DC, USA, 16th edition, 1995.

[26] S. P. McGrath and C. H. Cubliffe, "A simplified method for the extraction of metals Fe, Zn, Cu, Ni, Cd, Pb, Cr, Co and Mn from soils and sewage sludges," *Journal of the Science of Food and Agriculture*, vol. 36, pp. 794–798, 1985.

[27] T. A. Foglia, K. Petruso, and S. H. Feairheller, "Enzymatic interesterification of tallow-sunflower oil mixtures," *Journal of the American Oil Chemists' Society*, vol. 70, no. 3, pp. 281–285, 1993.

[28] C. Nergiz and S. Otles, "Chemical composition of *Nigella sativa* L. seeds," *Food Chemistry*, vol. 48, no. 3, pp. 259–261, 1993.

[29] A. R. El-Mahdy and L. A. El-Sebaiy, "Changes in phytate and minerals during germination and cooking of fenugreek seeds," *Food Chemistry*, vol. 9, no. 3, pp. 149–158, 1982.

[30] M. T. Sultan, M. S. Butt, F. M. Anjum, A. Jamil, S. Akhtar, and M. Nasir, "Nutritional profile of indigenous cultivar of black cumin seeds and antioxidant potential of its fixed and essential oil," *Pakistan Journal of Botany*, vol. 41, no. 3, pp. 1321–1330, 2009.

14

Bedside Calculation of Energy Expenditure Does Not Guarantee Adequate Caloric Prescription in Long-Term Mechanically Ventilated Critically Ill Patients: A Quality Control Study

Elisabeth De Waele,[1] Herbert Spapen,[1] P. M. Honoré,[1] Sabrina Mattens,[2] Thomas Rose,[1] and Luc Huyghens[1]

[1] *Department of Intensive Care Medicine, University Hospital, Vrije Universiteit Brussel, Laarbeeklaan 101, 1090 Brussels, Belgium*
[2] *Department of Dietetics, University Hospital, Vrije Universiteit Brussel, 1090 Brussels, Belgium*

Correspondence should be addressed to Elisabeth De Waele, elisabeth.dewaele@uzbrussel.be

Academic Editors: F. Catena, Y.-C. Huang, and C. Weissman

Nutrition is essential in critically ill patients, but translating caloric prescriptions into adequate caloric intake remains challenging. Caloric prescriptions (P), effective intake (I), and caloric needs (N), calculated with modified Harris-Benedict formulas, were recorded during seven consecutive days in ventilated patients. Adequacy of prescription was estimated by P/N ratio. I/P ratio assessed accuracy of translating a prescription into administered feeding. I/N ratio compared delivered calories with theoretical caloric needs. Fifty patients were prospectively studied in a mixed medicosurgical ICU in a teaching hospital. Basal and total energy expenditure were, respectively, 1361 ± 171 kcal/d and 1649 ± 233 kcal/d. P and I attained 1536 ± 602 kcal/d and 1424 ± 572 kcal/d, respectively. 24.6% prescriptions were accurate, and 24.3% calories were correctly administered. Excessive calories were prescribed in 35.4% of patients, 27.4% being overfed. Caloric needs were underestimated in 40% prescriptions, with 48.3% patients underfed. Calculating caloric requirements by a modified standard formula covered energy needs in only 25% of long-term mechanically ventilated patients, leaving many over- or underfed. Nutritional imbalance mainly resulted from incorrect prescription. Failure of "simple" calculations to direct caloric prescription in these patients suggests systematic use of more reliable methods, for example, indirect calorimetry.

1. Background

Delivering a correct amount of calories to critically ill patients is considered to be of cardinal importance [1, 2]. Indeed, inadequate nutrition (i.e., under- or overfeeding) in this population has distinct effects on immuno-inflammatory pathways, is associated with increased morbidity, and may impair survival [3, 4]. Underfeeding disturbs the regeneration of respiratory epithelium and causes respiratory muscle dysfunction [5] which may prolong ventilator dependence [6]. Even when present subclinically, it is responsible for reduced superficial and deep wound healing [7]. Also, failure to provide more than 25% of recommended calories significantly increases the risk of bloodstream infection [8]. In contrast, overfeeding is more likely to cause metabolic disturbances (hypertriglyceridemia, hyperglycemia, and azotemia) but may also be at the origin of organ (hepatic, respiratory) dysfunction [9, 10].

Still, discrepancies between theoretical energy requirements and actual delivery of nutrition in intensive care unit (ICU) patients are more rule than exception [10, 11]. Moreover, studies evaluating whether quality of nutrition matches current ICU feeding guidelines remain scarce, particularly in specific patients such as those receiving prolonged mechanical ventilation [12].

We therefore prospectively studied whether feeding prescriptions were translated into adequate caloric intake within the scope of a "real-life," guideline-oriented nutritional approach in a population of mechanically ventilated critically ill patients.

2. Methods

The study was approved by the hospital's Ethical Committee. Due to its observational nature, the need for informed consent was waived.

During a 4-month period, we included all patients older than 18 years admitted to our medicosurgical ICU when intubated and expected to receive mechanical ventilation for at least seven days. Patients were ventilated in pressure- or volume-controlled modes under continuous analgesic sedation with remifentanil and midazolam. Whenever possible, intravenous dextrose infusions were avoided. Insulin was infused to maintain a target blood glucose level of 80–110 mg/dL. All subjects received enteral and/or parenteral feeding, as part of their standard treatment. Feeding was provided according to a dedicated nutritional care plan. The used protocol closely reflected current evidence-based, easy-to-use feeding algorithms indicating amount, composition and route of delivery.

Gender, age, weight, height, and type of pathology were recorded at study entry. For obese patients, optimal caloric intake was calculated for a theoretical weight corresponding to a body mass index of 30 kg/m^2 [13]. Total caloric need (N, kcal/d) was assessed by multiplying basal energy expenditure, calculated with a modified Harris-Benedict equation as follows: male: resting energy expenditure (REE) (kcal/d) = 66.47 + 13.75 (wt) + 5.003 (ht) − 6.755 (a) (years); female: REE (kcal/d) = 655.1 + 9.563 (wt) + 1.850 (ht) − 4.676 (a) (years), where wt denotes weight, ht represents height and a refers to age [14], which was, daily adjusted for weight and stress. For uncomplicated and complicated surgery, a stress factor of, respectively, 1.1 and 1.3 was used. Fractures and polytrauma were given, respectively, 1.1 and 1.3. Patients with an uncomplicated infection received a correction factor of 1.1, but sepsis was attributed 1.3.

Attending ICU physicians, unaware of the study, based their daily caloric prescriptions on the expert-recommended 25 kcal/kg/d regimen [15]. For seven consecutive days, prescriptions (P, kcal/d) and effective intake (I, kcal/d) were recorded. A dedicated nutrition team measured caloric requirements with the "stress-adapted" Harris-Benedict formulas and estimated correctness of the prescription by calculating the P/N ratio. The accuracy of translating a prescription into really administered feeding was assessed by the I/P ratio. Finally, the I/N ratio was calculated to compare the amount of delivered calories with the theoretical caloric need. The latter was set at 100%, and both prescriptions and actual feeding were expressed as proportional to this percentage. A prescription was considered to be adequate when it covered 90 to 110% of total caloric need. Prescriptions not attaining 90% were considered to be "underestimated" whilst those exceeding 110% were said to be "overestimated."

Statistical analysis used SPSS 12.0 for Windows (Chicago, IL, USA). Results were expressed as means ± standard deviation and medians (range). Means between groups were compared with the Student's t-test. Statistical significance was accepted at a P value < 0.05.

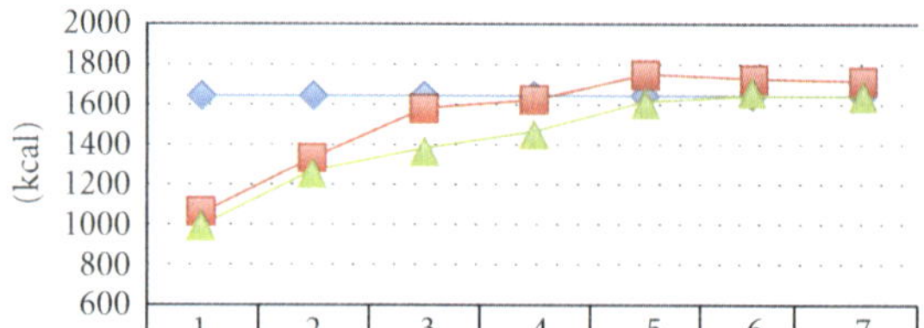

	1	2	3	4	5	6	7
Need	1649	1649	1649	1649	1649	1649	1649
Prescription	1065	1331	1579	1622	1747	1721	1719
Intake	992	1251	1369	1452	1609	1632	1636

(Day)

FIGURE 1: Evolution in time of caloric need, prescription and intake over the study period.

3. Results

579 patients were admitted to the ICU during the study period. 231 subjects were mechanically ventilated. Of the 81 patients meeting enrolment criteria, thirty-one were excluded from analysis. Reasons for exclusion were extubation before day 7 (n = 14), tracheostomy (n = 6), do-not-resuscitate order given (n = 3), and death (n = 8). Finally, fifty patients, 28 males and 22 females, representing a total of 350 nutrition days, were studied. Mean age was 65 (range 34–84) years. Mean body weight and length were, respectively, 76.9 ± 18.3 kg and 169.6 ± 9.7 cm. Twelve patients were obese. Mean APACHE II score was 28 ± 12. Mean resting energy expenditure for all studied patients was 1361 ± 171 kcal/d. Thirteen patients were allocated a stress factor 1.1, 18 patients received 1.2, and 19 subjects were assigned a factor 1.3. This resulted in a mean total energy expenditure of 1649 ± 233 kcal/d.

The mean daily amount of calories prescribed during the 350 study days reached 1536 ± 602 kcal. In average, 1424 ± 572 kcal/d were actually delivered to the patient. P and I varied with time (Figure 1). During the study period, median P/N ratio was 0.97 (range 0.0–1.80), mean I/N ratio 0.91 (range 0.0–1.84), and mean I/P ratio, or delivery rate, 0.95 (range 0.08–7.20).

24.6% of the 350 nutritional prescriptions correctly estimated the need. In 40.0% of cases, nutritional needs were insufficiently covered. Overestimation occurred in the remaining 35.4%.

Using similar cutoff percentages to evaluate effective feeding, patients were, respectively, correctly, over-, or underfed in 24.3%, 27.4%, and 48.3% of the nutrition days. Underfeeding was more frequent on the first as compared to the next 6 ventilation days (Figure 2). In fact, either no nutritional prescription was found in the medical records or feeding was started without a formal prescription.

The amount of effectively administered calories varied with time. Caloric prescription resulted in accurate delivery in 56.0% of cases. However, effective feeding was not met in 32.6% of prescriptions, and in 9.14% actual feeding surpassed the prescribed amount by more than 10%.

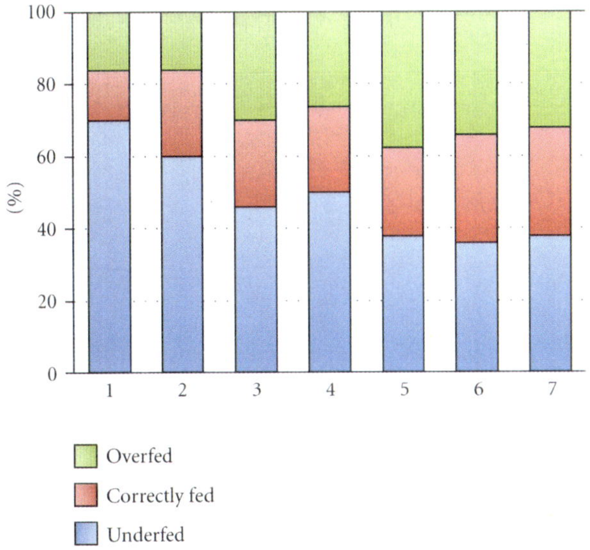

FIGURE 2: Feeding status per day.

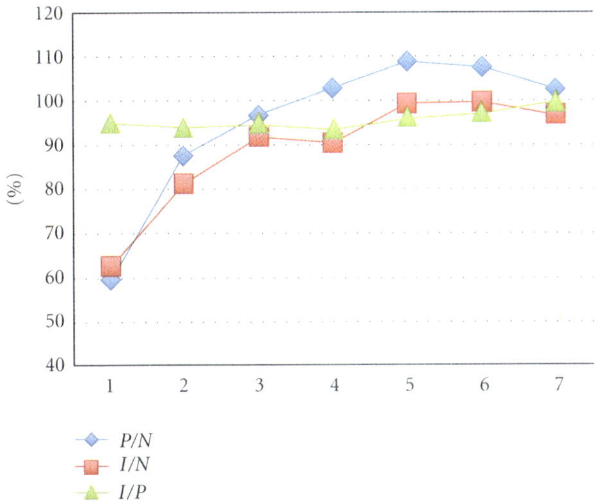

FIGURE 3: Evolution in time of median P/N, I/N, and I/P ratio.

Mean P/N ratio rose from 59.3 on day 1 to 102.7 on day 7, whilst the median I/N ratio increased from 62.6 to 97 during the same period. Thus, both estimation of needs and actually administered feeding improved with time. The delivery rate did not vary significantly during the observation period (Figure 3).

4. Discussion

Nutrition is an indispensable part of overall treatment in critically ill patients. Fundamental goals of nutritional support in the ICU are to meet energy requirements of (hyper)metabolic processes, to prevent nutrient deficiencies and to minimize protein catabolism. Whilst inadequate nutrition, in general, is known to significantly compromise outcome in the critically ill, its unwarranted effects may be even more pronounced in mechanically ventilated patients. Indeed, animals submitted to fasting or receiving long-term hypocaloric feeding in both aerobe and anaerobe conditions experienced muscle decay and dysfunction which incompletely recovered after realimentation [16, 17]. It is conceivable that these findings may translate into enhanced and/or prolonged respiratory failure and thus longer ventilator-dependency in humans.

Throughout the literature, most discussion regarding nutrition in mechanically ventilated patients is focused on type, composition, and caloric/nitrogen content of available feeding liquids. However, evaluating adequate, that is, correct and effective, feeding in this population remains challenging. The present study confirms that energetic requirements in critically ill, mechanically ventilated patients differ considerably in accordance to the severity of the underlying pathology. In general, energetic needs were well anticipated by the attending physicians, yet variations were large. 25% of the caloric prescriptions were correct, but a stunning 75% resulted in under- or overfeeding. Effective administration of calories followed the same trend as the prescription. However, energetic requirements were met in only 24% of the feeding days. The discrepancy between caloric prescription and intake caused underfeeding in nearly half and overfeeding in 27% of the study days. Our findings also highlighted that nutritional prescription was fairly well translated into effective feeding in the majority of patients but that extreme variations in intake/prescription ratio (up to 720% !) could occur. A possible explanation is that oral nutrition orders were executed without being recorded in the patient's files. Our results, demonstrating (a) > 90% I/P and P/N ratio after 72 hours, are in agreement and even better than those reported recently by Quenot et al. [18]. However, these authors only studied enteral nutrition aiming at a minimal caloric supply of 25 kcal/kg/day and did not calculate stress-adjusted energy requirements. Interestingly, they found that the I/P ratio was significantly influenced by gastric residual volume measurement [18].

Thirty years ago, Driver and LeBrun described iatrogenic malnutrition in more than 80% of mechanically ventilated patients [19]. Although nutrition policy in the ICU has considerably improved since, de Jonghe et al. recently reported that energetic needs still remained inadequately covered in more than 20% of ICU patients [11]. McClave et al. reported correct estimation of energetic needs in 29%, overestimation in 58%, and underestimation in 12% of cases. Fifty-eight percent of the patients were overfed, and 39% received too much calories. Correct feeding was provided in 25% of nutrition days which corresponds very well with the 24% incidence observed in our study [10]. Kan et al. reported adequate feeding in 37% and overfeeding in 35% critically ill ventilated patients [6], which also matches our results. Interestingly, physicians in our ICU tended to prescribe fewer calories than needed whereas in the above-mentioned studies caloric needs were generally overestimated, resulting in overfeeding. Traditionally, it is accepted that overfeeding produces higher CO_2 blood levels resulting in increased minute ventilation [20]. Nonetheless, McClave et al. found an inverse relationship between the amount of nutrition and minute ventilation in mechanically ventilated subjects.

However, this study is different from ours since patients were given only enteral feeding [10].

Nutritional care of critically ill patients is complicated. Patients form heterogeneous groups that are prone to significant and continuous metabolic fluctuations induced by type, severity, and evolution of the disease process. In addition, confounding variables such as over- or underweight, resuscitation edema, and concomitant medication (e.g., sedation) may all hamper correct estimation of metabolic demands [21, 22]. Indirect calorimetry definitely is the gold standard for determination of resting energy expenditure, but, when not available, specific prediction equations have up to now been widely accepted as an alternative [15]. To account for levels of disease or injury severity and complications, the so-called stress factors have been introduced. These corrective factors were obtained by comparing direct calorimetry measurements between hospitalized patients and healthy volunteers and are, by definition, arbitrary in the critically ill. Of note is that specific correction factors for ventilated patients are scarce. Casati et al. multiplied basal energy expenditure by 1.20, 1.28, or 1.50 in, respectively, nonsurgical/nonseptic conditions, complicated surgery, and severe infection/multiple trauma [23]. Cheng et al. applied a stress factor of 1.25 in all mechanically ventilated patients [14]. Kan et al. reported that at least 120% of resting energy requirement had to be administered to meet caloric needs in ventilated patients [6]. We used a modified Harris-Benedict equation attempting to anticipate on daily stress and injury events in a particular patient. Though considered to be an unreliable predictor of caloric needs in critically ill patients [24, 25], the Harris-Benedict formula proved to be relatively accurate in this population when a factor of 1.1 was multiplied to the equation [26]. Moreover, in a cohort of mechanically ventilated ICU patients, a modified Harris-Benedict equation (i.e., multiplied by a factor 1.2 and incorporating actual body weight) was found to be within 15% of measured energy expenditure determined by indirect calorimetry [27].

Our study has several shortcomings. First, calculations of caloric intake did not account for caloric content of eventually administered dextrose-containing infusions. Second, caloric requirements ideally should be measured by indirect calorimetry. Feeding near-target energy requirements based on repeated calorimetric measurements was associated with lower hospital mortality [28]. However, indirect calorimetry is not widely available or affordable. It is time consuming, requires dedicated equipment and staff, and only reflects the short-time window during which the patient is studied. Some guidelines for nutrition support in mechanically ventilated, critically ill adult patients do not even recommend its use [29]. Our approach using "corrected" Harris-Benedict equations to calculate energy requirements was motivated by the wide acceptance of this easy method for bedside assessment of nutritional therapy in ICU patients and is supported by the ESPEN guidelines on parenteral nutrition in an ICU setting [30]. Third, we did not assess outcome in our patients. Major reasons are the small study sample and the lack of correction for baseline differences in severity of disease. Moreover, the feeding protocol used in this study does not allow coping with the recently roused controversy regarding parenteral nutrition and outcome [31, 32]. Finally, the observational nature of our study obviously has inherent limitations though not altering the key message that basic directives obtained in well-controlled research settings do not easily translate in providing "quality" nutrition in daily ICU practice.

5. Conclusion

This prospective quality control study demonstrated an important dissimilarity between the amount of calories prescribed according to current nutritional guidelines and the caloric need calculated by a stress-corrected Harris-Benedict equation in critically ill mechanically ventilated patients. This was due to inadequate prescription and, to a lesser degree, to inappropriate conversion of correct prescriptions into "true" feeding. Repeated evaluation of caloric needs and administration using best evidence measurement tools and continuous feedback to all involved health care workers are critical issues for providing optimal nutritional care in these patients. In this context, a dedicated nutrition support team may play an important role [33]. Our observations add support to a more systematic use of indirect calorimetry in long-term mechanically ventilated patients.

Abbreviations

P: Prescriptions
I: Intake (effective)
N: Needs (caloric)
ICU: Intensive care unit.

Conflict of Interests

The authors hereby declare that the paper is original, is not under consideration for publication anywhere else, and has not been previously published. Moreover, the authors declare no potential or actual personal, political, or financial interest in the material, information, or techniques described in the paper.

Authors' Contribution

E. De Waele and H. Spapen designed the study' paper EDW executed the study, analysed the data, and drafted the paper. S. Mattens assisted with data collection. H. Spapen, P. M. Honoré and T. Rose cowrote the paper. L. Huyghens was responsible for the provision of practical support. All authors have read and approved the final manuscript. The authors declare no conflict of interest.

Acknowledgments

The authors would like to thank Dr. Boudewijn De Waele for his practical and mental support.

References

[1] P. Jolliet, C. Pichard, G. Biolo et al., "Enteral nutrition in intensive care patients: a practical approach," *Intensive Care Medicine*, vol. 24, no. 8, pp. 848–859, 1998.

[2] American Society for Parenteral and Enteral Nutrition, "Guidelines for the use of parenteral and enteral nutrition in adults and pediatric patients," *Journal of Parenteral and Enteral Nutrition*, vol. 17, no. 4, pp. 20SA–21SA, 1993.

[3] L. S. Harbige, "Nutrition and immunity with emphasis on infection and autoimmune disease," *Nutrition and Health*, vol. 10, no. 4, pp. 285–312, 1996.

[4] R. J. M. Strack van Schijndel, P. J. M. Weijs, R. H. Koopmans, H. P. Sauerwein, A. Beishuizen, and A. R. J. Girbes, "Optimal nutrition during the period of mechanical ventilation decreases mortality in critically ill, long-term acute female patients: a prospective observational cohort study," *Critical Care*, vol. 13, no. 4, article R132, 2009.

[5] J. Askanazi, C. Weissman, S. H. Rosenbaum, A. I. Hyman, J. Milic-Emili, and J. M. Kinney, "Nutrition and the respiratory system," *Critical Care Medicine*, vol. 10, no. 3, pp. 163–172, 1982.

[6] M. N. Kan, H. H. Chang, W. F. Sheu, C. H. Cheng, B. J. Lee, and Y. C. Huang, "Estimation of energy requirements for mechanically ventilated, critically ill patients using nutritional status," *Critical Care*, vol. 7, pp. R108–R115, 2003.

[7] H. Silberman, *Parenteral and Enteral Nutrition*, East Norwalk Connecticut, Appleton & Lange, 1989.

[8] L. Rubinson, G. B. Diette, X. Song, R. G. Brower, and J. A. Krishnan, "Low caloric intake is associated with nosocomial bloodstream infections in patients in the medical intensive care unit," *Critical Care Medicine*, vol. 32, no. 2, pp. 350–357, 2004.

[9] C. J. Klein, G. S. Stanek, and C. E. Wiles III, "Overfeeding macronutrients to critically ill adults: metabolic complications," *Journal of the American Dietetic Association*, vol. 98, no. 7, pp. 795–806, 1998.

[10] S. A. McClave, C. C. Lowen, M. J. Kleber et al., "Are patients fed appropriately according to their caloric requirements?" *Journal of Parenteral and Enteral Nutrition*, vol. 22, no. 6, pp. 375–381, 1998.

[11] B. de Jonghe, C. Appere-De-Vechi, M. Fournier et al., "A prospective survey of nutritional support practices in intensive care unit patients: what is prescribed? What is delivered?" *Critical Care Medicine*, vol. 29, no. 1, pp. 8–12, 2001.

[12] A. Frutiger, R. Moreno, L. Thijs, and J. Carlet, "A clinician's guide to the use of quality terminology," *Intensive Care Medicine*, vol. 24, no. 8, pp. 860–863, 1998.

[13] N. Barak, E. Wall-Alonso, and M. D. Sitrin, "Evaluation of stress factors and body weight adjustments currently used to estimate energy expenditure in hospitalized patients," *Journal of Parenteral and Enteral Nutrition*, vol. 26, no. 4, pp. 231–238, 2002.

[14] C. H. Cheng, C. H. Chen, Y. Wong, B. J. Lee, M. N. Kan, and Y. C. Huang, "Measured versus estimated energy expenditure in mechanically ventilated critically ill patients," *Clinical Nutrition*, vol. 21, no. 2, pp. 165–172, 2002.

[15] K. G. Kreymann, M. M. Berger, N. E.P. Deutz et al., "ESPEN guidelines on enteral nutrition: intensive care," *Clinical Nutrition*, vol. 25, no. 2, pp. 210–223, 2006.

[16] M. L. Nishio and K. N. Jeejeebhoy, "Effect of malnutrition on aerobic and anaerobic performance of fast- and slow-twitch muscles of rats," *Journal of Parenteral and Enteral Nutrition*, vol. 16, no. 3, pp. 219–225, 1992.

[17] A. M. de la Torre, A. Madapallimattam, A. Cross, R. L. Armstrong, and K. N. Jeejeebhoy, "Effect of fasting, hypocaloric feeding, and refeeding on the energetics of stimulated rat muscle as assessed by nuclear magnetic resonance spectroscopy," *Journal of Clinical Investigation*, vol. 92, no. 1, pp. 114–121, 1993.

[18] J. P. Quenot, G. Plantefeve, J. L. Baudel et al., "Bedside adherence to clinical practice guidelines for enteral nutrition in critically ill patients receiving mechanical ventilation: a prospective, multi-centre, observational study," *Critical Care*, vol. 14, no. 2, article R37, 2010.

[19] A. G. Driver and M. LeBrun, "Iatrogenic malnutrition in patients receiving ventilatory support," *Journal of the American Medical Association*, vol. 244, no. 19, pp. 2195–2196, 1980.

[20] P. C. Amene, R. N. Sladen, T. W. Feeley, and R. Fisher, "Hypercapnia during total parenteral nutrition with hypertonic dextrose," *Critical Care Medicine*, vol. 15, no. 2, pp. 171–172, 1987.

[21] C. Weissman, M. Kemper, and J. Askanazi, "Resting metabolic rate of the critically ill patient: measured versus predicted," *Anesthesiology*, vol. 64, no. 6, pp. 673–679, 1986.

[22] C. Weissman, M. Kemper, and D. H. Elwyn, "The energy expenditure of the mechanically ventilated critically ill patient: an analysis," *Chest*, vol. 89, no. 2, pp. 254–259, 1986.

[23] A. Casati, S. Colombo, C. Leggieri, S. Muttini, T. Capocasa, and G. Gallioli, "Measured versus calculated energy expenditure in pressure support ventilated ICU patients," *Minerva Anestesiologica*, vol. 62, no. 5, pp. 165–170, 1996.

[24] R. N. Walker and R. A. Heuberger, "Predictive equations for energy needs for the critically ill," *Respiratory Care*, vol. 54, no. 4, pp. 509–521, 2009.

[25] D. Frankenfield, M. Hise, A. Malone, M. Russell, E. Gradwell, and C. Compher, "Prediction of resting metabolic rate in critically Ill adult patients: results of a systematic review of the evidence," *Journal of the American Dietetic Association*, vol. 107, no. 9, pp. 1552–1561, 2007.

[26] J. Boullata, J. Williams, F. Cottrell, L. Hudson, and C. Compher, "Accurate determination of energy needs in hospitalized patients," *Journal of the American Dietetic Association*, vol. 107, no. 3, pp. 393–401, 2007.

[27] E. Alexander, G. M. Susla, A. H. Burstein, D. T. Brown, and F. P. Ognibene, "Retrospective evaluation of commonly used equations to predict energy expenditure in mechanically ventilated, critically ill patients," *Pharmacotherapy*, vol. 24, no. 12, pp. 1659–1667, 2004.

[28] P. Singer, R. Anbar, J. Cohen et al., "The tight calorie control study (TICACOS): a prospective, randomized, controlled pilot study of nutritional support in critically ill patients," *Intensive Care Medicine*, vol. 37, no. 4, pp. 601–609, 2011.

[29] D. K. Heyland, R. Dhaliwal, J. W. Drover, L. Gramlich, and P. Dodek, "Canadian clinical practice guidelines for nutrition support in mechanically ventilated, critically ill adult patients," *Journal of Parenteral and Enteral Nutrition*, vol. 27, no. 5, pp. 355–373, 2003.

[30] P. Singer, M. M. Berger, G. van den Berghe et al., "ESPEN guidelines on parenteral nutrition: intensive care," *Clinical Nutrition*, vol. 28, no. 4, pp. 387–400, 2009.

[31] J. Kutsogiannis, C. Alberda, L. Gramlich et al., "Early use of supplemental parenteral nutrition in critically ill patients: results of an international multicenter observational study," *Critical Care Medicine*, vol. 39, no. 12, pp. 2691–2699, 2011.

[32] M. P. Casaer, D. Mesotten, G. Hermans et al., "Early versus late parenteral nutrition in critically ill adults," *The New England Journal of Medicine*, vol. 365, no. 6, pp. 506–517, 2011.
[33] P. Frost and D. Bihari, "The route of nutritional support in the critically Ill: physiological and economical considerations," *Nutrition*, vol. 13, no. 9, supplement, pp. S58–S63, 1997.

15

Effect of Polyunsaturated Fatty Acids on Homocysteine Metabolism through Regulating the Gene Expressions Involved in Methionine Metabolism

Tao Huang,[1,2,3] Xiaojie Hu,[1,2] Nicholas Khan,[3] Jing Yang,[1,2] and Duo Li[1,2]

[1] *Department of Food Science and Nutrition, Zhejiang University, 866 Yu-Hang-Tang Road, Hangzhou 310059, China*
[2] *APCNS Centre of Nutrition and Food Safety, Hangzhou, China*
[3] *Department of International Health, Johns Hopkins Bloomberg School of Public Health, Baltimore, MD 21205, USA*

Correspondence should be addressed to Duo Li; duoli@zju.edu.cn

Academic Editors: Y.-C. Huang and N. Parletta

The objective was to investigate the regulatory effect of polyunsaturated fatty acids (PUFAs) on mRNA expression of key genes involved in homocysteine (Hcy) metabolism. Eighty male Sprague Dawley rats were randomly divided into eight groups. The oils were orally administered daily for 8 weeks. Plasma Hcy, phospholipids fatty acids, and mRNA expression were determined. Compared with the control group, plasma Hcy was significantly decreased in the 22:6*n*-3 and conjugated linoleic acid (CLA) groups; mRNA expression of *Mthfr* was significantly upregulated in the 22:6*n*-3, 20:5*n*-3, and 18:3*n*-3 groups and downregulated in the 18:2*n*-6 and stearolic acid (SO) groups. *Mat1a* was upregulated in the 22:6*n*-3, 20:5*n*-3, 18:3*n*-3, and CLA groups. In addition, *Cbs* was upregulated in the 22:6*n*-3, 20:5*n*-3, 18:3*n*-3 and CLA groups while downregulated in 18:2*n*-6 and SO groups. Dietary 22:6*n*-3 and CLA decrease the plasma concentration of Hcy. mRNA expression of *Mthfr, Mat1a, Cbs* and *Pemt, Gnmt, Mtrr,* and *Bad* is upregulated by *n*-3 PUFA and downregulated by *n*-6 PUFA. CLA upregulates mRNA expression of *Mat1a* and *Cbs*.

1. Introduction

Homocysteine (Hcy) is a sulfur-containing amino acid and a by-product of methionine metabolism [1]. Elevated plasma Hcy has been implicated as an independent risk factor for cardiovascular disease (CVD) [2].

Intracellular Hcy can be irreversibly degraded to cysteine through the transsulfuration pathway, a process primarily found in cells of the liver and kidneys. Two enzymes in this pathway, cystathionine b-synthase (CBS) and cystathionine gamma-lyase (CSE), are dependent on pyridoxal-5-phosphate, a biologically active form of vitamin B_6, as a cofactor. Hcy can also be remethylated to methionine by the enzyme methionine synthase (MS). This enzyme uses methylcobalamin, a biologically active form of vitamin B_{12}, as a cofactor. The methyl group for the latter reaction is donated by 5-methyl-tetrahydrofolate (5-methyl-THF). This form of folate is produced by the enzyme 5,10-methylenetetrahydrofolate reductase (MTHFR), which in turn uses flavin adenine dinucleotide, a biologically active form of vitamin B_2, as a cofactor. In most cases, disturbances in intracellular Hcy metabolism leads to elevated Hcy concentrations. Genetically determined functional deficiencies in enzymes integral to Hcy metabolism, like CBS, have a significant impact on Hcy concentration.

Numerous studies have investigated the effects of environmental factors on plasma Hcy metabolism since McCully hypothesized that elevated Hcy in blood was a risk factor for atherosclerosis [3]; some recent systematic reviews have described the impact of lifestyle and dietary factors on levels of plasma Hcy [1, 4]. Dietary intake of fish oil rich in *n*-3 polyunsaturated fatty acid (PUFA) leads to increased levels of *n*-3 PUFA in tissues [5, 6], which is associated with a protective effect on the cardiovascular system. We have previously demonstrated that increased total *n*-3 PUFA and

n-3/n-6 PUFA in platelet phospholipids (PL) is associated with decreased plasma Hcy [7, 8]. One study demonstrated that n-3 PUFA supplementation decreases plasma Hcy in diabetic dyslipidemia treated with a statin-fibrate combination [9]. Further, plasma Hcy concentration is significantly decreased in acute myocardial infarction patients after one year of n-3 PUFA treatment [10]. Based on the previous inconsistent results from the intervention studies, our meta-analysis demonstrated that high consumption of n-3 PUFA decreases plasma Hcy concentration [11].

Our animal study suggested that 22:6n-3 decreases plasma Hcy concentration through regulating critical gene expression and enzyme activity [12]. Our population studies found that dietary fatty acids interact with methylenetetrahydrofolate reductase (*MTHFR*) and methionine adenosyltransferase I, alpha (*MAT1A*) genetic variants in determining plasma Hcy concentration [13, 14]. Recently an intervention study also demonstrated that consumption of n-3 PUFA supplements (3 g/day) for 2 months decreases the levels of Hcy in those with type 2 diabetes mellitus [15].

However, the mechanism by which n-3 PUFA and plasma Hcy levels are associated is not yet fully understood. Therefore, to explore the potential mechanisms by which PUFA might regulate Hcy metabolism, we conducted an animal study to investigate the regulatory effects of different PUFA-rich oils on the mRNA expression of key genes involved in Hcy metabolism.

2. Materials and Methods

2.1. Animal Study Design. All procedures were approved by the Ethics Committee of the College of Biosystems Engineering & Food Science at Zhejiang University. Eighty male Sprague Dawley (SD) rats aged 3 weeks, weighing 120 ± 10 g, were purchased from the Zhejiang Laboratory Animal Center (Hangzhou, China). The rats were housed in a room under a 12/12 h light/dark cycle at 22°C. Two weeks later, the rats were randomly divided into eight groups of 10 rats (n-10 each group) and were fed a regular diet supplemented with different oils: a control group with no oil supplements (CC); an olive oil group (18:1) fed olive oil (0.5 mL); a tuna oil group (22:6n-3) fed a mix of oils (tuna oil 100 mg/kg BW + olive oil = 0.5 mL); a salmon oil group (20:5n-3) fed a mix of oils (salmon oil 100 mg/kg BW + olive oil = 0.5 mL); a group fed linseed oil (18:3n-3) (linseed oil 100 mg/kg BW + olive oil = 0.5 mL); a group fed corn oil (18:2n-6) (corn oil 100 mg/kg BW + olive oil = 0.5 mL); a group fed conjugated linoleic acid (CLA) oil (conjugated linoleic acid oil 100 mg/kg BW + olive oil = 0.5 mL); a group fed stearolic acid (SO) (stearolic acid oil 100 mg/kg BW + olive oil = 0.5 mL).

All rats were allowed free access to water and regular diet. The oil was orally administered using a stomach tube every day. The rats were killed at eight weeks, and blood (5 mL) was drawn from the abdominal vein. The liver and lungs were rapidly removed, weighed, frozen in liquid nitrogen, and stored at −70°C.

2.2. Plasma Measurements. The blood was centrifuged at 2000 rpm for 15 minutes, and the plasma was collected. Total plasma Hcy was determined by polarized fluorescence immunoassay in an AXSYM system [16]. Plasma folate and vitamin B_{12} were measured using immulite chemiluminescent kits according to the manufacturer's instructions (Diagnostic Products Corporation/Siemens, Los Angeles, CA).

2.3. Assay of Phospholipids n-3 PUFA in Tissues. Total lipid content of plasma was extracted with solvents, the PL fraction was separated by thin lay chromatography (TLC), and the fatty acid methyl esters were prepared and separated by gas-liquid chromatography as previously described [17].

2.4. Assay of mRNA Expression of Critical Genes Involved in Methionine Metabolism

2.4.1. Quantitative Real Time PCR Measurements. Total RNA from the livers was extracted using the Trizol reagent (Shingene, Shanghai, China). The first strand cDNA was synthesized using cDNA synthesis kit (Shinegene, Shanghai, China), the Real Time PCR were conducted on iCycler PCR using the HotStart DNA Master SYBR Green I kit (Takara, Dalian, China) [18]. Primers used are listed in Table 1. All PCR tests were carried out in duplicate with a final volume of 20 μL containing cDNA. Thermal cycling conditions were set as follows: an initial DNA denaturation step at 95°C for 5 seconds, followed by 40 cycles of denaturation at 95°C for 5 seconds, primer annealing at optimal temperature for 20 s, extension at 72°C for 30 s, and an additional incubation step at 80–85°C for 30 s to measure SYBR Green I fluorescence. Finally, melt curve analysis was performed by slowly cooling the PCR from 95 to 60°C (0.5°C per cycle) with simultaneous measurement of the SYBR Green I signal intensity. Gene expression was quantified using the comparative C(t) method [18].

2.5. Statistical Analysis. The data analyses were performed using an SPSS version 12 (SPSS Inc., Chicago, IL, USA) software program. All data are expressed as mean ± SD. Statistical analysis was performed using one-way ANOVA; differences between treatments were considered to be statistically significant at $P < 0.05$.

3. Results

3.1. The Effects of Oils on Plasma Phospholipids Fatty Acids Composition in Rats. After 8 weeks of treatment, plasma PL 22:6n-3, 20:5n-3, CLA, 18:2n-6, and 18:3n-3 were significantly increased in groups supplemented with 22:6n-3, 20:5n-3, CLA, 18:2n-6, and 18:3n-3 oils, respectively (Table 2).

3.2. The Effects of Oils on Plasma Biochemical Measurements in Rats. Plasma glucose and uric acid were significantly decreased, while total protein was significantly increased in the 22:6n-3 group. Plasma low-density lipoprotein (LDL), total cholesterol (TC), glucose, and aspartate aminotransferase (AST) were significantly decreased in the 20:5n-3 group.

Table 1: The primers used in real time PCR.

GenBank Acc.	Symbol	Primer	
NM_030850.1	*Bhmt*	F: TGCGCAGTGCGTTTGGTAA	R: AGGGCGTGGCTCATCAAGTAAG
NM_019179.1	*Tyms*	F: AAGAATCATCATGTGTGCCTGGAA	R: TCCTGACCGCTGGTAAAGCTG
NM_017201.1	*Sahh*	F: TGTGGACCCACCCAGACAAATA	R: CAGCTTGGTCAGCTTGACGTTC
NM_017127.1	*Chka*	F: GGACCAGTTCCACATCAGTGTCA	R: GAGGTTCATCACCAACACTGGCTA
NM_017084.1	*Gnmt*	F: GCCAGCGACAAGATGCTGAA	R: GACAGCGTCAAAGCCATCTCC
NM_017074.1	*Cse*	F: CAGTGATGTTGTCATGGGCTTAGTG	R: CATCCGGATCTGCAGTGTCTTC
NM_013003.1	*Pemt*	F: AGGAGTCCAGAGTGACCACATTTC	R: CACGTAGACGAGTGCCACCA
NM_012860.2	*Mat1a*	F: CCGAGCGAGAGCTACTAGAGGTTG	R: CCGAAATGACCATAGCATGCAG
NM_012522.2	*Cbs*	F: TGCATTATCGTGATGCCTGAGAA	R: GGGAATCGAATCTGGCGTTG
NM_001107894.1	*Etnk1*	F: TGAGTTTATCCAGGGTGAAGCTTTG	R: TCCAGCCATTGTGTGCATGA
NM_001039003.1	*Mtrr*	F: CAAAGTATGTGCAAGACAACCTCCA	R: TGATTTCTACAAGGGCGTCGTG
NM_001009349.1	*Mthfs*	F: AATCACATGGACATGGTGAGGCTA	R: CAGCCGGTTGCCATCTTTG
NM_001007699.1	*Ceptl*	F: TGCAAGGATACTGGGAATGGCTA	R: AGGCGATGTAAGCCCACAGAG
NM_198731.2	*Chdh*	F: CATCCCTGTGGTGTGCCATC	R: TGTGTGCAAGCATGCTGAATGTA
NM_030864.1	*Mtr*	F: ACTTGCGCAAACTCCGCTATG	R: TGCCAAGGATTCTGTCAACCTG
NM_022698.1	*Bad*	F: GGCAGCCAATAACAGTCATCA	R: GGTACGAACTGTGGCGACTC
XM_342975.4	*Mthfr*	F: AGCTTGAAGCCACCTGGACTGTAT	R: AGACTAGCGTTGCTGGGTTTCAGA
NM_031144.2	*Actb*	F: GGAGATTACTGCCCTGGCTCCTA	R: GACTCATCGTACTCCTGCTTGCTG

Mthfr: methylenetetrahydrofolate reductase; *Sahh*: S-adenosylhomocysteine hydrolase; *Bhmt*: betaine-homocysteine methyltransferase; *Cbs*: cystathionine beta synthase; *Mat1a*: methionine adenosyltransferase I, alpha; *Pemt*: phosphatidylethanolamine N-methyltransferase; *Cse*: cystathionine gamma-lyase; *Chka*: choline kinase alpha; *Tyms*: thymidylate synthetase; *Chdh*: choline dehydrogenase; *Gnmt*: glycine N-methyltransferase; *Mthfs*: 5,10-methenyltetrahydrofolate synthetase; *Mtr*: 5-methyltetrahydrofolate-homocysteine methyltransferase; *Ceptl*: choline/ethanolamine phosphotransferase 1; *Mtrr*: 5-methyltetrahydrofolate-homocysteine methyltransferase reductase; *Bad*: betaine aldehyde dehydrogenase; *Etnk1*: ethanolamine kinase 1.

Table 2: Changes of plasma phospholipids fatty acids in rats after supplementations.

PL fatty acids, %	CC	18:1	22:6*n*-3	20:5*n*-3	18:3*n*-3	18:2*n*-6	CLA	SO
18:1*n*-9	6.62 ± 0.32	10.40 ± 0.34	7.84 ± 0.31	8.30 ± 0.32	7.93 ± 0.36	11.21 ± 0.31	10.50 ± 0.30	9.84 ± 0.31
18:1*n*-7	1.06 ± 0.67	1.12 ± 1.69	0.91 ± 0.66	1.05 ± 0.67	0.77 ± 0.71	0.92 ± 0.22	0.92 ± 0.21	0.91 ± 0.16
18:2*n*-6	27.89 ± 3.87	26.63 ± 3.89	24.22 ± 3.86	27.33 ± 3.87	24.82 ± 3.91	28.29 ± 3.50	32.94 ± 3.49	28.52 ± 2.86
18:3*n*-6	0.82 ± 0.12	1.13 ± 0.16	2.01 ± 0.13	1.52 ± 0.14	0.90 ± 0.23	0.65 ± 0.14	0.48 ± 0.13	0.91 ± 0.13
18:3*n*-3	0.83 ± 0.16	0.96 ± 0.08	0.90 ± 0.05	0.83 ± 0.06	1.23 ± 0.19	0.93 ± 0.07	1.12 ± 0.07	0.90 ± 0.15
20:00	1.12 ± 0.11	1.03 ± 0.16	2.13 ± 0.13	1.78 ± 0.14	0.93 ± 0.23	0.77 ± 0.14	0.15 ± 0.17	1.13 ± 0.13
20:1*n*-9	0.30 ± 0.17	0.28 ± 0.19	0.38 ± 0.16	0.50 ± 0.17	0.25 ± 0.21	0.24 ± 0.17	0.51 ± 0.16	0.31 ± 0.16
20:2*n*-6	0.82 ± 0.61	0.86 ± 0.62	1.78 ± 0.59	0.98 ± 0.6	0.71 ± 0.69	0.55 ± 0.56	0.39 ± 0.55	0.78 ± 0.25
20:3*n*-6	0.30 ± 0.99	0.30 ± 2.01	0.37 ± 1.98	0.30 ± 1.99	0.25 ± 0.08	0.19 ± 1.81	0.35 ± 1.80	0.77 ± 1.91
20:4*n*-6	29.11 ± 3.80	25.43 ± 3.83	22.78 ± 3.81	22.75 ± 3.8	27.08 ± 3.91	23.53 ± 3.45	20.11 ± 3.44	24.78 ± 4.81
20:5*n*-3	0.89 ± 2.87	0.64 ± 2.90	1.20 ± 2.87	1.61 ± 2.87	0.71 ± 2.97	0.29 ± 0.61	0.17 ± 2.60	1.21 ± 0.92
22:1*n*-9	1.13 ± 1.03	0.89 ± 1.06	0.80 ± 1.03	1.98 ± 1.03	0.99 ± 0.13	0.48 ± 0.95	1.51 ± 0.94	0.97 ± 0.13
22:2*n*-6	0.89 ± 0.25	0.64 ± 0.30	1.33 ± 0.27	1.98 ± 0.25	0.99 ± 0.27	0.48 ± 0.27	1.51 ± 0.26	1.13 ± 0.21
22:4*n*-6	0.39 ± 0.52	0.37 ± 0.57	0.52 ± 0.54	0.43 ± 0.53	0.78 ± 0.52	0.18 ± 0.51	0.28 ± 0.50	0.42 ± 0.55
22:5*n*-6	0.42 ± 0.27	0.32 ± 0.31	0.90 ± 0.28	0.91 ± 0.27	0.66 ± 0.21	0.17 ± 0.28	0.14 ± 0.27	0.72 ± 0.27
22:5*n*-3	0.83 ± 0.51	0.71 ± 0.63	0.56 ± 0.62	0.80 ± 0.59	0.71 ± 0.58	0.27 ± 0.57	0.78 ± 0.56	0.52 ± 0.72
22:6*n*-3	3.86 ± 1.42	4.53 ± 1.44	5.87 ± 1.41	5.36 ± 1.4	5.27 ± 1.39	3.47 ± 1.30	4.76 ± 1.29	5.81 ± 2.40
SFA	3.46 ± 3.23	24.29 ± 3.67	24.96 ± 3.64	28.13 ± 3.63	25.07 ± 3.62	26.27 ± 3.30	27.57 ± 3.29	24.67 ± 5.67
MUFA	9.53 ± 5.38	9.53 ± 5.33	13.15 ± 5.33	10.77 ± 5.28	12.42 ± 5.28	10.60 ± 4.80	13.90 ± 4.79	13.25 ± 2.13
PUFA	67.07 ± 4.61	62.52 ± 4.69	62.43 ± 4.66	64.49 ± 4.65	64.13 ± 4.61	59.01 ± 4.22	63.03 ± 4.21	64.41 ± 6.61
n-3 PUFA	6.42 ± 3.71	6.85 ± 3.25	8.51 ± 3.22	8.30 ± 3.21	7.93 ± 3.2	4.96 ± 2.93	6.84 ± 2.92	7.51 ± 1.21
n-6 PUFA	60.64 ± 3.41	55.68 ± 3.95	53.91 ± 3.92	56.19 ± 3.91	56.19 ± 3.9	54.05 ± 3.56	56.19 ± 3.55	54.91 ± 5.92
n-3:*n*-6	0.11 ± 0.09	0.12 ± 0.09	0.16 ± 0.06	0.15 ± 0.05	0.14 ± 0.12	0.09 ± 0.08	0.12 ± 0.07	0.14 ± 0.16

Sample size in each group: $n = 10$, data was expressed as mean ± SD. CC: control group; CLA: conjugated linoleic acid; SO: stearolic acid. SFA: saturated fatty acids, MUFA: monounsaturated fatty acids, PUFA: polyunsaturated fatty acids; PL: phospholipids.

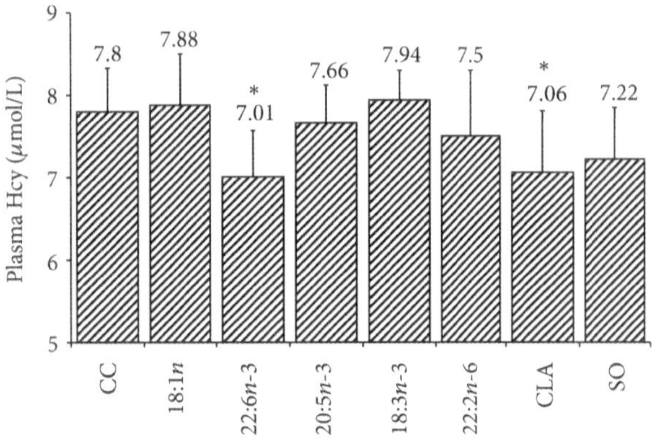

Figure 1: The effect of fatty acids on plasma Hcy concentration. n-10, data was expressed as mean ± SD. *indicate significant difference when compared with 18 : 1 group. CC: control group; SO: stearolic acid.

Plasma HDL was significantly increased, while plasma glucose was decreased in the 18:3n-3 group (Table 3).

3.3. The Effects of Oils on Plasma Hcy and Vitamin B_{12} and Folate in Rats. The oils differential effects on plasma Hcy concentration in rats. Plasma Hcy concentration was significantly decreased in the 22:6n-3 and CLA groups, while plasma Hcy concentration was not significantly affected in other groups (Figure 1). In addition, plasma vitamin B_{12} and folate concentration were not significantly affected in treatment groups (Table 2).

3.4. Effects of Oil on the Expression of Critical Genes Involved in Hepatic Hcy Metabolism. mRNA expression of *Mthfr* was significantly upregulated in the 22:6n-3, 20:5n-3, and 18:3n-3 groups and down-regulated in the 18:2n-6 and SO groups. *Bhmt* was significantly upregulated in the 20:5n-3, 18:3n-3, and 18:2n-6 groups. *Mat1a* was significantly upregulated in the 22:6n-3, 20:5n-3, 18:3n-3, and CLA groups. In addition, *Cbs* was significantly upregulated in the 22:6n-3, 20:5n-3, 18:3n-3, and CLA groups, while down-regulated in the 18:2n-6 and SO groups. *Pemt* was significantly upregulated in the 20:5n-3 and 18:3n-3 groups, and downregulated in the SO group. However, the different oil supplements did not significantly affect the mRNA expression of *Sahh*. Other critical gene expression (*Bhmt, Cse, Chka, Tyms, Chdh, Gnmt, Mthfs, Mtr, Cept1, Mtrr, Etnk1,* and *Bad*) involved in Hcy and phospholipids metabolism was also regulated by the different oils (Table 4).

4. Discussion

In the present study, we found that oils rich in 22:6n-3 and CLA significantly decreased plasma Hcy concentration. These oils have different regulatory effects on the mRNA expression of a critical gene involved in Hcy metabolic pathway.

n-3 PUFAs are essential for normal growth and development and for the prevention and treatment of coronary heart disease [19, 20], hypertension [21], and type 2 diabetes mellitus [22, 23]. Previous studies suggested that n-3 PUFAs play an important role in Hcy metabolism [13, 14]. The possible mechanism by which n-3 PUFA regulate Hcy metabolism was also investigated [12, 24]; Piolot reported the apparent interaction of n-3 PUFA and NO on Hcy metabolism in healthy people [24]. They suggested a probable mechanism by which n-3 PUFA supplementation can reduce the production of Hcy. The reduced Hcy concentrations observed in their study are attributed to possible oxidative stress induction by n-3 PUFA and stimulation of the oxidative catabolism of Hcy [25]. Investigators have previously reported increased susceptibility to oxidative stress due to n-3 PUFA supplementation [26]. Our animal and population studies have also investigated the potential mechanisms [12–14] (Figure 2). In our animal study, we found that plasma Hcy was significantly decreased by tuna oil rich in 22:6n-3. MAT activity was significantly increased, and MAT mRNA expression was significantly upregulated by 22:6n-3; CSE mRNA expression was significantly upregulated by 22:6n-3. We have suggested that 22:6n-3 decreases the concentration of Hcy despite increasing MAT activity and upregulation of MAT mRNA expression through compensatory CSE mRNA expression, both of which are involved in Hcy metabolism [12].

However, the determination of Hcy concentration is multifactorial shaped by gene-environment interactions. Thus, genetic variants involved in the Hcy metabolic pathway may modify the effect of dietary fatty acids on plasma Hcy in humans. Our population studies found an interaction between dietary fatty acids and genetic variants *MTHFR* and *MAT1A* in determining plasma Hcy concentration [13, 14]. Two functional *MTHFR* variants, 1298A > C and 677C > T, which were not in linkage disequilibrium, were significantly associated with hypertension. Importantly, the variants exhibited significant interactions with intakes of total and n-6 PUFA and a dietary n-3 : n-6 PUFA ratio in determining plasma Hcy concentration. In addition, participants with combined genotypes of both SNP (677 TT with 1298 AC or CC) who consumed high levels of n-3 PUFA (>0.66% energy) had lower plasma Hcy compared with those who had the same genotype and consumed low levels of n-3 PUFA (</=0.66% energy). It was thus suggested that dietary PUFA intake modulates the effect of *MTHFR* variants on plasma Hcy [14]. Moreover, genetic variant *MAT1A* 3U1510 displayed a significant interaction with dietary n-3 : n-6 PUFA ratio in determining plasma Hcy. 3U1510G homozygotes had significantly lower plasma Hcy concentration than major allele homozygotes and heterozygotes (AA + AG) when the n-3 : n-6 ratio was >0.09. Two other *MAT1A* variants (d18777 and i15752) also showed significant interactions with different constituents of dietary fat in influencing Hcy concentration. Further, haplotypes consisting of three variants displayed a strong interaction with one's n-3 : n-6 ratio in influencing Hcy concentrations [13].

Taken together, the studies by Noga et al. [27] and Jacobs et al. [28] provide strong evidence that phosphatidylethanolamine N-methyltransferase (PEMT) plays a significant role in the regulation of plasma Hcy concentrations. Noga et al. utilized PEMT-/- knockout mice and McArdle RH-7777 cells

ABLE 3: Changes of biochemical measurements in the rats after the supplementation.

	CC	18:1	22:6n-3	20:5n-3	18:3n-3	18:2n-6	CLA	SO
LDL-C, mmol/L	0.22 ± 0.12	0.21 ± 0.11	0.21 ± 0.12	0.18 ± 0.10*	0.20 ± 0.23	0.26 ± 0.11	0.19 ± 0.12	0.28 ± 0.13
TG, mmol/L	0.91 ± 0.76	1.07 ± 0.70	1.07 ± 0.75	1.08 ± 0.74	1.04 ± 0.87	0.73 ± 0.71*	1.06 ± 0.73	0.86 ± 0.84
HDL-C, mmol/L	0.98 ± 0.69	0.98 ± 0.63	1.00 ± 0.68	0.94 ± 0.67	1.11 ± 0.80*	0.98 ± 0.64	0.86 ± 0.67	0.96 ± 0.76
TC, mmol/L	1.82 ± 0.78	1.83 ± 0.72	1.84 ± 0.77	1.72 ± 0.75*	1.94 ± 0.89	1.82 ± 0.73	1.65 ± 0.75	1.80 ± 0.86
Glucose, mmol/L	5.98 ± 2.18	6.01 ± 2.01	5.49 ± 2.16*	4.94 ± 2.14*	4.82 ± 2.27*	5.44 ± 2.03	6.19 ± 2.11	5.15 ± 2.40*
Uric acid, μmol/L	49.02 ± 8.68	44.88 ± 7.99	39.34 ± 8.59*	43.00 ± 8.57	52.12 ± 8.71	48.50 ± 8.08	44.64 ± 8.39	43.92 ± 9.55
ALT,U/L	55.80 ± 9.12	61.20 ± 8.39	56.57 ± 9.03	49.80 ± 9.01	57.60 ± 9.12	58.80 ± 8.49	58.60 ± 8.82	47.40 ± 10.03*
AST, U/L	184.20 ± 26.74	231.40 ± 21.60	168.86 ± 26.48	159.40 ± 26.45*	181.20 ± 26.56	192.40 ± 24.89	190.00 ± 25.86	140.80 ± 29.41*
Creatinine, μmol/L	63.00 ± 10.21	61.78 ± 9.39	63.21 ± 10.11	59.30 ± 10.09*	62.90 ± 10.20	59.78 ± 9.51	57.34 ± 9.87*	56.58 ± 11.23*
BUN, mmol/L	5.95 ± 2.19	6.33 ± 2.01	6.50 ± 2.17	5.81 ± 2.15	5.85 ± 2.26	6.08 ± 2.04	5.83 ± 2.12	5.52 ± 2.41*
Alb, g/L	45.34 ± 9.19	46.12 ± 8.45	45.70 ± 9.10	45.72 ± 9.08	46.22 ± 9.21	45.56 ± 8.56	45.64 ± 8.89	44.60 ± 10.11
Glob, g/L	24.50 ± 7.12	23.20 ± 6.55	27.30 ± 7.05	22.24 ± 7.03*	28.26 ± 7.14	24.00 ± 6.63	23.96 ± 6.89	24.54 ± 7.83
A : G	1.87 ± 0.78	2.00 ± 0.72	1.69 ± 0.77	2.06 ± 0.75	1.67 ± 0.89	1.91 ± 0.73	1.91 ± 0.75	1.84 ± 0.86
TP, g/L	69.84 ± 9.91	69.32 ± 9.12	73.00 ± 9.81*	67.96 ± 9.79	74.48 ± 9.90*	69.56 ± 9.23	69.60 ± 9.58	69.14 ± 10.90
VitaminB_{12}, ng/mL	688 ± 78	691 ± 89	690 ± 101	695 ± 70	691 ± 84	690 ± 120	690 ± 97	688 ± 89
Folate, pmol/L	26.8 ± 7.9	26.3 ± 6.1	27.0 ± 5.8	26.9 ± 6.8	27.1 ± 7.3	26.2 ± 5.7	26.0 ± 8.5	26.5 ± 7.1

Sample size in each group: $n = 10$, data was expressed as mean ± SD.

*indicates significant difference when compared with 18:1 group.

CC: control group; CLA: conjugated linoleic acid; SO: stearolic acid; TC: total cholesterol; TG: total triglyceride; HDL-C: high density cholesterol; LDL-C: low density cholesterol; A : G: Alb : Glob; ALT: alanine transaminase; AST: aspartate aminotransferase; TP: total protein; BUN: blood urea nitrogen.

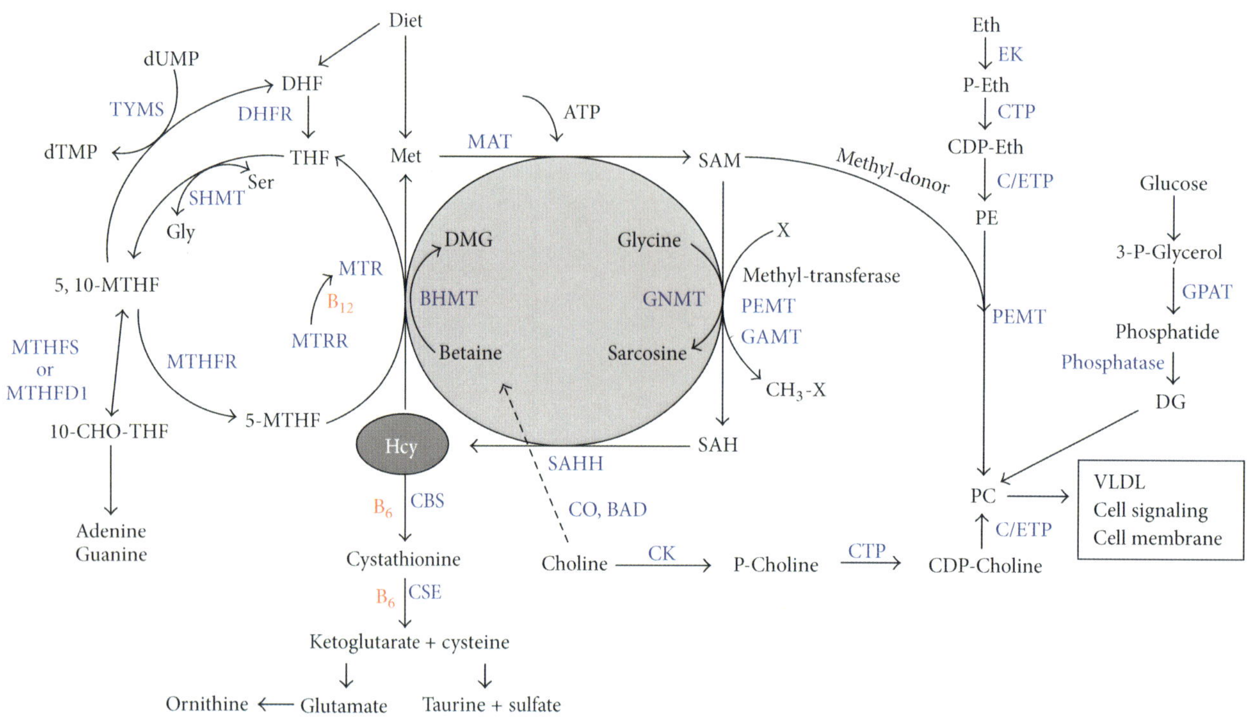

FIGURE 2: Homocysteine metabolism. *Mthfr*:methylenetetrahydrofolate reductase; *Sahh*:S-adenosylhomocysteine hydrolase; *Bhmt*:betaine-homocysteine methyltransferase; *Cbs*: cystathionine beta synthase; *Mat1a*: methionine adenosyltransferase I, alpha; *Pemt*: phosphatidylethanolamine N-methyltransferase; *Cse*: cystathionine gamma-lyase; *Chka*: choline kinase alpha; *Tyms*: thymidylate synthetase; *Chdh*: choline dehydrogenase; *Gnmt*: glycine N-methyltransferase; *Mthfs*: 5,10-methenyltetrahydrofolate synthetase; *Mtr*: 5-methyltetrahydrofolate-homocysteine methyltransferase; *Ceptl,* choline/ethanolamine phosphotransferase 1; *Mtrr*: 5-methyltetrahydrofolate-homocysteine methyltransferase reductase; *Bad*: betaine aldehyde dehydrogenase; *Etnk1*: ethanolamine kinase 1.

TABLE 4: Gene expression of the critical genes involved in Hcy and phospholipids metabolism pathway.

Gene	CC	18:1	22:6*n*-3	20:5*n*-3	18:3*n*-3	18:2*n*-6	CLA	SO
Mthfr	1.0	1.1	**2.4**	**2.2**	**2.9**	**0.3**	1.1	0.4
Sahh	1.0	**0.5**	0.8	0.9	0.8	0.8	1.3	0.8
Bhmt	1.0	0.8	1.1	**2.1**	**2.7**	**3.2**	1.9	0.8
Mat1a	1.0	1.1	**2.0**	**2.0**	**2.6**	0.6	**2.3**	0.7
Cbs	1.0	1.6	**2.3**	**2.6**	**4.2**	**0.5**	**2.2**	0.5
Pemt	1.0	1.5	1.7	**2.7**	**4.1**	0.8	1.8	0.4
Cse	1.0	0.7	1.5	1.2	0.9	0.6	0.6	0.8
Chka	1.0	1.0	1.4	**3.4**	**3.2**	1.2	1.4	**0.2**
Tyms	1.0	0.6	1.2	0.6	1.2	**0.2**	0.6	**0.2**
Chdh	1.0	0.8	0.6	1.1	1.0	**0.1**	1.1	**0.2**
Gnmt	1.0	0.8	1.8	**2.4**	**3.3**	0.6	1.4	**0.3**
Mthfs	1.0	0.9	1.4	1.8	**2.9**	1.0	1.6	**0.3**
Mtr	1.0	0.9	0.9	**2.6**	**2.1**	0.8	1.0	0.3
Ceptl	1.0	1.1	**0.3**	**0.3**	**0.3**	0.6	**0.2**	**0.1**
Mtrr	1.0	0.7	0.7	**2.1**	**2.4**	0.7	1.7	0.5
Etnk1	1.0	0.9	**0.3**	**0.4**	0.6	0.7	**0.4**	**0.1**
Bad	1.0	0.6	0.7	**2.8**	**3.5**	0.7	1.4	**0.3**

transfected with PEMT to study the contribution of PEMT to Hcy levels. Plasma Hcy concentrations in the Pemt-/- knockout mice were 50% of those in the wild-type mice. Furthermore, when McArdle RH-7777 cells with negligible PEMT activity were transfected to stably express PEMT, there was more than a 2-fold increase in Hcy secretion compared with cells that were transfected with the vector alone. These studies illustrate the potential for PEMT to regulate plasma Hcy or to be a major determinant of Hcy concentration [29]. The PEMT pathway primarily contains PUFA, such as 20:4*n*-6 and 22:6*n*-3 [30], but PEMT also has an important role in the distribution of fatty acids to tissues [30]. An animal study showed that 22:6*n*-3 in plasma phosphatidylcholine may be a potential marker for in vivo PEMT activity in humans [30]. We try to examine the effect of fatty acids on gene expression of *Pemt* in the present study, but did not observe a significant regulatory effect of 22:6*n*-3 on *Pemt* expression, though 20:5*n*-3 and 18:3*n*-3 significantly upregulated the expression of *Pemt*. A recent paper by Ratnam et al. presented convincing evidence that betaine-homocysteine S- methyltransferase (BHMT) plays an essential role in lowering plasma Hcy levels in a diabetic state [31]. Jacobs et al. noted that there was increased activity and abundance of BHMT and MAT, leaving the possibility that BHMT would be able to compensate for the increased Hcy production [28]. The present study showed that *Bhmt* was significantly upregulated in the 20:5*n*-3, 18:3*n*-3, and 18:2*n*-6 groups.

However, considering the significance of *n*-3 PUFA in decreasing plasma Hcy levels and protecting from CVD, more cell cultures, animal studies, and population studies should be conducted to investigate the potential mechanism by which *n*-3 PUFA decreases plasma Hcy concentration. In addition, the genetic variation of some critical genes among populations could account for the difference in the results of intervention studies; nutrigenomics may be essential in identifying interactions between the genetic variants and dietary fatty acids in determining plasma Hcy concentration.

In summary, dietary intake of 22:6*n*-3 and CLA decrease the plasma concentration of Hcy. Different PUFAs have different effects on the mRNA expression of key genes involved in Hcy metabolism; *n*-3 PUFA upregulates expression, while *n*-6 PUFA down-regulates mRNA expression of *Mthfr*, *Mat1a*, *Cbs*, *Pemt*, *Gnmt*, *Mtrr*, and *Bad*. *n*-3 PUFA and CLA down-regulate mRNA expression of *Cept1*, *Etnk1*, and CLA upregulates mRNA expression of *Mat1a* and *Cbs*.

Conflict of Interests

The authors have no financial/commercial conflict of interests in this work.

Authors' Contribution

T. Huang, X. Hu, N. Khan, and J. Yong carried out the studies, analyzed data, and drafted the paper; T. Huang and D. Li participated in the project design. All authors read and approved the final paper.

Acknowledgment

This work was supported by a Grant from National High Technology Research and Development Program of China (no. N20080753), the National Natural Science Foundation of China (no. 30972464), and the National Basic Research Program of China (973 Program: 2011CB504002).

References

[1] A. de Bree, W. M. M. Verschuren, D. Kromhout, L. A. J. Kluijtmans, and H. J. Blom, "Homocysteine determinants and the evidence to what extent homocysteine determines the risk of coronary heart disease," *Pharmacological Reviews*, vol. 54, no. 4, pp. 599–618, 2002.

[2] T. Huang, G. Yuan, Z. Zhang, Z. Zou, and D. Li, "Cardiovascular pathogenesis in hyperhomocysteinemia," *Asia Pacific Journal of Clinical Nutrition*, vol. 17, no. 1, pp. 8–16, 2008.

[3] K. S. McCully and R. B. Wilson, "Homocysteine theory of arteriosclerosis," *Atherosclerosis*, vol. 22, no. 2, pp. 215–227, 1975.

[4] H. J. Blom, "Determinants of plasma homocysteine," *The American Journal of Clinical Nutrition*, vol. 67, no. 2, pp. 188–189, 1998.

[5] F. B. Hu, M. J. Stampfer, J. E. Manson et al., "Dietary intake of α-linolenic acid and risk of fatal ischemic heart disease among women," *American Journal of Clinical Nutrition*, vol. 69, no. 5, pp. 890–897, 1999.

[6] H. Iso, K. M. Rexrode, M. J. Stampfer et al., "Intake of fish and omega-3 fatty acids and risk of stroke in women," *Journal of the American Medical Association*, vol. 285, no. 3, pp. 304–312, 2001.

[7] D. Li, X. M. Yu, H. B. Xie et al., "Platelet phospholipid n-3 PUFA negatively associated with plasma homocysteine in middle-aged and geriatric hyperlipaemia patients," *Prostaglandins Leukotrienes and Essential Fatty Acids*, vol. 76, no. 5, pp. 293–297, 2007.

[8] D. Li, N. J. Mann, and A. J. Sinclair, "A significant inverse relationship between concentrations of plasma homocysteine and phospholipid docosahexaenoic acid in healthy male subjects," *Lipids*, vol. 41, no. 1, pp. 85–89, 2006.

[9] M. Zeman, A. Zak, M. Vecka, E. Tvrzicka, A. Pisarikova, and B. Stankova, "N-3 fatty acid supplementation decreases plasma homocysteine in diabetic dyslipidemia treated with statin-fibrate combination," *Journal of Nutritional Biochemistry*, vol. 17, no. 6, pp. 379–384, 2006.

[10] H. Grundt, D. W. T. Nilsen, M. A. Mansoor, Ø. Hetland, and A. Nordøy, "Reduction in homocysteine by n-3 polyunsaturated fatty acids after 1 year in a randomised double-blind study following an acute myocardial infarction: no effect on endothelial adhesion properties," *Pathophysiology of Haemostasis and Thrombosis*, vol. 33, no. 2, pp. 88–95, 2003.

[11] T. Huang, J. Zheng, Y. Chen, B. Yang, M. L. Wahlqvist, and D. Li, "High consumption of omega-3 polyunsaturated fatty acids decrease plasma homocysteine: a meta-analysis of randomized, placebo-controlled trials," *Nutrition*, vol. 27, no. 9, pp. 863–867, 2011.

[12] T. Huang, M. L. Wahlqvist, and D. Li, "Docosahexaenoic acid decreases plasma homocysteine via regulating enzyme activity and mRNA expression involved in methionine metabolism," *Nutrition*, vol. 26, no. 1, pp. 112–119, 2010.

[13] T. Huang, K. Tucker, Y. Lee et al., "MAT1A variants modulate the effect of dietary fatty acids on plasma homocysteine concentrations," *Nutrition, Metabolism & Cardiovascular Diseases*, vol. 22, no. 4, pp. 362–368, 2010.

[14] T. Huang, K. L. Tucker, Y. C. Lee et al., "Methylenetetrahydrofolate reductase variants associated with hypertension and cardiovascular disease interact with dietary polyunsaturated fatty acids to modulate plasma homocysteine in Puerto Rican adults," *Journal of Nutrition*, vol. 141, no. 4, pp. 654–659, 2011.

[15] S. Pooya, M. D. Jalali, A. D. Jazayery, A. Saedisomeolia, M. R. Eshraghian, and F. Toorang, "The efficacy of omega-3 fatty acid supplementation on plasma homocysteine and malondialdehyde levels of type 2 diabetic patients," *Nutrition, Metabolism and Cardiovascular Diseases*, vol. 20, pp. 326–331, 2010.

[16] G. Vizcaíno, M. Diez-Ewald, F. H. Herrmann, G. Schuster, E. Torres-Guerra, and M. Arteaga-Vizcaíno, "Homocysteinemia and its relationship with the methylentetrahydrofolate reductase polymorphism in various ethnic groups from western Venezuela," *Investigacion Clinica*, vol. 46, no. 4, pp. 347–355, 2005.

[17] N. J. Mann, D. Li, A. J. Sinclair et al., "The effect of diet on plasma homocysteine concentrations in healthy male subjects," *European Journal of Clinical Nutrition*, vol. 53, no. 11, pp. 895–899, 1999.

[18] E. O. Uthus and H. M. Brown-Borg, "Methionine flux to transsulfuration is enhanced in the long living Ames dwarf mouse," *Mechanisms of Ageing and Development*, vol. 127, no. 5, pp. 444–450, 2006.

[19] M. L. Burr, A. M. Fehily, J. F. Gilbert et al., "Effects of changes in fat, fish, and fibre intakes on death and myocardial reinfarction:

diet and reinfarction trial (DART)," *The Lancet*, vol. 2, no. 8666, pp. 757–761, 1989.

[20] T. Huang, J. S. Andrew, S. Lirong, B. Yang, and D. Li, "Comparative effects of tuna oil and salmon oil on liver lipid metabolism and fatty acid concentrations in rats," *Journal of Food Lipids*, vol. 16, no. 4, pp. 436–451, 2009.

[21] L. J. Appel, E. R. Miller III, A. J. Seidler, and P. K. Whelton, "Does supplementation of diet with 'fish oil' reduce blood pressure? A meta-analysis of controlled clinical trials," *Archives of Internal Medicine*, vol. 153, no. 12, pp. 1429–1438, 1993.

[22] T. Huang, S. Bhulaidok, Z. Cai et al., "Plasma phospholipids n-3 polyunsaturated fatty acid is associated with metabolic syndrome," *Molecular Nutrition and Food Research*, vol. 54, no. 11, pp. 1628–1635, 2010.

[23] T. Huang, M. L. Wahlqvist, T. Xu, A. Xu, A. Zhang, and D. Li, "Increased plasma n-3 polyunsaturated fatty acid is associated with improved insulin sensitivity in type 2 diabetes in China," *Molecular Nutrition and Food Research*, vol. 54, supplement 1, pp. S112–S119, 2010.

[24] A. Piolot, D. Blache, L. Boulet et al., "Effect of fish oil on LDL oxidation and plasma homocysteine concentrations in health," *The Journal of Laboratory and Clinical Medicine*, vol. 141, no. 1, pp. 41–49, 2003.

[25] P. Durand, M. Prost, N. Loreau, S. Lussier-Cacan, and D. Blache, "Impaired homocysteine metabolism and atherothrombotic disease," *Laboratory Investigation*, vol. 81, no. 5, pp. 645–672, 2001.

[26] A. Saedisomeolia, L. G. Wood, M. L. Garg, P. G. Gibson, and P. A. B. Wark, "Lycopene enrichment of cultured airway epithelial cells decreases the inflammation induced by rhinovirus infection and lipopolysaccharide," *Journal of Nutritional Biochemistry*, vol. 20, no. 8, pp. 577–585, 2009.

[27] A. A. Noga, L. M. Stead, Y. Zhao, M. E. Brosnan, J. T. Brosnan, and D. E. Vance, "Plasma homocysteine is regulated by phospholipid methylation," *The Journal of Biological Chemistry*, vol. 278, pp. 5952–5955.

[28] R. L. Jacobs, L. M. Stead, C. Devlin et al., "Physiological regulation of phospholipid methylation alters plasma homocysteine in mice," *Journal of Biological Chemistry*, vol. 280, no. 31, pp. 28299–28305, 2005.

[29] C. S. Hartz and K. L. Schalinske, "Phosphatidylethanolamine N-methyltransferase and regulation of homocysteine," *Nutrition Reviews*, vol. 64, no. 10, pp. 465–467, 2006.

[30] K. A. da Costa, L. M. Sanders, L. M. Fischer, and S. H. Zeisel, "Docosahexaenoic acid in plasma phosphatidylcholine may be a potential marker for *in vivo* phosphatidylethanolamine A/-methyltransferase activity in humans," *American Journal of Clinical Nutrition*, vol. 93, no. 5, pp. 968–974, 2011.

[31] S. Ratnam, E. P. Wijekoon, B. Hall, T. A. Garrow, M. E. Brosnan, and J. T. Brosnan, "Effects of diabetes and insulin on betaine-homocysteine S-methyltransferase expression in rat liver," *American Journal of Physiology—Endocrinology and Metabolism*, vol. 290, no. 5, pp. E933–E939, 2006.

16

Dietary Available Phosphorus Affected Growth Performance, Body Composition, and Hepatic Antioxidant Property of Juvenile Yellow Catfish *Pelteobagrus fulvidraco*

Qin Tang,[1] Chunfang Wang,[1] Congxin Xie,[1] Jiali Jin,[1] and Yanqing Huang[2]

[1] *College of Fisheries, Huazhong Agricultural University, Wuhan 430070, China*
[2] *East China Sea Fisheries Research Institute, Chinese Academy of Fishery Sciences, Shanghai 200090, China*

Correspondence should be addressed to Chunfang Wang, cfwang@mail.hzau.edu.cn

Academic Editors: D. Benke and V. Dilis

An 8-week feeding trial was carried out with juvenile yellow catfish to study the effects of dietary available phosphorus (P) on growth performance, body composition, and hepatic antioxidant property. Six pellet diets were formulated to contain graded available P levels at 0.33, 0.56, 0.81, 1.15, 1.31, and 1.57% of dry matter, respectively. Triplicate tanks with each tank containing 60 juveniles (3.09 ± 0.03 g) were fed one of the six experimental diets for 8 weeks. Specific growth rate, feeding rate, and protein efficiency ratio were significantly higher at 0.81% dietary available P. Efficiency of P utilization distinctly decreased with increasing P level. Body lipid content significantly decreased while body ash and feces P content significantly increased with increasing P level. Quadratic regression analysis indicated that vertebrae P content was maximized at 1.21% dietary available P. Fish fed 1.57% dietary available P had highest activity of hepatic superoxide dismutase and catalase and malonaldehyde content. In conclusion, decreasing dietary available P increased P utilization efficiency and body lipid content while decreased vertebrae P content. Juvenile yellow catfish were subjected to oxidative damage under the condition of high dietary P content (1.57%), and the damage could not be eradicated by their own antioxidant defense system.

1. Introduction

Phosphorus (P) is an important constituent of nucleic acids and cell membranes and is directly involved in all energy-producing cellular reactions [1, 2]. Fish must obtain P from their food because of the low concentration of phosphate in natural waters [3]. P deficiency or P excess could probably affect the production of ATP, the synthesis of nucleic acids, and the complement of cell membranes, thus cause anorexia, transient lethargy, reduced growth, and dark coloration [4]. In most fish, the main signs of P deficiency include poor growth, poor feed efficiency, and bone mineralization [1].

Phosphorus deficiency enhanced lipid peroxidation and induced oxidative stress in plants [5], such as, bean [6], barley [7], and oilseed rape [8]. With the decrease of inorganic phosphate concentration in tissues, lipid peroxidation increased in cells [6]. Normally, generation of reactive oxygen species (ROS) is kept under control by antioxidant defense system that includes antioxidative enzymes, superoxide dismutase (SOD), catalase (CAT), peroxidase (POD), and glutathione peroxidase (GPX) and enzymes of Halliwell-Asada pathway and antioxidative molecules: ascorbates, α-tocopherol, carotenoids, flavonoids, and glutathione [9–11]. Overproduction of ROS results in oxidative stress, a deleterious process that can be an important mediator of damage to cell structures, including lipids and membranes, proteins, and DNA [12]. In the process of eliminating the free radicals, SOD, GSH-Px, and CAT are the major indirect free radical scavengers [12]. In unfavorable circumstance, the balance between the activities and the intracellular levels of these antioxidants is broken, and the imbalance will result in the accumulation of malonaldehyde (MDA) and finally lead to oxidative damage to cell [13].

Therefore, appropriate P is critical for organisms to maintain both structural and functional roles and to form an intricate and interwoven system regulating the healthy functioning [5]. P starvation is an abiotic stress that imposes an oxidative stress in plant root cells [6]. However, there was no clear report about the relationship between dietary P deficiency or P excess and oxidative responses in animals. Three types of metabolic control of oxidative metabolism observed in the various living tissues of animals had been reported: in skeletal muscle by ADP (or Pi/phosphocreatine), in cardiac tissue a coordinated control of substrate delivery that may involve Ca^{2+} and inorganic P control of NADH, and control of O_2 delivery [14]. Also, in rheumatoid arthritis patients, oxidative metabolism within the cell had been altered and oxygen free radicals were generated, which altered calcium and phosphorus levels in skeletal muscle cells [15].

Yellow catfish (*Pelteobagrus fulvidraco*) is a freshwater species native to Asian-Pacific waters, which is now becoming one of the major commercial species cultured by farmers in China. The annual production of yellow catfish reached 163,556 tons in the year of 2009, an increase of 21.65% over the year 2008 [16]. Most farmers use commercial feed to produce high output. However, these feeds are usually high in phosphorus content (about 20 to 25 kg $Ca(H_2PO_4)_2 \cdot H_2O$ per ton feed). Large amounts of uneaten feed and feces released into the aquatic environment lead to eutrophication and cause a serious threat to the sustainable aquaculture of this species. P is the limiting nutrient for algae growth in freshwater ecosystem [17]. The effect of P is immediate and broad, causing both environmental concern and possible economic inefficiencies in the production systems due to increased costs associated with the biological and chemical processing of the waste [1].

Therefore, a need exists to determine the effects of dietary P content on fish performance and health functioning in the aquaculture setting, to balance the desire for high fish production with protection of the aquatic environment. Little research on dietary P, especially hepatic antioxidant property under dietary P stress, has been conducted on yellow catfish. In the present study, six diets were formulated to contain low to high levels of P by adding $Ca(H_2PO_4)_2 \cdot H_2O$ into the basal diet. $Ca(H_2PO_4)_2 \cdot H_2O$ was chosen as the source of P due to two reasons: first, reports showed that dietary calcium concentration or calcium-phosphorus (Ca/P) imbalance has no effect on P requirement of catfish [18–20]; second, in the same growth trial, the expression of NaPi-IIb cotransporter was needed to be detected in the intestine, which transports inorganic P from lumen to blood when dietary P content is pretty low in lumen (in another manuscript) and probably would be affected if we chose $NaH_2PO_4 \cdot H_2O$ or $KH_2PO_4 \cdot H_2O$.

The purpose of this study was to investigate the effects of different dietary P levels on growth performance, body composition, and hepatic antioxidant property of juvenile yellow catfish.

2. Materials and Methods

2.1. Diet Preparation. Six experimental diets were formulated to contain graded levels of available P (0.33, 0.56, 0.81, 1.15, 1.31, and 1.57 g 100 g^{-1} feed, resp., and alpha cellulose used as filler). Formulation and chemical composition of the diets are presented in Table 1. P content in each ingredient was as follows (as % dry matter): casein 0.74, blood meal 0.44, gelatin 0.08, squid meal 0.97, and wheat flour 0.01. Chromic (III) oxide (Cr_2O_3) was added (1.0%) to the diets as an inert digestion marker.

All the ingredients were finely ground to pass through 60 mesh sieve (250 μm) and weighed. The dry ingredients were mixed one by one manually for at least 20 min. Then fish oil and soy bean oil were added and mixed-in for another 20 min. Finally the mixture was transferred to a mixer and homogenized for about 20 min. Distilled water was added to the mixture to achieve a proper pelleting consistency, and then the mixture was extruded through a 2.0 mm diameter die to form pellets. After that, diets were dried in an oven at 60°C until the moisture was reduced to less than 10%, then stored in a freezer at −20°C until use. A representative sample was taken for proximate analysis. The stability of P in diets was tested by measuring the total P content in the diets before and after immersed in water for 30 min, and the result showed that the experimental diets held 97.35% total P after immersed in water for 30 min.

2.2. Growth Trial. About 1400 yellow catfish larvae were obtained from Southlake hatchery based in Wuhan (Hubei, China) and then were stocked in 18 indoor fiberglass tanks (water volume, 395 L) in aquaculture center of The College of Fisheries, Huazhong Agricultural University. Before starting the experiment, all the larvae were acclimatized to laboratory conditions for four weeks; for the first two weeks, the larvae were fed with Tubificidae and the next two weeks were fed with the basal diet (diet 1) (Table 1). Prior to the feeding trial, all fish were starved for 24 h. Altogether 1080 fish with similar size (3.09 ± 0.03 g) were distributed into 18 indoor fiberglass tanks (395 L) at a stocking density of 60 fish per tank. Fifty fish with similar size around 3 g were anaesthetized in MS 222 (Sigma) solution (100 mg L^{-1}) and then kept at −20°C as initial samples for proximate analysis. Each diet was fed for eight weeks (from August to October in 2010) to triplicate groups of fish. During the experiment, water flow was maintained constant at 1.5 L min^{-1}, water temperature was 27 ± 0.4°C, dissolved oxygen was about 8 mg L^{-1}, and pH was 7.84 ± 0.03. During the experiment, the diurnal cycle was 12-h light/12-h dark.

Every morning about one hour before feeding, about 25% of the water from each tank was drained and replaced with fresh water. Feed was distributed to fish at 08:00 and 16:00 to apparent satiation, and each feeding period lasted for about 2 h. The fish were fed every 30 min and altogether 4 times for each feeding period. Since yellow catfish was active in feed intake, this feeding strategy was to ensure fish in each tank eating up almost all the feed in about 30 min. Apparent satiation was assessed by the feeding behavior of yellow catfish: when we threw the feed into the tanks, fish were not interested in the feed and did not swim quickly to get the feed actively. Uneaten feed was collected after the fourth feeding during each feeding period and complete feces were collected by siphoning after 2 h of feeding from the second week. The uneaten feed was dried to constant

TABLE 1: Formulation and chemical composition of the experimental diets (g kg^{-1} dry matter).

Ingredients	Diets					
	1	2	3	4	5	6
Casein	350.0	350.0	350.0	350.0	350.0	350.0
Blood meal	100.0	100.0	100.0	100.0	100.0	100.0
Gelatin	20.0	20.0	20.0	20.0	20.0	20.0
Squid meal	70.0	70.0	70.0	70.0	70.0	70.0
Wheat flour	210.0	210.0	210.0	210.0	210.0	210.0
Fish oil	60.0	60.0	60.0	60.0	60.0	60.0
Soy bean oil	30.0	30.0	30.0	30.0	30.0	30.0
Vitamin premix[1]	5.0	5.0	5.0	5.0	5.0	5.0
Mineral premix (P free)[2]	27.5	27.5	27.5	27.5	27.5	27.5
Vitamin C	5.0	5.0	5.0	5.0	5.0	5.0
Choline chloride	2.5	2.5	2.5	2.5	2.5	2.5
Cr_2O_3	10.0	10.0	10.0	10.0	10.0	10.0
$Ca(H_2PO_4)_2 \cdot H_2O$	0.0	12.0	24.0	36.0	48.0	60.0
α-cellulose	110.0	98.0	86.0	74.0	62.0	50.0
Chemical composition (per kg dry matter)						
Moisture (g)	83.9	98.6	78.3	71.0	92.5	99.6
Crude protein (g)	455.9	452.9	447.5	446.1	457.5	444.1
Crude lipid (g)	62.8	62.6	65.4	60.1	63.3	62.7
Ash (g)	48.2	52.3	59.1	69.6	77.0	87.0
Total phosphorus (g)	3.8	6.3	8.9	12.2	14.2	17.1
Available phosphorus (g)	3.3	5.6	8.1	11.5	13.1	15.7

[1]Vitamin Premix was bought from Fulong Feed Company in Wuhan (Hubei province, China) and contained the following vitamins (mg kg^{-1} feed): vitamin K_3, 20; niacin, 250; riboflavin, 50; pyridoxine, 25; thiamin, 25; D-calcium pantothenate, 100; biotin, 1.5; foliacin, 10; vitamin B_{12}, 0.125; ascorbic acid, 250; inositol, 750; (IU kg^{-1} feed): vitamin A, 17500; vitamin D_3, 2500; vitamin E, 175.
[2]Mineral premix (P free) contained the following minerals (mg kg^{-1} feed): NaCl, 275; $MgSO_4 \cdot 7H_2O$, 4125; Na_2SO_4, 6270; K_2SO_4, 5638; $CaCl_2 \cdot 2H_2O$, 3218; $FeSO_4$, 688; Calcium lactate, 963; $ZnSO_4 \cdot 7H_2O$, 97; $MnSO_4 \cdot 4H_2O$, 45; $CuSO_4 \cdot 5H_2O$, 8.53; $CoSO_4$, 0.28; KI, 0.83.

weight at 60°C in an oven and weighed to determine daily feed consumption. Pooled feces of each tank were also dried at 60°C. Mortality was checked daily. The cultured water was disinfected periodically by chlorine dioxide to prevent diseases.

2.3. Sample Collection and Analysis. At the end of the experiment, all fish were starved for 24 h, counted, bulk weighed by tank for the calculation of survival rate and growth rate, and then returned to each tank. Ten fish were randomly selected from each tankanaesthetized in MS 222 (Sigma) (200 mg L^{-1}) and then kept at −20°C for whole body proximate composition and mineral analysis.

Five fish from each tank were selected randomly, anaesthetized (MS 222, 200 mg L^{-1}), and then kept at −20°C for vertebrae samples. Vertebrae were removed from fish after heating fish in a microwave oven for 120 s, then lightly scrubbed and washed with distilled water to remove surrounding tissues and muscles, dried in an oven at 105°C for 6 h, extracted with 20 mL chloroform and methanol (1 : 1, v/v) for 12 h to remove lipid, and then dried.

Three fish from each tank were selected randomly, anaesthetized (MS 222, 200 mg L^{-1}) first, and then liver samples of these three fish from each tank were frozen immediately in liquid nitrogen and kept at −80°C until use. Before measuring the activity of antioxidative enzymes, the pooled livers by tank were manually homogenized in a glass homogenizer with 0.7% NaCl (w/v) to 10% homogenate.

Chemical compositions of the dried whole fish, experimental diets, pretreated vertebrae and feces were examined using the following procedure: body ash content and vertebrae ash content by incinerating samples at 550°C for 18 h in a muffle furnace, then wet digested with HCl and HNO_3 subsequently for the analysis of P content by the molybdovanadate method [21]; crude protein (N × 6.25) by the Kjeldahl method [21]; crude lipid by extraction with petroleum ether for 12 h in a Soxhlet extractor [21]; moisture content by drying to constant weight at 105°C for 6 h [21]. Body calcium and vertebrae calcium contents were analyzed by atomic absorption spectrophotometer (Varian AA240FS Fast Sequential AA Spectrometer, USA). Chromium content of experimental diets and feces was determined using the procedure of Bolin et al. [22].

Activities of liver superoxide dismutase (SOD), catalase (CAT), and glutathione peroxidase (GSH-Px) and content of malonaldehyde (MDA) were all analyzed spectrophotometrically using diagnostic reagent kits (Nanjing Jiancheng Bioengineering Institute, China).

2.4. Calculation and Statistical Analysis. Growth parameters were calculated according to the following equations:

$$\text{Specific growth rate } \left(\text{SGR \% day}^{-1}\right) = 100 \times \frac{[\text{Ln(final weight)} - \text{Ln(initial weight)}]}{\text{duration (days)}},$$

$$\text{Feed efficiency (FE \%)} = 100 \times \frac{\text{wet weight gain}}{\text{dry feed intake}},$$

$$\text{Feeding rate } \left(\text{FR \% BW day}^{-1}\right) = 100 \times \frac{\text{dry feed intake}}{[\text{days} \times (\text{FBW} + \text{IBW})/2]},$$

$$\text{Survival (\%)} = 100 \times \frac{\text{final numbers of fish}}{\text{initial numbers of fish}},$$

$$\text{Protein efficiency ratio (PER \%)} = \frac{\text{weight gain}}{\text{crude protein intake}},$$

$$\text{Protein retention efficiency (PRE \%)} = 100 \times \left(\frac{\text{protein retained in fish body}}{\text{protein intake}}\right),$$

$$\text{Apparent digestibility coefficient of dry matter (ADCd \%)} = 100 \times \left[1 - \left(\frac{Cr_2O_3 \text{ in the diet}}{Cr_2O_3 \text{ in the feces}}\right)\right],$$

$$\text{Apparent digestibility coefficient of protein (ADCp \%)} = 100 \times \left[1 - \left(\frac{Cr_2O_3 \text{ in the diet}}{Cr_2O_3 \text{ in the feces}}\right) \times \left(\frac{\text{crude protein in feces}}{\text{crude protein in the diet}}\right)\right],$$

$$\text{Apparent digestibility coefficient of P (ADCph \%)} = 100 \times \left[1 - \left(\frac{Cr_2O_3 \text{ in the diet}}{Cr_2O_3 \text{ in the feces}}\right) \times \left(\frac{\text{P in feces}}{\text{P in the diet}}\right)\right],$$

$$\text{Efficiency of phosphorus (P) utilization (\%)} = 100 \times \left[\frac{\text{(final phosphorus fish content)}}{\text{phosphorus intake}} - \frac{\text{(initial phosphorus fish content)}}{\text{phosphorus intake}}\right],$$

$$\text{Available P content of the diets} = \text{total P content} \times \text{apparent digestibility coefficient of P (ADCph) of the diets.} \quad (1)$$

Since we wanted to compare the levels of the dietary available P to see if change in the levels leads to a significant change in the response, we chose the model of one-way analysis of variance (ANOVA) to analyze all the relative responses. When differences among levels were identified, Duncan's multiple-range tests were used to determine the significant differences among different level treatment means of dietary available P at $\alpha = 0.05$ (Statistica 8.0 software, StatSoft Inc, Tulsa, Oklahoma). The data were presented as means ± SE.

To estimate maximum vertebrae P, we fitted a quadratic regression line to vertebrae P as a function of dietary available P level using SPSS 16.0 (SPSS Inc, Chicago, Ill, USA).

3. Results

3.1. Apparent Digestibility, Efficiency of P Utilization, and Feces P. Apparent digestibility coefficient of P (ADCph), dry matter and protein digestibility was shown in Table 2. There was no significant difference in dry matter and protein digestibility (ADCd and ADCp) ($P > 0.05$) among all treatments. Apparent digestibility of P (ADCph) significantly increased with increasing dietary available P up to the 0.81% level ($P < 0.05$) and then plateaued with further increases in dietary available P. Efficiency of P utilization decreased ($P < 0.05$) and feces P content increased with the increase of the dietary P level (Table 2).

3.2. Growth Performance. Effects of dietary available P on growth performance were shown in Table 3. The final body weight (FBW), specific growth rate (SGR), and feeding rate (FR) were all significantly improved by dietary available P up to 0.81% ($P < 0.05$) and then significantly decreased compared to the 0.81% dietary group ($P < 0.05$). The protein efficiency ratio (PER) of the 0.81% and 1.57% groups was significantly higher than that of the other groups ($P < 0.05$). However, dietary available P had no significant effects on feed efficiency (FE), protein retention efficiency (PRE), and survival rate.

3.3. Body Composition. Dietary available P level significantly affected yellow catfish whole body crude lipid, ash, Ca, vertebrae P, Ca, and ash content ($P < 0.05$) (Table 4). With the increase of dietary available P, body crude lipid content significantly decreased ($P < 0.05$). Body ash, vertebrae ash, and vertebrae P content increased until available P reached 1.31% ($P < 0.05$), then decreased. Quadratic regression analysis showed that the maximum vertebrae P accumulation occurred at a dietary available P of 1.21% (Figure 1).

3.4. Antioxidant Property. Dietary available P content significantly affected hepatic SOD and CAT activity and MDA content ($P < 0.05$) (Table 5). Fish in the highest dietary available P content (1.57%) group had higher SOD, CAT activity, and MDA content than all the other groups ($P < 0.05$). There was no significant difference in GSH-Px activity among all the groups ($P > 0.05$).

4. Discussion

In the present study, we found the efficiency of P utilization increased with decreasing dietary available P. There are two patterns for P absorption in animals. When the concentration of inorganic P is high in the lumen, passive

TABLE 2: Effects of dietary available P level on apparent digestibility coefficient (ADC), P utilization efficiency, and feces P content in yellow catfish fed experimental diets for eight weeks (Mean ± SE, $n = 3$).

Available P in diet (%)	0.33	0.56	0.81	1.15	1.31	1.57
Dry matter (ADCd, %)	87.21 ± 2.94	83.21 ± 2.58	87.17 ± 1.37	89.29 ± 1.29	88.08 ± 2.69	88.21 ± 0.04
Protein (ADCp, %)	98.22 ± 0.41	96.89 ± 0.43	97.48 ± 0.13	97.80 ± 0.36	97.38 ± 0.65	97.47 ± 0.06
P (ADCph, %)	87.01 ± 3.40^{b}	89.43 ± 1.26^{bc}	90.47±0.67^{abc}	94.18 ± 0.50^{a}	92.57 ± 1.59^{ac}	92.06 ± 0.20^{ac}
Efficiency of P utilization (%)	77.46 ± 7.45^{a}	57.99 ± 5.37^{ab}	54.45 ± 3.81^{b}	46.38 ± 7.43^{b}	37.51 ± 3.41^{b}	45.18± 10.30^{b}
Feces P (g kg^{-1} dry matter)	0.38 ± 0.01^{d}	0.40 ± 0.02^{d}	0.67 ± 0.03^{c}	0.67 ± 0.03^{c}	0.89 ± 0.01^{b}	1.15 ± 0.03^{a}

Note: values with different letters within the same row are significantly different ($P < 0.05$).

TABLE 3: The growth performance of yellow catfish under different dietary treatments for eight weeks (Mean ± SE, $n = 3$).

Available P in diet (%)	0.33	0.56	0.81	1.15	1.31	1.57
IBW (g)	3.02 ± 0.05	3.10 ± 0.03	3.03 ± 0.09	3.00 ± 0.07	3.14 ± 0.06	3.23 ± 0.01
FBW (g)	6.08 ± 0.09^{bc}	6.44 ± 0.08^{b}	7.51 ± 0.36^{a}	5.45 ± 0.23^{c}	6.19 ± 0.36^{bc}	6.58 ± 0.21^{b}
SGR (% day^{-1})	1.25 ± 0.01^{bc}	1.31 ± 0.02^{b}	1.62 ± 1.10^{a}	1.06 ± 0.04^{c}	1.21 ± 0.08^{bc}	1.27 ± 0.06^{b}
FR (% BW day^{-1})	1.74 ± 0.08^{b}	1.70 ± 0.02^{b}	1.93 ± 0.02^{a}	1.46 ± 0.06^{c}	1.57 ± 0.04^{c}	1.54 ± 0.01^{c}
FE (%)	64.40 ± 1.81	68.57 ± 1.07	73.04 ± 3.69	64.92 ± 4.05	69.45 ± 2.59	76.31 ± 3.83
PER (%)	1.36 ± 0.04^{b}	1.45 ± 0.04^{b}	1.56 ± 0.11^{ab}	1.35 ± 0.10^{b}	1.45 ± 0.04^{b}	1.70 ± 0.09^{a}
PRE (%)	17.63 ± 0.94	19.26 ± 3.29	21.33 ± 1.72	21.75 ± 1.02	19.91 ± 1.96	21.59 ± 2.61
Survival rate (%)	92.22 ± 0.56	91.67 ± 1.67	89.44 ± 2.00	90.56 ± 2.00	92.78 ± 2.42	96.11 ± 0.56

Note: IBW: initial body weight; FBW: final body weight; SGR: specific growth rate; FR: feeding rate; FE: feed efficiency; PER: protein efficiency ratio; PRE: protein retention efficiency.
Values with different letters within the same row are significantly different ($P < 0.05$).

TABLE 4: Effects of dietary available P level on body composition of yellow catfish for eight weeks (Mean ± SE, $n = 3$).

Available P in diet (%)	Initial	0.33	0.56	0.81	1.15	1.31	1.57
Whole body (% of wet weight)							
Moisture	76.95 ± 0.60	74.20 ± 1.62	75.73 ± 1.48	74.26 ± 0.78	74.44 ± 0.99	75.07 ± 1.00	76.89 ± 1.35
Crude protein	12.79 ± 0.40	12.93 ± 0.50	13.01 ± 1.00	13.28 ± 0.23	14.10 ± 0.65	13.24 ± 0.68	12.75 ± 0.67
Crude lipid	3.83 ± 0.21^{c}	6.49 ± 0.70^{a}	4.57 ± 0.60^{bc}	5.47 ± 0.61^{ab}	4.43 ± 0.26^{bc}	4.44 ± 0.25^{bc}	3.62 ± 0.43^{c}
Ash	3.36 ± 0.13^{bd}	3.27 ± 0.16^{d}	3.63 ± 0.12^{bd}	3.97 ± 0.23^{abc}	4.31 ± 0.19^{a}	4.46 ± 0.34^{a}	4.14 ± 0.17^{ab}
Body P	0.64 ± 0.07	0.63 ± 0.02	0.66 ± 0.02	0.71 ± 0.04	0.81 ± 0.05	0.80 ± 0.04	0.81 ± 0.09
Body Ca	0.26 ± 0.02^{c}	0.30 ± 0.03^{bc}	0.33 ± 0.01^{ab}	0.37 ± 0.03^{a}	0.38 ± 0.01^{a}	0.38 ± 0.01^{a}	0.38 ± 0.01^{a}
Vertebrae (P and Ca, g kg^{-1}; ash, % of dry matter)							
P	72.00	59.58 ± 2.92^{c}	64.66±0.30^{bc}	66.99±1.74^{ab}	69.28±2.07^{ab}	72.26 ± 1.72^{a}	67.46 ± 0.86^{ab}
Ca	38.78	28.51 ± 1.19^{b}	34.09 ± 0.93^{a}	33.67 ± 2.13^{a}	34.15 ± 0.79^{a}	35.67 ± 2.36^{a}	35.84 ± 0.96^{a}
Ash	38.35	28.49 ± 1.10^{c}	34.63 ± 0.21^{b}	35.60 ± 0.98^{b}	37.11±0.86^{ab}	39.08 ± 0.68^{a}	36.58 ± 0.48^{ab}

Note: values with different letters within the same row are significantly different ($P < 0.05$).

TABLE 5: Effects of dietary available P level on hepatic biochemical indicators of yellow catfish for eight weeks (Mean ± SE, $n = 3$).

% P in diet	0.33	0.56	0.81	1.15	1.31	1.57
SOD (U mgpro^{-1})	33.94 ± 2.27^{c}	37.09 ± 4.07^{bc}	46.19 ± 5.37^{ab}	37.74 ± 0.69^{bc}	39.98 ± 3.47^{bc}	56.46 ± 4.92^{a}
CAT (U mgpro^{-1})	4.87 ± 0.54^{b}	4.75 ± 0.44^{b}	5.68 ± 0.42^{ab}	4.59 ± 0.27^{b}	4.79 ± 0.32^{b}	6.97 ± 0.63^{a}
MDA (nmol mgpro^{-1})	0.48 ± 0.06^{b}	0.50 ± 0.04^{b}	0.77 ± 0.06^{a}	0.45 ± 0.03^{b}	0.54 ± 0.07^{b}	0.89 ± 0.11^{a}
GSH-Px (U)	2.02 ± 0.44	2.66 ± 0.61	1.89 ± 0.50	1.47 ± 0.58	2.18 ± 0.33	2.43 ± 0.56

Note: values in the same row with different letters are significantly different ($P < 0.05$).
SOD: superoxide dismutase; CAT: catalase; GSH-Px: glutathione peroxidase; MDA: malonaldehyde.

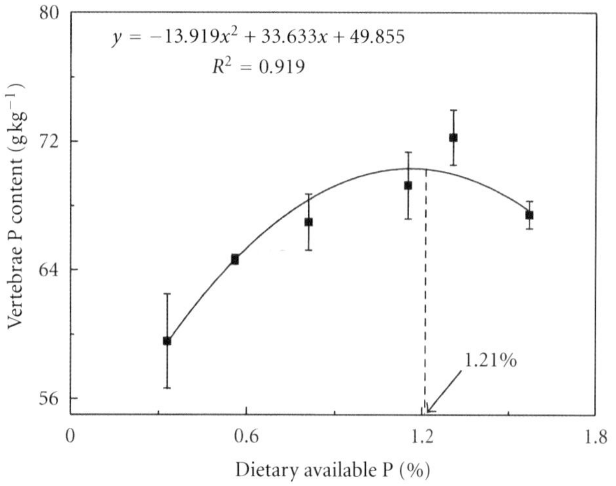

FIGURE 1: Effect of dietary available P level on vertebrae P content of juvenile yellow catfish. The predicted maximum level occurred at dietary available P equal to 1.21%, based on quadratic regression analysis.

transportation of P is predominant; when the concentration of P is low, active transportation of P via NaPi cotransporter is predominant [23]. The present study showed that lower dietary P level led to higher P utilization; similar results were observed in rainbow trout [24] and black sea bream [25]. However, these authors didn't give any explanation on this observed phenomenon. We inferred that low dietary P content stimulated the active transportation of P in the intestine and thus increased P absorption.

Effects of dietary P level on growth performance were reported in many fish species. Improved growth was seen in common carp [26], juvenile haddock [2], juvenile silver perch [27], and juvenile black sea bream [26]. However, other studies reported that dietary P level did not change the growth of sea bass [28] and Atlantic salmon [29]. Animal growth depends on several factors, including age, stage of development, diet composition, duration of experiment, health, and rearing condition. Young animals were more sensitive to nutrient deficiency than those at a later stage of development [2]. In the current study, juvenile yellow catfish (average initial body weight was about 3 g) were sensitive to dietary P content and showed different growth performance under different dietary P treatments. However, the improved growth performance was only observed until the dietary available P level reached 0.81%, indicating that juvenile yellow catfish needed about 0.8% dietary available P to obtain maximum growth. There were several reports about catfish dietary available P requirements based on channel catfish (*Ictalurus punctatus*). Andrews et al. [18] reported that the P requirement of catfish is 0.8 percent of available P in practical-type diets. However, Lovell [19] and Wilson et al. [20] reevaluated the P requirement using chemically defined diets and estimated it to be approximately 0.42 percent available P. NRC [1] recommended the appropriate dietary available P to be 0.45 percent for channel catfish. However, in the present study, this small omnivorous fish gained highest growth at 0.81% dietary available P. The difference between yellow catfish and channel catfish was probably due to the species specific, different growth rate, and ingredients content of the diets or the culture system.

Dietary P level had no effects on fish whole body moisture and crude protein content in the present study, which was similar to findings in red sea bream [30] and European sea bass [31]. However, crude lipid content decreased with increasing level of dietary P in our experiment. An inverse relationship between whole body crude lipid content and dietary P was also reported in channel catfish [32], red sea bream [30, 33], common carp [34], juvenile haddock [2], Japanese sea bass [35], large yellow croaker [36], and juvenile black sea bream [25]. Since P plays an important role in energy metabolism and lipid beta oxidation, P deficiency will cause cellular hypoxia and thus produce more lipid. The reduction in the lipid content of the fish fed higher levels of P may be due to enhancement of P oxidation of fatty acids, increase in glycogenesis or some type of repartitioning effect, resulting in increased deposition of protein and reduced deposition of lipid [32].

The whole-body or vertebrae ash and P levels had been commonly used as indicators of dietary P status in fish nutrition studies [4, 25, 36–38]. Signs of P deficiency are poor bone mineralization and bad growth performance. Dietary available P levels greatly affected the ash, calcium, and P contents both of the whole body and vertebrae of carp [39]. In our study, whole-body ash, vertebrae, ash and vertebrae P content of juvenile yellow catfish increased until dietary available P level reached 1.31% and then decreased at the 1.57% dietary available P level. Quadratic analysis based on vertebrae P contents indicated maximum vertebrae P at a dietary available P of 1.21%, higher than the requirement of 0.81% dietary available P for maximum growth. Similar findings were reported in large yellow croaker [36] and black sea bream [25]. The minimum available P requirement for maximum growth of large yellow croaker was 0.70%; however, based on the P content in either vertebrae or whole body, the requirements were 0.89% and 0.91%, respectively. In black sea bream, maximum weight gain was obtained at dietary available P concentration of 0.55%; however, quadratic analysis based on P content in vertebrae indicated that the requirement was 0.87%. The dietary P requirement for bone mineralization was usually higher than that for maximum growth [32, 40]. Differences among empirically established P requirements may be due in part to differences in the choice of response variable used [41]. The requirement must depend on what is considered a physiologically, economically, or environmentally important trait [32]. Thus, in the present study, if growth rate is used as a marker the requirement is 0.8%, but if maximum vertebrae P content is applied the requirement is 1.2%. If the dietary available P level is higher than 0.8% the growth is reduced. Considering the economic cost and environmental cost, dietary available P level of 0.8% is recommended for young yellow catfish.

Only a few preliminary researches have been reported about the roles of minerals in the antioxidant system of aquatic animals, including selenium [42], iron [43], and zinc [44], no research concerns the role of phosphorus in antioxidant defense systems in fish. Since P is important in energy metabolism and lipid beta oxidation, lipid peroxidation is supposed to be susceptible to dietary P level. In order to elaborate the basic oxidative functional responses of yellow catfish under different dietary P treatments so to determine whether they could be used as indicators of the stimulatory activity of dietary P, we measured hepatic SOD, CAT, and GPx activities and the content of MDA. We found hepatic SOD, CAT, and MDA contents except GPx activities were significantly affected by dietary available P level. Unlike in plant, no antioxidant responses were observed in low P groups (0.33% and 0.56%) compared to high P groups (1.57%).

The effect of oral P exposure was reported in the form of white phosphorus [45]. LD_{50} values of 4.82 mg kg^{-1} and 4.85 mg kg^{-1} were reported for female and male mice, respectively [46]. Fish fed with the highest dietary available P (1.57%) had the highest hepatic SOD and CAT activities and highest MDA content. The SOD in fish is known to be induced in those tissues that are suffering from oxidative stress [47]. Ou et al. [48] claimed that the induction of these antioxidant enzymes is an important protective mechanism to minimize cell oxidative damage in unfavorable environments. In our study, high-level dietary P induced the antioxidative responses in juvenile yellow catfish. It is possible that the fish in this study were under an oxidative stress at the high levels of dietary available P which no longer served as a required nutrient but tended to be a stressor. Since SOD and CAT play the major role in the process of eliminating the free radicals [12], hepatic SOD and CAT were upregulated in juvenile yellow catfish in order to reduce free radicals produced by high dietary P. However, upregulated levels of SOD and CAT were not enough to eliminate the free radicals in fish fed 1.57% dietary available P, which led to the accumulation of the final product of lipid peroxidation, and finally the damage of cell membrane could not be restored in this group of fish.

5. Conclusions

This was the first study to show that dietary available P level affected hepatic antioxidant responses in fish. The current study indicated that the decrease of dietary available P increased the efficiency of P utilization and the body lipid content. However, vertebrae P also decreased, which could affect the bone mineralization of juvenile yellow catfish. Juvenile yellow catfish were subjected to oxidant damage and could not be reduced or eradicated by their own antioxidant defense system under the condition of high dietary P content. Therefore, as an essential nutrient for growth, bone mineralization, and maintaining the antioxidant property of this species, it is very important to optimize the dietary P content. In order to achieve the maximum growth rate, the optimal dietary available P of juvenile yellow catfish were estimated to be 0.81%. Based on maximum vertebrae P content, the optimal dietary available P of juvenile yellow catfish were estimated to be 1.21%.

Acknowledgments

This research was funded by the National Natural Science Foundation of China (Project no. 4004-094102) and the State Key Laboratory of Freshwater Ecology and Biotechnology (Project no. 2010FB11). The authors also thanked Dr. Min Xue from Chinese Academy of Agricultural Sciences for the help in feed formulation and Xuewen Lei, Chaofan Wang, and Qiao Liu for their great help during feeding trial and sample analysis.

References

[1] NRC, *Nutrient Requirements of Fish and Shrimp*, The National Academies Press, Washington, DC, USA, 2011.

[2] P. K. Roy and S. P. Lall, "Dietary phosphorus requirement of juvenile haddock (*Melanogrammus aeglefinus L.*)," *Aquaculture*, vol. 221, no. 1–4, pp. 451–468, 2003.

[3] R. M. Coloso, S. P. Basantes, K. King et al., "Effect of dietary phosphorus and vitamin D3 on phosphorus levels in effluent from the experimental culture of rainbow trout (*Oncorhynchus mykiss*)," *Aquaculture*, vol. 202, no. 1-2, pp. 145–161, 2001.

[4] R. W. Hardy, W.T. Fairgrieve, and T. M. Scott, "Periodic feeding of low-phosphorus diet and phosphorus retention in rainbow trout *Oncorhynchus mykiss*," in *Fish Nutrition Practice*, S. J. Kauchik and P. Luquet, Eds., no. 61, pp. 403–412, Les Colloques, INRA, Paris, France, 1993.

[5] R. K. Tewari, P. Kumar, N. Tewari, S. Srivastava, and P. N. Sharma, "Macronutrient deficiencies and differential antioxidant responses—influence on the activity and expression of superoxide dismutase in maize," *Plant Science*, vol. 166, no. 3, pp. 687–694, 2004.

[6] I. Juszczuk, M. Malusa, and A. Rychter, "Phosphate deficiency induced oxidative stress in bean (*Phaseolus vulgaris L.*)," in *Development in Plant and Soil Sciences*, W. J. Horst, M.K. Schenk, A. Bürkert et al., Eds., vol. 92 of *Plant Nutrition—Food Security and Sustainability of Agro-Ecosystems*, pp. 148–149, Kluver Academic Publishers, Dordecht, The Netherlands, 2002.

[7] O. T. Zribi, C. Abdelly, and A. Debez, "Interactive effects of salinity and phosphorus availability on growth, water relations, nutritional status and photosynthetic activity of barley (*Hordeum vulgare L.*)," *Plant Biology*, vol. 13, no. 6, pp. 872–880, 2011.

[8] Y. Yao, H. Sun, F. Xu, X. Zhang, and S. Liu, "Comparative proteome analysis of metabolic changes by low phosphorus stress in two *Brassica napus* genotypes," *Planta*, vol. 233, no. 3, pp. 523–537, 2011.

[9] R. G. Alscher, J. L. Donahue, and C. L. Cramer, "Reactive oxygen species and antioxidants: relationships in green cells," *Physiologia Plantarum*, vol. 100, no. 2, pp. 224–233, 1997.

[10] C. H. Foyer, H. Lopez-Delgado, J. F. Dat, and I. M. Scott, "Hydrogen peroxide- and glutathione-associated mechanisms of acclimatory stress tolerance and signalling," *Physiologia Plantarum*, vol. 100, no. 2, pp. 241–254, 1997.

[11] G. Noctor and C. H. Foyer, "Ascorbate and glutathione: keeping active oxygen under control," *Annual Review of Plant Biology*, vol. 49, pp. 249–279, 1998.

[12] M. Valko, D. Leibfritz, J. Moncol, M. T. D. Cronin, M. Mazur, and J. Telser, "Free radicals and antioxidants in normal physiological functions and human disease," *International Journal of Biochemistry and Cell Biology*, vol. 39, no. 1, pp. 44–84, 2007.

[13] I. Ahmad, T. Hamid, M. Fatima et al., "Induction of hepatic antioxidants in freshwater catfish (*Channa punctatus Bloch*) is a biomarker of paper mill effluent exposure," *Biochimica et Biophysica Acta*, vol. 1523, no. 1, pp. 37–48, 2000.

[14] B. Chance, J. S. Leigh, and J. Kent, "Multiple controls of oxidative metabolism in living tissues as studied by phosphorus magnetic resonance," *Proceedings of the National Academy of Sciences of the United States of America*, vol. 83, no. 24, pp. 9458–9462, 1986.

[15] S. D. Walwadkar, A. N. Suryakar, R. V. Katkam, K. M. Kumbar, and R. D. Ankush, "Oxidative stress and calcium-phosphorus levels in rheumatoid arthritis," *Indian Journal of Clinical Biochemistry*, vol. 21, no. 2, pp. 134–137, 2006.

[16] *China Fishery Statistical Yearbook*, Fishery Bureau of Ministry of Agriculture, China Agriculture Press, 2010.

[17] H. J. Wang, X. M. Liang, P. H. Jiang, J. Wang, S. K. Wu, and H. Z. Wang, "TN : TTP ratio and planktivorous fish do not affect nutrient-chlorophyll relationships in shallow lakes," *Freshwater Biology*, vol. 53, no. 5, pp. 935–944, 2008.

[18] J. W. Andrews, T. Murai, and C. Campbell, "Effects of dietary calcium and phosphorus on growth, food conversion, bone ash and hematocrit levels of catfish," *Journal of Nutrition*, vol. 103, no. 5, pp. 766–771, 1973.

[19] R. T. Lovell, "Dietary phosphorus requirement of channel catfish (*Ictalurus punctatus*)," *Transactions of the American Fisheries Society*, vol. 107, no. 4, pp. 617–621, 1978.

[20] R. P. Wilson, E. H. Robinson, D. M. Gatlin, and W. E. Poe, "Dietary phosphorus requirement of channel catfish," *Journal of Nutrition*, vol. 112, no. 6, pp. 1197–1202, 1982.

[21] AOAC, *Official Methods of Analysis*, Association of Official Analytical Chemists, Washington, DC, USA, 16th edition, 1998.

[22] D. W. Bolin, R. P. King, and E. W. Klosterman, "A simplified method for the determination of chromic oxide (Cr_2O_3) when used as an index substance," *Science*, vol. 116, no. 3023, pp. 634–635, 1952.

[23] S. H. Sugiura and R. P. Ferraris, "Contributions of different NaPi cotransporter isoforms to dietary regulation of P transport in the pyloric caeca and intestine of rainbow trout," *Journal of Experimental Biology*, vol. 207, no. 12, pp. 2055–2064, 2004.

[24] E. M. Avila, H. Tu, S. Basantes, and R. P. Ferraris, "Dietary phosphorus regulates intestinal transport and plasma concentrations of phosphate in rainbow trout," *Journal of Comparative Physiology. B*, vol. 170, no. 3, pp. 201–209, 2000.

[25] Q. Shao, J. Ma, Z. Xu, W. Hu, J. Xu, and S. Xie, "Dietary phosphorus requirement of juvenile black seabream, *Sparus macrocephalus*," *Aquaculture*, vol. 277, no. 1-2, pp. 92–100, 2008.

[26] B. Hepher and S. Sandbank, "The effect of phosphorus supplementation to common carp diets on fish growth," *Aquaculture*, vol. 36, no. 4, pp. 323–332, 1984.

[27] S. D. Yang, T. S. Lin, F. G. Liu, and C. H. Liou, "Influence of dietary phosphorus levels on growth, metabolic response and body composition of juvenile silver perch (*Bidyanus bidyanus*)," *Aquaculture*, vol. 253, no. 1–4, pp. 592–601, 2006.

[28] M. Boonyaratpalin, "Effects of ash and inorganic phosphorus in diets on growth and mineral composition of seabass *Lates calcarifer* (Bloch)," *Aquaculture Research*, vol. 32, supplement 1, pp. 53–59, 2001.

[29] J. Vielma and S. P. Lall, "Control of phosphorus homeostasis of Atlantic salmon (*Salmo salar*) in fresh water," *Fish Physiology and Biochemistry*, vol. 19, no. 1, pp. 83–93, 1998.

[30] S. Sakamoto and Y. Yone, "Effects of dietary phosphorus level on chemical composition of red sea bream," *Bulletin of the Japanese Society of Scientific Fisheries*, vol. 44, pp. 227–229, 1978.

[31] A. Oliva-Teles and A. Pimentel-Rodrigues, "Phosphorus requirement of European sea bass (*Dicentrarchus labrax L.*) juveniles," *Aquaculture Research*, vol. 35, no. 7, pp. 636–642, 2004.

[32] J. C. Eya and R. T. Lovell, "Available phosphorus requirements of food-size channel catfish (*Ictalurus punctatus*) fed practical diets in ponds," *Aquaculture*, vol. 154, no. 3-4, pp. 283–291, 1997.

[33] S. Sakamoto and Y. Yone, "A principal source of deposited lipid in phosphorus deficient Red Sea bream," *Bulletin of the Japanese Society of Scientific Fisheries*, vol. 46, pp. 1227–1230, 1980.

[34] M. Takeuchi and J. Nakazoe, "Effect of dietary phosphorus on lipid content and its composition in carp," *Bulletin of the Japanese Society of Scientific Fisheries*, vol. 47, pp. 347–352, 1981.

[35] C. Zhang, K. Mai, Q. Ai et al., "Dietary phosphorus requirement of juvenile Japanese seabass, *Lateolabrax japonicus*," *Aquaculture*, vol. 255, no. 1–4, pp. 201–209, 2006.

[36] K. Mai, C. Zhang, Q. Ai et al., "Dietary phosphorus requirement of large yellow croaker, *Pseudosciaena crocea* R," *Aquaculture*, vol. 251, no. 2-4, pp. 346–353, 2006.

[37] D. I. Skonberg, L. Yogev, R. W. Hardy, and F. M. Dong, "Metabolic response to dietary phosphorus intake in rainbow trout (*Oncorhynchus mykiss*)," *Aquaculture*, vol. 157, no. 1-2, pp. 11–24, 1997.

[38] Z. Luo, X. Y. Tan, X. Liu, and W. M. Wang, "Dietary total phosphorus requirement of juvenile yellow catfish *Pelteobagrus fulvidraco*," *Aquaculture International*, vol. 18, no. 5, pp. 897–908, 2010.

[39] C. Ogino and H. Takeda, "Mineral requirements in fish. III. Calcium and phosphorus requirements in carp," *Bulletin of the Japanese Society of Scientific Fisheries*, vol. 42, pp. 793–799, 1976.

[40] P. P. Ketaren, E. S. Batterham, E. Belinda, E. B. Dettmann, and D. J. Farrell, "Phosphorus studies in pigs. 2. Assessing phosphorus availability for pigs and rats," *British Journal of Nutrition*, vol. 70, no. 1, pp. 269–288, 1993.

[41] T. Åsgård and K. D. Shearer, "Dietary phosphorus requirement of juvenile Atlantic salmon, *Salmo salar* L," *Aquaculture Nutrition*, vol. 3, no. 1, pp. 17–23, 1997.

[42] Y. H. Lin and S. Y. Shiau, "Dietary selenium requirements of juvenile grouper, *Epinephelus malabaricus*," *Aquaculture*, vol. 250, no. 1-2, pp. 356–363, 2005.

[43] F. Andersen, B. Lygren, A. Maage, and R. Waagbø, "Interaction between two dietary levels of iron and two forms of ascorbic acid and the effect on growth, antioxidant status and some non-specific immune parameters in Atlantic salmon (*Salmo salar*) smolts," *Aquaculture*, vol. 161, no. 1–4, pp. 437–451, 1998.

[44] Z. Kucukbay, H. Yazlak, N. Sahin et al., "Zinc picolinate supplementation decreases oxidative stress in rainbow trout (*Oncorhynchus mykiss*)," *Aquaculture*, vol. 257, no. 1–4, pp. 465–469, 2006.

[45] Sciences International Inc., *Toxicological Profile for White Phosphorus*, CAS no. 7723-14-0, US Department of Health and Human Services, Public Health Service, Agency for Toxic Substances and Disease Registry, 1997.

[46] C. C. Lee, J.V. Dilley, J.R. Hodgson, D.O. Helton, and W. J. Wiegand, "Mammalian toxicity of munition compounds.

Phase I. Acute oral toxicity primary skin and eye irritation, dermal sensitization, and disposition and metabolism," Contract DAMD17-74-C-4073, US Army Medical Research and Development Command, Washington, DC, USA, 1975.

[47] T. Sakai, H. Murata, K. Y. Sekiya, and M. Ukawa, "Effects of dietary lipid peroxides contents on in vitro lipid peroxidation, α-tocopherol contents and superoxide dismutase and glutathione peroxidase activities in the liver of yellowtail," *Bulletin of the Japanese Society of Scientific Fisheries*, vol. 58, no. 8, pp. 1483–1486, 1992.

[48] M. M. Ou, Y. Wang, and W. M. Cai, "Physiological and biochemical changes in *Microcystis aeruginosa Qutz.* in phosphorus limitation," *Journal of Integrative Plant Biology*, vol. 47, no. 6, pp. 692–702, 2005.

17

Comparing the Effect of Oral Supplementation of Vitamin E, Injective Vitamin E and Selenium or Both during Late Pregnancy on Production and Reproductive Performance and Immune Function of Dairy Cows and Calves

Farokh Kafilzadeh,[1] Habibollah Kheirmanesh,[1] Hamed Karami Shabankareh,[1] Mohhamad Reza Targhibi,[1] Elaheh Maleki,[1] Mahdi Ebrahimi,[2] and Goh Yong Meng[2,3]

[1] *Department of Animal Science, Faculty of Agriculture, Razi University, Kermanshah, Iran*
[2] *Department of Veterinary Preclinical Sciences, Faculty of Veterinary Medicine, Universiti Putra Malaysia (UPM), 43400 Serdang, Selangor, Malaysia*
[3] *Institute of Tropical Agriculture, Universiti Putra Malaysia, 43400 Serdang, Selangor, Malaysia*

Correspondence should be addressed to Goh Yong Meng; ymgoh@upm.edu.my

Academic Editor: Joaquin Sanchez

The object of this study was to determine the effect of prepartum supplementation of vitamin E with or without injective vitamin E and selenium (Se) on productive and reproductive performances and immune function in dairy cows. Sixty multiparous Holstein dairy cows were divided randomly into three groups at the end of gestation. Cows in each group received one of three treatments: (1) a single intramuscular (im) injection of vit. E + selenium 3 weeks prepartum; (2) daily supplementation of oral vit. E given from 3 weeks prepartum to parturition; (3) injective vit. E + Se with daily supplementation of oral vit. E. Blood samples were collected from cows at calving and from calves at 0 and 7 days of age. Concentration of IgG in serum of cows and calves as well as in colostrum was determined. No significant differences among treatments occurred in the concentrations of IgG, animal, and calf production and reproduction performance. Due to the lack of significant difference between injection and oral supplementation, it is recommended to replace the injection with oral supplementation.

1. Introduction

Most diseases in dairy cows occur at or just after calving, which is a period associated with immune suppression, resulting in an increased susceptibility to infections [1, 2]. Prepartum immune suppression is multifactorial but is associated with endocrine changes and decreased intake of critical nutrients [3]. Vitamin E is a fat-soluble vitamin and is not synthesized in the rumen. The vitamin E requirement must therefore be provided in the field. However, the vitamin E content of the basal diet is highly variable and is not known in most situations. Although vitamin E content is high in fresh grass, it markedly reduces during storage and conservation [4]. Therefore, NRC [5] recommends that the total vitamin E requirement should be given via dietary supplements when conserved forages are fed and that extra supplementation may be useful during periods of immune suppression, such as around calving. Vitamin E and Se are essential micronutrients that share a common biological role as antioxidants [6, 7]. The vitamin E (α-tocopherol) status of dairy cows is one important component of a well-functioning immune system because of its antioxidant effects on cows [8–10] and young dairy calves [11, 12]. At parturition, plasma concentrations of vitamin E were found to decrease by 47% [13], because of secretion of the vitamin into the udder during colostrogenesis, decreased dry matter intake (DMI) at calving, and an increased need for antioxidants during this time [13–15]. Passive transfer of colostral immunoglobulins is vital to short-term health and survival of neonates, and limited data suggest that inadequate transfer occurs in 10 to 25% of newborn beef calves [16]. Low serum immunoglobulins in young calves were related to increased incidence of disease [17]. Previous investigations have revealed that serum IgG concentrations decreased at parturition [18, 19].

Antioxidants are necessary to prevent some disorders in female reproduction [20]. Effects of Se, vitamin E, or their combination on fertility have been variable, with some studies reporting no effect [21] or an increase in fertility [22, 23]. Retained fetal membranes (RFM) occur when the placenta has not been shed within a short time after parturition. Cows with RFM have increased risks for metritis [24, 25] and mastitis [26] during early lactation. Some researchers [27] have observed a reduction in the incidence of RFM with a single injection of Se and vitamin E given approximately 21 d prepartum. In contrast, other researchers [23, 28, 29] have found no benefit of vitamin E or Se.

Smith et al. [30] were the first to report a beneficial effect of vit. E supplementation on incidence of mastitis. Feeding vit. E during dry periods until 30 days after calving resulted in 80% decrease in clinical mastitis and 60% reduction in intramammary infections [31] while Batra et al. [32] found no benefit of vit. E supplementation.

Lacetera et al. [33] reported that milk yield was higher in cows treated with Se and vitamin E than nontreated cows, but Weiss and Spears [10] showed no beneficial effect of Se or vitamin E supplementation on milk production.

Effects of Se and/or vitamin E on calf weight have been variable, with some studies reporting benefit effect [34, 35] and some reporting no effect [36, 37].

It is a common practice in all dairy farms in Iran to give an injective dose of vitamin E and Se 21 days prior to calving. Previous study [37] from our colleagues indicated a beneficial effect of double injection of vitamin E and Se (each mL contained 0.5 mg Se as sodium selenite and 50 IU of d-l-α-tocopheryl acetate) over a single injection 21 days prepartum. However, it was not clear whether that was due to the extra vitamin E, selenium, or both. The objectives of this study were to determine the effect of prepartum dietary supplementation of vitamin E in addition to or without injective vitamin E + selenium during late pregnancy on production and reproduction performance and immune system of multiparous cows and their calves.

2. Materials and Methods

This study was conducted in a large commercial dairy farm in Kermanshah province in the west of Iran. The research protocol was approved by Razi University Animal Care and Use Committee. Sixty multiparous Holstein dairy cows in late gestation were randomly assigned into three groups. Cows in each group received one of three treatments: (1) a single intramuscular injection of 20 mL vit. E + selenium, 3 weeks prepartum (each mL contained 0.5 mg Se as sodium selenite and 50 IU of d-l-α-tocopheryl acetate); (2) oral supplementation of vit. E (4000 IU vit. E from d-l-α-tocopherol acetate) given from 3 weeks prepartum to parturition; (3) injective vit. E + Se plus oral vit. E. Animals were fed a total mixed ration (TMR) containing alfalfa hay, corn silage, and concentrate according to NRC [5] (Table 1).

Table 1: Nutrient composition of precalving and postcalving experimental diets.

Item	Precalving	Postcalving
NE_l (Mcal/Kg DM)	1.52	1.69
CP (%)	15.3	19.3
RDP (%)	10.5	12.1
NDF (%)	41.8	33.9
NFC (%)	36	39.5
Ca (%)	0.71	0.95
P (%)	0.32	0.4

NE_l: net energy for lactation; CP: crude protein, RDP: ruminant degradable protein; NDF: neutral detergent fiber, NFC: nonfiber carbohydrate.

The calves were separated immediately after birth (within 15 min) and received 2 L of colostrum followed by feeding another 2 L in 8–10 hours by a nursing bottle tube. Blood samples were collected from cows at calving and from calves at 0 and 7 days of age. All blood samples were centrifuged for serum collection and then stored at −20°C. Concentrations of IgG in serum and colostrum were determined by sandwich ELISA.

After parturition, the animals were moved in with the lactating herd. Monthly milk productions of animals were recorded every 15 days until 90 DIM. Calf birth weight, the mean daily gain, and weaning weights, calving to placenta expulsion, were recorded. The case definition for RFM was failure to pass the fetal membranes by 12 h after calving and for clinical mastitis was a producer diagnosis of abnormal milk or swelling of the udder, including cows with systemic illness attributed to mastitis, within 3 months after calving.

Duncan's multiple range tests were used to test differences between means once a significant effect of treatment was indicated by ANOVA. All statistical analyses were performed using SPSS package 16 [38]. The model used is described as follows:

$$X_{ij} = \mu + T_j + \varepsilon_{ij}, \quad (1)$$

where X_{ij} is dependent variable, μ is the overall mean, T_j is the effect of treatment, and ε_{ij} is the random error.

3. Results and Discussion

No significant differences among treatments occurred in the concentrations of IgG in serum and colostrum of dairy cows (Table 2). Reddy et al. [39] observed a trend for greater titer values for those given 125 IU of vitamin E daily compared with cattle receiving no vitamin E. But Lacetera et al. [33] found that administration of 5 mg of Se in sodium selenite form and 25 IU of vitamin E/100 kg of body weight of cows did not affect plasma IgG concentrations in cows. Similarly, no change in IgG was observed when ewes were supplemented with vitamin E [40].

TABLE 2: Effect of oral supplementation of vitamin E with or without injective vitamin E on immunoglobin concentrations (mg/dL) in blood and colostrums.

Immunoglobulin concentration (mg/dL)	Treatments		
	Injection	Injections + oral	Oral
Cattles blood serum at parturition	2039 ± 39	2128 ± 40	2118 ± 38
Calves blood serum at birth	132 ± 17	153 ± 22	129 ± 22
Calves blood serum at day 7	1312 ± 27	1279 ± 22	1216 ± 22
Colostrum at parturition	6097 ± 32	6012 ± 31	6346 ± 34

Because of placenta layer in cattle, there was no placental transfer of immunoglobulin, and the newborn calf is dependent upon colostrum for passive immunity [39]. The lack of difference in serum IgG of calves, in the present study, supplemented with both forms of vit. E could probably be due to the variation in absorptive ability among calves or to the sufficiency of vit. E used in only injective or oral supplemented groups, which could have partially masked the enhancing effect. A previous report from the same farm showed no significant differences in concentration of IgG in serum and colostrum. No change in colostral IgG to vit. E supplementation has been reported by others in ewes [40] and in cows [33, 41].

Effect of treatment on birth weight, daily gain, and weaning weight was not significant because of the sufficiency of vitamin E and Se level in all experimental groups (Table 3). Cohen et al. [42] reported that precalving Se and vitamin E injections had no effect on calf birth weight, daily gain, and weaning weight compared with control, when cows were in marginal (95 μg/L) selenium status. Other investigators have also reported no significant impact of Se and/or vit. E supplementation of dams on body weight gain of their calves [21, 36, 37].

There was no effect of treatment on milk yield, fat percentage and yield, and the incidence of clinical mastitis (Tables 4 and 5). It is generally accepted that the performance of lactating dairy cows can be affected by vitamin E and Se status during the parturient period [33, 43]. Lacetera et al. [33] reported that milk production increased by 10% in cows supplemented with 25 IU of vitamin E and 5 mg Se per 100 kg of body weight. Moeini et al. [37] also showed that milk production during 8 weeks of lactation was higher when a double injection of vitamin E and Se (each injection contained 1000 IU vitamin E and 10 mg Se) was given, but this effect was not observed when milk yield during 12 weeks was compared between cows that received a single or double dose or injective vitamin E and Se. Weiss and Spears [10] and Bourne et al. [44] found no significant effect on milk production due to vit. E supplementation.

Days open and services per conception did not differ between experimental groups (Table 5). Reports on the effects of Se, vitamin E, or their combination with fertility are variable, with some studies reporting an increase in fertility [2, 22, 34] and some reporting no effect [37, 44].

TABLE 3: Effect of oral supplementation of vitamin E with or without injective vitamin E on body weight of calves.

Item	Treatments		
	Injection	Injections + oral	Oral
Birth weight	43.35 ± 3.71	42.55 ± 4.34	42.86 ± 4.08
Weaning weight	94.18 ± 9.19	89.56 ± 12.81	97.35 ± 9.84
Body weight gain	50.82 ± 9.36	50.18 ± 14.73	53.30 ± 11.7
Daily body weight gain	0.564 ± 0.10	0.557 ± 0.16	0.592 ± 0.13

TABLE 4: Effect of oral supplementation of vitamin E with or without injective vitamin E on milk yield in multiparous dairy cows.

Item	Treatments		
	Injection	Injections + oral	Oral
Milk production			
First month	31.44 ± 9.31	35.33 ± 8.83	36.63 ± 7.59
Second month	32.16 ± 9.68	34.53 ± 8.90	34.79 ± 7.06
Third month	31.29 ± 7.74	30.07 ± 6.24	33.64 ± 7.63
Fat (percentage)			
First month	2.728 ± 0.64	2.37 ± 0.57	2.483 ± 0.55
Second month	2.681 ± 0.10	2.573 ± 0.10	2.501 ± 0.06
Third month	2.721 ± 0.53	2.819 ± 0.43	2.680 ± 0.62
FCM			
First month	24.65 ± 4.93	26.11 ± 4.71	27.81 ± 4.15
Second month	24.91 ± 5.53	26.41 ± 4.36	26.58 ± 3.79
Third month	24.78 ± 4.67	24.40 ± 3.50	26.40 ± 3.97

The reasons of these discrepancies could be related to the level of Se, interaction of Se-vit. E, and other nutrition factors as protein, energy, Ca, Mg, and P intake that might also influence reproduction rates [45]. Differences between studies in the amount of vit. E and/or Se administered, the period of administration, and nutritional status of the experimental animals with respect to vit. E and Se intake could explain some of these differential results [2].

4. Conclusions

Due to the lack of significant difference between treatments and ease of use of oral supplements, oral supplementation is recommended to replace the injection. No advantage of oral supplementation plus injective vitamin E compared to either of them alone could be due to the sufficiency of vitamin E in all treatments. As discussed above, the illnesses suffered after birth were suitable indicators showing good nutritional and other management conditions under which the dairy herd was kept.

TABLE 5: Effect of oral supplementation of vitamin E with or without injective vitamin E on reproductive performance in multiparous dairy cows.

Item	Treatments		
	Injection	Injections + oral	Oral
Mastitis	2	1	2
Metritis	2	0	0
Retained placenta	0	0	1
Open days	118.41 ± 46.08	143.06 ± 47.62	118.36 ± 40.90
Service per conception	2.00 ± 1.28	3.07 ± 1.75	2.36 ± 1.21

Conflict of Interests

The authors declare that there is no conflict of interests regarding the publication of this paper.

References

[1] B. A. Mallard, J. C. Dekkers, M. J. Ireland et al., "Alteration in immune responsiveness during the peripartum period and its ramification on dairy cows and calf health," *Journal of Dairy Science*, vol. 81, no. 2, pp. 589–595, 1998.

[2] K. Persson Waller, "Mammary gland immunology around parturition. Influence of stress, nutrition and genetics," *Advances in Experimental Medicine and Biology*, vol. 480, pp. 3488–3497, 2000.

[3] J. P. Goff and R. L. Horst, "Physiological changes at parturition and their relationship to metabolic disorders," *Journal of Dairy Science*, vol. 80, no. 7, pp. 1260–1268, 1997.

[4] K. Persson Waller, C. H. Sandgren, U. Emanuelson, and S. K. Jensen, "Supplementation of RRR-α-tocopheryl acetate to periparturient dairy cows in commercial herds with high mastitis incidence," *Journal of Dairy Science*, vol. 90, no. 8, pp. 3640–3646, 2007.

[5] NRC, *Nutrient Requirements of Dairy Cattle*, National Academy Press, Washington, DC, USA, 7th edition, 2001.

[6] A. Bendich, "Antioxidant micronutrients and immune responses," *Annals of the New York Academy of Sciences*, vol. 587, pp. 168–180, 1990.

[7] J. S. Hogan, W. P. Weiss, K. L. Smith, L. M. Sordillo, and S. N. Williams, "α-tocopherol concentrations in milk and plasma during clinical *Escherichia coli* mastitis," *Journal of Dairy Science*, vol. 79, no. 1, pp. 71–75, 1996.

[8] J. S. Hogan, W. P. Weiss, and K. L. Smith, "Role of vitamin E and selenium in host defense against mastitis," *Journal of Dairy Science*, vol. 76, no. 9, pp. 2795–2803, 1993.

[9] I. Politis, N. Hidiroglou, J. H. White et al., "Effects of vitamin E on mammary and blood leukocyte function, with emphasis on chemotaxis, in periparturient dairy cows," *American Journal of Veterinary Research*, vol. 57, no. 4, pp. 468–471, 1996.

[10] W. P. Weiss and J. W. Spears, "Vitamin and trace mineral effects on immune function of ruminants," in *Ruminant Physiology. Digestion, Metabolism and Impact of Nutrition on Gene Expression, Immunology and Stress*, K. Sejrsen, T. Hvelplund, and M. O. Nielsen, Eds., pp. 473–496, Wageningen Academic Publishers, Wageningen, The Netherlands, 2006.

[11] J. E. Cipriano, J. L. Morrill, and N. V. Anderson, "Effect of dietary vitamin E on immune responses of calves," *Journal of Dairy Science*, vol. 65, no. 12, pp. 2357–2365, 1982.

[12] S. D. Eicher-Pruiett, J. L. Morrill, F. Blecha, J. J. Higgins, N. V. Anderson, and P. G. Reddy, "Neutrophil and lymphocyte response to supplementation with vitamins C and E in young calves," *Journal of Dairy Science*, vol. 75, no. 6, pp. 1635–1642, 1992.

[13] J. P. Goff and J. R. Stabel, "Decreased plasma retinol, α-tocopherol, and zinc concentration during the periparturient period: effect of milk fever," *Journal of Dairy Science*, vol. 73, no. 11, pp. 3195–3199, 1990.

[14] W. P. Weiss, D. A. Todhunter, J. S. Hogan, and K. L. Smith, "Effect of duration of supplementation of selenium and vitamin E on periparturient dairy cows," *Journal of Dairy Science*, vol. 73, no. 11, pp. 3187–3194, 1990.

[15] G. E. Meglia, S. K. Jensen, C. Lauridsen, and K. P. Waller, "α-Tocopherol concentration and stereoisomer composition in plasma and milk from dairy cows fed natural or synthetic vitamin E around calving," *Journal of Dairy Research*, vol. 73, no. 2, pp. 227–234, 2006.

[16] L. J. Perino, "A guide to colostrum management in beef cows and calves," *Veterinary Medicine*, vol. 92, no. 1, pp. 75–82, 1997.

[17] A. D. McEwan, E. W. Fisher, and I. E. Selman, "Observations on the immune globulin levels of neonatal calves and their relationship to disease," *Journal of Comparative Pathology*, vol. 80, no. 2, pp. 259–265, 1970.

[18] J. C. Detilleux, M. E. Kehrli Jr., J. R. Stabel, A. E. Freeman, and D. H. Kelley, "Study of immunological dysfunction in periparturient Holstein cattle selected for high and average milk production," *Veterinary Immunology and Immunopathology*, vol. 44, no. 3-4, pp. 251–267, 1995.

[19] M. E. Kehrli Jr. and J. P. Goff, "Periparturient hypocalcemia in cows: effects on peripheral blood neutrophil and lymphocyte function," *Journal of Dairy Science*, vol. 72, no. 5, pp. 1188–1196, 1989.

[20] J. Fujii, Y. Iuchi, and F. Okada, "Fundamental roles of reactive oxygen species and protective mechanisms in the female reproductive system," *Reproductive Biology and Endocrinology*, vol. 3, article 43, 2005.

[21] S. A. Gunter, P. A. Beck, and J. M. Phillips, "Effects of supplementary selenium source on the performance and blood measurements in beef cows and their calves," *Journal of Animal Science*, vol. 81, no. 4, pp. 856–864, 2003.

[22] C. F. Arrehiga, O. Ortiz, and P. J. Hansen, "Effect of prepartum injection of vitamin E and selenium on postpartum reproductive function of dairy cattle," *Theriogenology*, vol. 41, no. 6, pp. 1251–1258, 1994.

[23] E. C. Segerson, G. J. Riviere, H. L. Dalton, and M. D. Whitacre, "Retained placenta of Holstein cows treated with selenium and vitamin E," *Journal of Dairy Science*, vol. 64, no. 9, pp. 1833–1836, 1981.

[24] U. Emanuelson, P. A. Oltenacu, and Y. T. Gröhn, "Nonlinear mixed model analyses of five production disorders of dairy cattle," *Journal of Dairy Science*, vol. 76, no. 9, pp. 2765–2772, 1993.

[25] M. T. Correa, H. Erb, and J. Scarlett, "Path analysis for seven postpartum disorders of Holstein cows," *Journal of Dairy Science*, vol. 76, no. 5, pp. 1305–1312, 1993.

[26] P. H. Bendixen, B. Vilson, I. Ekesbo, and D. B. Åstrand, "Disease frequencies in dairy cows in Sweden. v. mastisis," *Preventive Veterinary Medicine*, vol. 5, no. 4, pp. 263–274, 1988.

[27] S. Eger, D. Drori, I. Kadoori, N. Miller, and H. Schindler, "Effects of selenium and vitamin E on incidence of retained placenta," *Journal of Dairy Science*, vol. 68, no. 8, pp. 2119–2122, 1985.

[28] M. Hidiroglou, "Mammary transfer of vitamin E in dairy cows," *Journal of Dairy Science*, vol. 72, no. 4, pp. 1067–1071, 1989.

[29] E. C. Segerson Jr., F. A. Murray, A. L. Moxon, D. R. Redman, and H. R. Conrad, "Selenium/vitamin E: role in fertilization of bovine ova," *Journal of Dairy Science*, vol. 60, no. 6, pp. 1001–1005, 1977.

[30] K. L. Smith, J. H. Harrison, D. D. Hancock, D. A. Todhunter, and H. R. Conrad, "Effect of vitamin E and selenium supplementation on incidence of clinical mastitis and duration of clinical symptoms," *Journal of Dairy Science*, vol. 67, no. 6, pp. 1293–1300, 1984.

[31] W. P. Weiss, J. S. Hogan, D. A. Todhunter, and K. L. Smith, "Effect of vitamin E supplementation in diets with a low concentration of selenium on mammary gland health of dairy cows," *Journal of Dairy Science*, vol. 80, no. 8, pp. 1728–1737, 1997.

[32] T. R. Batra, K. H. Singh, S. K. Ho, and M. Hidiroglou, "Concentration of plasma and milk vitamin E and plasma beta-carotene of mastitic and healthy cows," *International Journal for Vitamin and Nutrition Research*, vol. 62, no. 3, pp. 233–237, 1992.

[33] N. Lacetera, U. Bernabucci, B. Ronchi, and A. Nardone, "Effects of selenium and vitamin E administration during a late stage of pregnancy on colostrum and milk production in dairy cows, and on passive immunity and growth of their offspring," *American Journal of Veterinary Research*, vol. 57, no. 12, pp. 1776–1780, 1996.

[34] J. J. Wichtel, A. L. Craigie, H. Varela-Alvarez, and N. B. Williamson, "The effect of intraruminal selenium pellets on growth rate, lactation and reproductive-efficiency in dairy cattle," *New Zealand Veterinary Journal*, vol. 42, no. 6, pp. 205–210, 1994.

[35] D. M. Castellan, J. P. Maas, I. A. Gardner, J. W. Oltjen, and M. L. Sween, "Growth of suckling beef calves in response to parenteral administration of selenium and the effect of dietary protein provided to their dams," *Journal of the American Veterinary Medical Association*, vol. 214, no. 6, pp. 816–821, 1999.

[36] M. Mohri, H. A. Seifi, and J. Khodadadi, "Effects of preweaning parenteral supplementation of vitamin E and selenium on hematology, serum proteins, and weight gain in dairy calves," *Comparative Clinical Pathology*, vol. 14, no. 3, pp. 149–154, 2005.

[37] M. M. Moeini, H. Karami, and E. Mikaeili, "Effect of selenium and vitamin E supplementation during the late pregnancy on reproductive indices and milk production in heifers," *Animal Reproduction Science*, vol. 114, no. 1–3, pp. 109–114, 2009.

[38] SPSS, *Base System Syntax Reference Guide, Release 16*, SPSS, Chicago, Ill, USA, 1993.

[39] P. G. Reddy, J. L. Morrill, H. C. Minocha, and J. S. Stevenson, "Vitamin E is immunostimulatory in calves," *Journal of Dairy Science*, vol. 70, no. 5, pp. 993–999, 1987.

[40] J. T. Daniels, P. G. Hatfield, D. E. Burgess, R. W. Kott, and J. G. P. Bowman, "Evaluation of ewe and lamb immune response when ewes were supplemented with vitamin E," *Journal of Animal Science*, vol. 78, no. 10, pp. 2731–2736, 2000.

[41] M. M. Moeini, A. Kiani, E. Mikaeili, and H. K. Shabankareh, "Effect of prepartum supplementation of selenium and vitamin e on serum Se, IgG concentrations and colostrum of heifers and on hematology, passive immunity and Se status of their offspring," *Biological Trace Element Research*, vol. 144, no. 1–3, pp. 529–537, 2011.

[42] R. D. Cohen, B. D. King, C. Guenther, and E. D. Janzen, "Effects of prepartum parenteral supplementation of pregnant beef cow with selenium/vitamin E on cow and calf plasma selenium and productivity," *The Canadian Veterinary Journal*, vol. 32, pp. 113–115, 1991.

[43] L. Pavlata, J. Prasek, A. Podhorsky, A. Pechova, and T. Haloun, "Selenium maternal transfer of selenium to newborn calves at different selenium concentrations in dams," *Acta Veterinaria Brno*, vol. 72, no. 4, pp. 639–646, 2003.

[44] N. Bourne, D. C. Wathes, K. E. Lawrence, M. McGowan, and R. A. Laven, "The effect of parenteral supplementation of vitamin E with selenium on the health and productivity of dairy cattle in the UK," *Veterinary Journal*, vol. 177, no. 3, pp. 381–387, 2008.

[45] J. E. Ramírez-Bribiesca, J. L. Tortora, M. Huerta, L. M. Hernández, R. López, and M. M. Crosby, "Effect of selenium-vitamin E injection in selenium-deficient dairy goats and kids on the Mexican plateau," *Arquivo Brasileiro de Medicina Veterinaria e Zootecnia*, vol. 57, no. 1, pp. 77–84, 2005.

Evaluation of the Nutritive and Organoleptic Values of Food Products Developed by Incorporated *Catharanthus roseus* (*Sadabahar*) Fresh Leaves Explore Their Hypoglycemic Potential

Gita Bisla,[1] Shailza Choudhary,[1] and Vijeta Chaudhary[2]

[1] *Department of Food Science and Nutrition, Banasthali University, Rajasthan 304022, India*
[2] *Department of Commerce, V.M.L.G College, Ghazibad, Uttar Pradesh, India*

Correspondence should be addressed to Gita Bisla; gitabisla@gmail.com

Academic Editors: A. Chicco and N. Vikram

Diabetes becomes a real problem of public health in developing countries, where its prevalence is increasing steadily. Diabetes mellitus can be found in almost every population in the world. Since the Ayurvedic practice started in India, plants are being used in the cure of diseases. Although the *Catharanthus roseus* have been used for their alleged health benefits and avail their hypoglycemic effect, used as medicine by diabetics. Medicinal plants have rarely been incorporated in food preparations. To fill these lacunae, food products were prepared by using *Catharanthus roseus* (*Sadabahar*) fresh leaves with hypoglycemic properties. Commonly consumed recipes in India are prepared for diabetic patients and were developed at different levels at 3 g, 4 g, and 6 g per serving. Food product development and their acceptability appraisal through organoleptic evaluation were carried out by semitrained panel comprising 15 trained panelists from the department of Food Science and Nutrition, Banasthali University. Seven products were developed by incorporating *Catharanthus roseus* fresh leaves. Nine point hedonic scale was used as a medium to know about the product acceptability at various variances. All products are moderately acceptable at different concentrations except product fare "6 g" which was more acceptable than the standard. Among the three variations of incorporating the *Catharanthus roseus* (*Sadabahar*) Leaves, 3 g variation is more acceptable than other variations.

1. Introduction

Diabetes mellitus is a chronic condition characterized by major derangements in glucose metabolism and abnormalities in fat and protein metabolism [1]. Patients use many products and modalities to treat diabetes or its comorbidities. People with diabetes are 1.6 times more likely to use a complementary and alternative medicine (CAM) treatment modality than those without diabetes [2].

The World Health Organization (WHO) estimates that currently more than 180 million people worldwide have diabetes and it is likely to double by 2030, with India, China, and the United States predicted to have the largest number of affected individuals [3]. Many plants and their active chemical compounds have demonstrated activity in the treatment of various disorders [4]. According to ethnobotanical information, more than 800 plants are used as traditional remedies in one or other form for the treatment of diabetes [5]. With the disturbing rise in the prevalence of this metabolic disease and associated healthcare cost, interest in alternative or complementary therapies has been grown. This interest is due to reasons such as ease of access, better culture acceptability and compatibility, cost effectiveness, and also the bid to "Go Natural".

A plant is a living organism able to convert inorganic material into organic molecules necessary for the life of the plant itself and serves as food, for example, insects, animals, and humans. Plants also provide medicines and many other commodities. However, our knowledge about plants with their enormous diversity is still limited in many aspects. Still many novel products might be obtained from plants; however, this is hampered by the rapid loss of plant diversity on earth due to, for example, deforestation. The sustainable exploitation of plants for food and medicines requires extensive knowledge about plants. As the world's population grows to an estimated 9 billion people in 2050, the availability of food and medicines for all people in the future should be a concern to all of us. Up to now, plants remain a primary source of medicines for most people in the world. Therefore, research in plant science is of great importance for human health, both for the production of healthier food and for development and production of medicines [6].

The important values of some plants have long been published but a large number of them remain unexplored. So, there is a necessity to explore their uses and to conduct pharmacognostic and pharmacological studies to ascertain their therapeutic properties. Despite considerable progress in the management of diabetes mellitus by synthetic drugs, the search for natural antidiabetic plant products for controlling diabetes is going on. There are many hypoglycemic plants known through the folklore but their introduction into the modern therapy system awaits the discovery of animal test system that is closely parallel to the pathological course of diabetes in human beings. Hypoglycemic activity has been reported in many plants during the last twenty years [7].

In India, herbal medicines date back several thousand years to the Rig-Veda, a collection of Hindu sacred verses, system of health care known as Ayurvedic medicine, which is still widely practiced in India today. *Catharanthus roseus* belongs to the family apocynaceae [8] *Catharanthus roseus* is commonly called as *Periwinkle*, *Madagascar periwinkle*, and *Sadabahar*. It grows throughout India and is found as an escape in waste places and sandy tracts. More than 130 different compounds have been reported including about 100 monoterpenoid indole alkaloids [9]. As an important medical plant, it has a good antioxidant potential throughout its parts under drought stress [10]. There are several health benefits of *Catharanthus roseus* leaves such as maintaining blood sugar [11], lowering high blood pressure [12], menstruation irregularities, Hodgkin's disease [13], and as antioxidant [14].

Recently there has been a shift in universal trend from synthetic to herbal medicine, which we can say "Return to Nature." Subsequently, with this background in mind, this study was embarking on the study of hypoglycemic effect of *Catharanthus roseus* fresh leaves in type II Diabetes Mellitus. Most of the people do not know *Catharanthus roseus* nutritional quality, health benefits, and how to use and what to use. They are not utilized to its full potential. So, the basic aim of this study is to create awareness about *Catharanthus roseus* leaves among the population. As many other herbal plants established in the indigenous system of medicine for their antidiabetic potentials and this plant has to be established in this indigenous system of medicines. Therefore, the present study was undertaken to develop commonly consumed food preparations for diabetics by incorporating *Catharanthus roseus* fresh leaves and evaluate their acceptability. Traditional foods reflect cultural inheritance and have left their imprints on contemporary dietary patterns [15].

2. Material and Methods

2.1. Sample Description. Catharanthus roseus fresh leaves were collected from the main campus of Banasthali University, Rajasthan, India. The leaves were washed thoroughly with tap water followed with sterilized distilled water for the removal of dust and sand particles. Commonly seven consumed recipes in India are prepared for diabetic patients were developed at different levels at 3 g, 4 g, and 6 g per serving.

2.2. Panel Selection and Training. Food product development and their acceptability appraisal through organoleptic evaluation carried out by a trained panel comprising 30 panelists from the department of Food Science and Nutrition, Banasthali University. They were preselected on the basis of good health conditions, time availability, no allergy plants products, any aversion to *Catharanthus roseus*, and willingness to participate. Panelists were then subjected to preliminary acuity tests to investigate their ability to recognize basic taste, basic aromas, and to describe basic attributes in prepared products by triangle method [16, 17]. After the screening process fifteen panelists were selected. Twelve panelists were female and three were male in the range of 20–35 years old of age. They went under training to perform the sensory evaluation of the products.

Training consisted of: (1) initial orientation session where panelists received detailed explanation about the organoleptic methodology; (2) group meetings for general description of the *Catharanthus roseus* fresh leaves incorporating food products development, which required 30 minutes to 1-hour sessions; (3) individual training during opening sessions panelists, took part in exercise. They were provided with the three samples (plain, salted, and sugary flavors in mango shake), which were diluted in 2% of cinnamon solution. They were asked to smell and taste them and list as many aromas and flavor terms as possible for each sample and discuss individual results to come up with a consensus.

2.3. Outcome Measures. The panelists performed organoleptic appraisal by 9 point hedonic test [18] to assess the overall products preferences. Evaluation of taste, flavor, color, texture, appearance, after taste, and overall acceptability were made in the scale. Two samples were during a 60-minute session and the evaluations were repeated two more times and they were asked to rinse their penchant well with water between samples. For this purpose, panelists used room-temperature drinking water.

2.4. Quality Control

(i) Panelist should be fit and free from tiredness to reduce the possibility of errors.

(ii) Ensure that there is sufficient light at the judgment site.

(iii) If too many people congregate, it may interfere with the sensory evaluation, site should be free from distraction.

(iv) Drink water between the evaluations of samples.

Table 1: Food preparations prepared with different methods of cooking by incorporating *Catharanthus roseus* fresh leaves.

Food preparations	Method of processing
Fure	Steaming
Rasam	Roasting and pressure cooking
Stuffed idli	Fermentation and steaming
Palak methi muthia	Steaming
Methi paratha	Stir frying
Coriander chutney	Grinding
Cucumber soup	Pressure cooking

(v) The panelists were instructed not to swallow the samples.

(vi) Proper weighing of the raw materials to be used in the cooking.

(vii) Area should be odor free.

(viii) There should be proper ventilation.

(ix) Instruction to the panelists should be understandable, concise, and appropriate to the test.

2.5. Standardization of Food Products and Nutritive Value of Food Products. Fresh leaves of medicinal plants, namely, *Catharanthus roseus*, leaves incorporating in food products, respectively, developed different levels at 3 g, 4 g, and 6 g per serving. Food preparations made by using different cooking methods (Table 1). Nutrient content per serving of the products incorporated *Catharanthus roseus* fresh leaves was calculated from the values given in nutritive value of Indian foods [19].

2.6. Statistical Analysis. The data were subjected to statistical analysis using Statistical Package for Social Sciences (SPSS) version 16.0. Mean ± SD was used to obtain the differences in organoleptic scores, within different levels of incorporation of *Catharanthus roseus* fresh leaves in food preparations. Level of significance was accepted at $P \leq 0.05$.

3. Results

3.1. Organoleptic Evaluation. All the food products incorporated with *Catharanthus roseus* (*Sadabahar*) fresh leaves were found to be organoleptically satisfactory at different variations. Comparing the food products at different variations with standard of the food products, respectively. Although the scores of standard was more acceptable than all the variations made at different concentrations. It was also observed that the concentration of *Catharanthus roseus* fresh leaves in the samples was inversely proportional to the acceptability scores except in product *fure* where the scores of "6 g" were better than all the variations made at different concentrations for all attributes. As the concentration was increased, the mean scores for appearance, Color, flavor, texture, taste, after taste, and overall acceptability were found to be increased.

In *Catharanthus roseus* (*Sadabahar*) fresh leaves incorporated food products (Table 2), namely, *fure,* the most acceptable level of incorporation was 6 g and the mean scores for overall acceptability were 8.63 ± 0.82. However, scores for all organoleptic characteristics of *fure* within 3 g and 4 g levels of incorporation were found to be nonsignificantly different.

Rasam and *Stuffed Idli* were moderately acceptable and the scores for their overall acceptability awarded by the panel of judges were 7.0 ± 1.23 at 3 g and 7.4 ± 0.06 at 4 g, respectively. Nonsignificant difference was noticed in scores for all organoleptic characteristics of *Rasam* and *Stuffed Idli* within variations of incorporation of *Catharanthus roseus* (*Sadabahar*) fresh leaves (Table 2). However, the acceptable level of incorporation varied in different food products. It has been found that when the level of incorporation of fresh leaves increased beyond the accepted levels in any food products,the mean scores for all organoleptic characteristics decreased.

For *palak methi muthia, methi parantha, coriander chutney,* and *cucumber soup* the most acceptable level of incorporation of *Catharanthus roseus* (*Sadabahar*) fresh leaves was 3 g per serving and the respective scores for overall acceptability ranged from 6.6 ± 0.07 (*palak methi muthia*) to 7.15 ± 0.09 (*cucumber soup*). Nonsignificant differences were found in scores for all organoleptic characteristics of food products (Table 2).

3.2. Nutritive Evaluation. Energy content of all the food products prepared by incorporating 3 g *Catharanthus roseus* (*Sadabahar*) fresh leaves per serving was varied from 13.31 Kcal of *cucumber soup* to 240.34 Kcal per serving of *methi parantha* (Table 3). Protein content was the highest in *fure* (12.51 g/serving) and the lowest in *cucumber soup* (0.34 g/serving). Fat content ranged between 0.03 g in *cucumber soup* and 12.51 g per serving in *fure.* Carbohydrate content of 3 g *Catharanthus roseus* (*Sadabahar*) fresh incorporated food products varied from 1.18 g of soup to 35.66 g per serving of *stuffed idli.* The highest fibre content was found in *coriander chutney* (0.75 g/serving) and minimum in soup was (0.05 g/serving). The hypoglycemic activity of *Catharanthus roseus* leaves may be due to the presence of alkaloid-like vincristine and vinblastine through stimulation of β cell activity leading to increased insulin production and release [20].

4. Conclusions

The scores of standard were more acceptable than all the variations made at different concentrations. It was also observed that the concentration of *Catharanthus roseus* fresh leaves, in the samples was inversely proportional to the acceptability scores. Three g per serving *Catharanthus roseus* freshleaves incorporation in food products developed was found to be organoleptically acceptable by the semitrained panel members. Amongst the incorporated food preparations, the mean scores for overall acceptability were highest for *fure* and lowest for methi parantha. Thus, this holds great promise for future research for the formulation of potent antidiabetic drug for the present plant.

TABLE 2: Organoleptic evaluation of food products developed by incorporation of *Catharanthus roseus* fresh leaves.

Food products	g/serving	Appearance	Color	Texture	After taste	Overall acceptability
Fure	Standard	8.2 ± 0.08	8.5 ± 0.61	8.5 ± 0.56	8.3 ± 0.03	8.25 ± 0.52
	3 g	8.6 ± 0.82	8.06 ± 1.25	8.4 ± 0.61	8.2 ± 0.09	8.3 ± 0.87
	4 g	8.6 ± 0.89	8.7 ± 0.56	8.4 ± 1.06	8.4 ± 0.76	8.4 ± 0.06
	6 g	8.7 ± 0.05	8.8 ± 0.59	8.5 ± 0.56	8.5 ± 0.53	8.63 ± 0.82
Rasam	Standard	7.2 ± 0.06	8.1 ± 0.71	7.52 ± 0.67	8.3 ± 0.06	8.2 ± 0.56
	3 g	7.2 ± 0.08	7.4 ± 0.93	7.2 ± 1.10	7.5 ± 0.89	7.0 ± 1.23
	4 g	7.8 ± 0.32	7.0 ± 0.04	6.1 ± 0.58	6.3 ± 0.79	6.7 ± 0.15
	6 g	7.0 ± 0.85	7.1 ± 0.88	5.42 ± 1.23	5.6 ± 0.40	6.02 ± 0.04
Stuffed idli	Standard	8.0 ± 0.54	7.5 ± 0.02	7.5 ± 0.08	8.5 ± 0.79	8.0 ± 0.63
	3 g	7.6 ± 0.80	7.9 ± 0.56	7.49 ± 1.61	7.21 ± 0.43	7.3 ± 0.32
	4 g	7.20 ± 0.34	7.7 ± 0.12	7.4 ± 0.06	6.4 ± 0.11	7.4 ± 0.06
	6 g	6.69 ± 0.84	6.7 ± 0.65	6.5 ± 1.23	6.5 ± 0.49	6.62 ± 0.98
Palak methi muthia	Standard	8.0 ± 0.23	7.1 ± 0.99	8.1 ± 0.72	7.9 ± 0.88	8.05 ± 0.66
	3 g	7.8 ± 0.04	6.43 ± 0.99	7.3 ± 1.01	6.3 ± 0.61	6.6 ± 0.07
	4 g	6.2 ± 0.63	6.0 ± 0.70	6.7 ± 0.85	6.31 ± 0.56	6.1 ± 0.51
	6 g	6.06 ± 0.78	6.11 ± 0.44	5.07 ± 0.45	6.6 ± 0.09	6.0 ± 0.74
Methi parantha	Standard	8.85 ± 0.80	8.06 ± 0.18	8.50 ± 0.66	7.5 ± 1.23	8.01 ± 0.36
	3 g	7.69 ± 0.55	6.61 ± 0.74	6.45 ± 0.17	6.22 ± 0.99	6.36 ± 0.47
	4 g	6.09 ± 0.22	6.2 ± 0.50	5.49 ± 0.75	6.24 ± 1.06	6.01 ± 0.89
	6 g	5.43 ± 0.68	5.38 ± 0.34	5.5 ± 0.32	5.5 ± 0.53	5.6 ± 0.62
Coriander chutney	Standard	8.5 ± 0.54	8.81 ± 0.28	8.15 ± 0.01	8.05 ± 0.54	8.42 ± 0.33
	3 g	8.3 ± 0.14	8.24 ± 0.39	8.34 ± 0.09	8.08 ± 0.37	8.1 ± 0.67
	4 g	8.09 ± 0.54	7.8 ± 0.04	7.5 ± 0.87	7.27 ± 0.01	7.08 ± 0.69
	6 g	8.0 ± 0.87	7.04 ± 0.88	6.98 ± 0.59	6.62 ± 0.37	7.03 ± 0.03
Cucumber soup	Standard	7.76 ± 0.54	8.0 ± 0.77	7.5 ± 1.32	8.3 ± 0.98	8.12 ± 0.59
	3 g	7.6 ± 0.82	6.07 ± 0.25	7.4 ± 0.36	7.2 ± 0.09	7.15 ± 0.09
	4 g	6.87 ± 0.03	6.55 ± 1.87	6.08 ± 0.43	5.29 ± 0.26	6.28 ± 0.37
	6 g	6.6 ± 0.54	5.9 ± 0.66	5.05 ± 0.67	5.76 ± 0.67	5.54 ± 0.51

All values are found to be Nonsignificant.

TABLE 3: Nutritive evaluation of food products developed by incorporation of 3 g *Catharanthus roseus* fresh leaves per serving.

Food products	Cooked weight/serving (g)	Energy (kcal)	Protein (g)	Fat (g)	Carbohydrate (g)	Fiber (g)
Fure	80	137.34	12.51	3.87	34.58	0.16
Rasam	244	80.2	3.43	3.58	17.1	0.69
Stuffed idli	78	142.76	7.07	0.84	35.66	0.58
Palak methi muthia	65	168.52	10.58	2.65	23.04	0.12
Methi paratha	92	240.34	11.32	7.98	29.65	0.11
Coriander chutney	46	55	1.67	0.07	3.5	0.75
Cucumber soup	185	13.31	0.34	0.03	1.18	0.05

Conflict of Interests

The authors declare that there is no conflict of interests regarding the publication of this paper.

References

[1] NOIC, *Diabetes Among African Americans*, National Diabetes Information Clearinghouse.

[2] L. E. Egede, X. Ye, D. Zheng, and M. D. Silverstein, "The prevalence and pattern of complementary and alternative medicine use in individuals with diabetes," *Diabetes Care*, vol. 25, no. 2, pp. 324–329, 2002.

[3] S. Wild, G. Roglic, A. Green, R. Sicree, and H. King, "Global prevalence of diabetes: estimates for the year 2000 and projections for 2030," *Diabetes Care*, vol. 27, no. 5, pp. 1047–1053, 2004.

[4] E. A. Palombo, "Phytochemicals from traditional medicinal plants used in the treatment of diarrhoea: modes of action and

effects on intestinal function," *Phytotherapy Research*, vol. 20, no. 9, pp. 717–724, 2006.

[5] F. J. Alarcon-Aguilara, R. Roman-Ramos, S. Perez-Gutierrez, A. Aguilar-Contreras, C. C. Contreras-Weber, and J. L. Flores-Saenz, "Study of the anti-hyperglycemic effect of plants used as antidiabetics," *Journal of Ethnopharmacology*, vol. 61, no. 2, pp. 101–110, 1998.

[6] G. A. Cordell, "Natural products in drug discovery—creating a new vision," *Phytochemistry Reviews*, vol. 1, no. 3, pp. 261–273, 2002.

[7] Z. Daniel and H. Maria, *Domestication of Plants in the Old World*, University Press, Oxford, UK, 3rd edition, 2000.

[8] C. A. Jaleel, "change in non enzymatic antioxidants and ajmalicine production in *Catharanthus roseus* with different soil salinity regimes," *Botany Research International*, vol. 2, no. 1, pp. 1–6, 2009.

[9] D. M. Pereira, J. Faria, P. Valentao, M. Sottomayor, and P. B. Andrade, "Exploiting *Catharanthus roseus* roots: source of antioxidants," *Journal of Food Chemistry*, vol. 6, pp. 235–242, 2010.

[10] N. Rasool, K. Rizwan, M. Zubair, K. U. R. Naveed, I. Imran, and V. U. Ahmed, "Antioxidant potential of different extracts and fractions of *Catharanthus roseus* shoots," *International Journal of Phytomedicine*, vol. 3, no. 1, pp. 108–114, 2011.

[11] S. Nammi, M. K. Boini, S. D. Lodagala, and R. B. S. Behara, "The juice of fresh leaves of *Catharanthus roseus* Linn. reduces blood glucose in normal and alloxan diabetic rabbits.," *BMC Complementary and Alternative Medicine*, vol. 3, no. 1, p. 4, 2003.

[12] N. Ara, M. Rashid, and M. D. S. Amran, "Comparison of hypotensive and hypolipidemic effects of *Catharanthus roseus* leaves extract with atenolol on adrenaline induced hypertensive rats," *Pakistan Journal of Pharmaceutical Sciences*, vol. 22, no. 3, pp. 267–271, 2009.

[13] P. R. H. Moreno, R. van der Heijden, and R. Verpoorte, "Effect of terpenoid precursor feeding and elicitation on formation of indole alkaloids in cell suspension cultures of *Catharanthus roseus*," *Plant Cell Reports*, vol. 12, no. 12, pp. 702–705, 1993.

[14] C. A. Jaleel, R. Gopi, P. Manivannan, M. Gomathinayagam, R. Sridharan, and R. Panneerselvam, "Antioxidant potential and indole alkaloid profile variations with water deficits along different parts of two varieties of *Catharanthus roseus*," *Colloids and Surfaces B*, vol. 62, no. 2, pp. 312–318, 2008.

[15] A. Trichopoulou, S. Soukara, and E. Vasilopoulou, "Traditional foods: a science and society perspective," *Trends in Food Science and Technology*, vol. 18, no. 8, pp. 420–427, 2007.

[16] A. J. Byer and D. A. Abram, "comparsion of triangular and two sample taste test method," *Food Technology*, vol. 7, article 185, 1953.

[17] M. A. Amerine, R. M. Pangborn, and E. B. Roessler, *Principles of Sensory Evaluation of Food*, Academic Press, New York, NY, USA, 1965.

[18] D. Peryam and N. F. Girardot, "Advanced taste test," *Food Engineering*, vol. 24, pp. 58–61, 1952.

[19] C. Gopalan, B. V. Ramasastri, S. C. Balasubramanian, B. S. Narasinga Rao, Y. G. Deosthale, and K. C. Pant, *Nutritive Value of Indian Foods*, National Institute of Nutrition (ICMR), Hyderabad, India, 2004.

[20] S. Ghosh and S. A. Suryawanshi, "Effect of Vinca rosea extracts in treatment of alloxan diabetes in male albino rats," *Indian Journal of Experimental Biology*, vol. 39, no. 8, pp. 748–759, 2001.

Individualized Tailor-Made Dietetic Intervention Program at Schools Enhances Eating Behaviors and Dietary Habits in Obese Hispanic Children of Low Socioeconomic Status

Leticia Elizondo-Montemayor,[1] Diana Moreno-Sànchez,[1] Norma G. Gutierrez,[1] Fabiola Monsivais-Rodriguez,[1] Ubaldo Martinez,[1] Ana C. Lamadrid-Zertuche,[1] and Martin M. Hernandez-Torre[2]

[1] *Clinical Nutrition and Obesity Research Center, School of Medicine and Health Sciences, Tecnológico de Monterrey, Avenue Morones Prieto 3000 Pte., Col. Los Doctores, 64710 Monterrey, NL, Mexico*
[2] *Tecnológico de Monterrey, Avenue Morones Prieto 3000 Pte., Col. Los Doctores, 64710 Monterrey, NL, Mexico*

Correspondence should be addressed to Leticia Elizondo-Montemayor; lelizond@itesm.mx

Academic Editors: Y.-C. Huang, T. A. Mori, and N. Vikram

Hispanic children and those from low-socioeconomic status are predisposed to unhealthy eating habits and obesity. *Aim.* to implement an individualized, face-to-face, parent supported, and school-partnership dietetic intervention to promote healthy eating habits and decrease body mass index. Prospective school year dietetic intervention of 101 obese, Hispanic, low-socioeconomic school-age children representative of Monterrey, Mexico, consisted of anthropometrics, dietetic assessment, energy-restriction tailor-made daily menus, and parental education every three weeks. Student's t-test was used for means comparison. A significant decrease was found in body mass index percentile (96.43 ± 3.32 to $93.42 \pm 8.12/P = 0.00$) and energy intake/day of −755.7 kcal/day ($P = 0.00$). Among other energy dense foods with significant decline in servings/day and servings/week were processed meats (3.13 ± 1.43 to $2.19 \pm 1.04/P = 0.00$ and 5.60 ± 1.75 to $4.37 \pm 2.10/P = 0.00$, resp.), saturated fat (1.47 ± 1.08 to $0.78 \pm 0.79/P = 0.00$ and 2.19 ± 2.18 to $1.1 \pm 1.36/P = 0.00$), sweetened beverages (2.79 ± 1.99 to 1.42 ± 1.21 and 6.21 ± 1.72 to $3.89 \pm 2.80/P = 0.00$), and desserts and refined-grain bakery (1.99 ± 1.54 to 1.32 ± 1.59 and 2.85 ± 2.54 to $1.57 \pm 2.20/P = 0.00$). There was a significant increase in servings/day and servings/week of water (2.98 ± 2.02 to 4.91 ± 2.37 and 6.62 ± 2.03 to $6.87 \pm 0.91/P = 0.00$, resp.) and nutrient dense foods such as fruits (1.31 ± 0.89 to 1.66 ± 0.96 and 3.34 ± 2.24 to $4.28 \pm 2.43/P = 0.00$) and fish and poultry (3.76 ± 2.15 to $4.54 \pm 2.25/P = 0.00$). This intervention created healthy eating habits and decreased body mass index in a high risk population. Trial registration number: NCT01925976.

1. Introduction

Obesity in children is a rapidly expanding disease across the world [1]. Currently, with a 32.8 percent of adult obesity rate, Mexico is just inches past the 31.8 percent obesity rate in the United States, according to a study released on June 4th, 2013 by the United Nations Food and Agricultural Organization. Mexico has one of the highest rates of obesity in the world [2]. However, the last national survey made in Mexico, in 2012, states that for adults, the combined prevalence of obesity and overweight in the country is 64.9%, and in school-aged children it reaches 34.4%, with a gender difference of 36.9% for boys and 32% for girls [3]. Childhood obesity carries great health risks for children; it is associated with insulin resistance and increased risk of developing cardiovascular disease, type 2 diabetes, hypertension, dyslipidemia, long-term vascular complications, and the metabolic syndrome [1, 4]. Furthermore, overweight and obese children are likely to become obese as adults and to develop cardiovascular and metabolic complications at a younger age [1].

Ethnicity also plays a role in predisposition to obesity. It has been demonstrated that Hispanic children and adolescents have greater proportion of visceral fat and obesity [5, 6]

and are likely to have less healthy eating habits [7, 8] than those that are not Hispanic. As well, socioeconomic status contributes to obesity rates and less healthy eating habits. It has been established that children from low socioeconomic status (LSE status) are also less likely to have healthy eating habits than those from higher income status, since it has been shown that they consume more energy dense (ED) and nutrient-poor diets [9, 10], which makes them even more prone to overweight and obesity [9, 11, 12].

The appropriate approach to decrease overweight and obesity prevalence, according to the Academy of Nutrition and Dietetics [13], the American Heart Association [1], and the American Academy of Pediatrics [14] is through change in dietary habits and physical activity. Studies find that parental food choices influence children's food preferences, dietary habits, and nutrient intakes [1, 15, 16], so parental education regarding healthy eating is of the upmost importance. National associations [13, 14] recommended that health providers should work with communities and schools to help individuals modify their health habits as part of their efforts to control obesity. Although some school-based interventions directed at curriculum modifications or changing school policies have had positive effects on improving healthy eating habits [16], some others have not [17, 18]. Many of these school-based studies had some significant limitations; they either neglected or poorly addressed the importance of parental support, or what children ate outside of school, or they were short-term and they were not carried out on an individualized basis. Currently, there is only limited available evidence about effective strategies to manage childhood obesity [1]; therefore, innovative dietetic interventions are needed. Few comprehensive dietetic intervention programs have been carried out with obese Hispanic children from LSE status, and no studies have used an individualized, tailor-made approach.

Therefore, the aims of this study were to implement an innovative, comprehensive, individualized, face-to-face with the registered dietitian, at school, and parent supported, school year dietetic intervention program aimed at promoting healthy eating in obese Hispanic children from LSE status to (1) decrease body mass index percentiles (BMI), (2) examine the modifications in energy intake, (3) identify variations in the consumption of macronutrients, (4) determine changes in the contribution of individual food groups to eating habits, and (5) detect gender differences regarding eating habits.

2. Materials and Methods

2.1. Study Population. This was a prospective interventional study. An open invitation was made to children ages 5–12 years from eight public schools of LSE status, representative of Monterrey, the second largest city in Mexico, to screen for overweight and obesity. From a total of 4300 children in these schools, 1300 children were randomly selected for screening for overweight and obesity using BMI percentiles with an error <1.4% for the sample. Overweight/obesity was found in 451 children, who were all invited to participate in the dietetic intervention program at no cost. From these, 125 children accepted to participate and 101 completed the school-year dietetic intervention program. The rest of the overweight/obese children's parents were not interested in the intervention program, or did not meet all of the inclusion criteria, but most of them were simply not concerned. Some of the reasons why 24 children dropped out of the program were due to change of school, lack of parent or caregiver attendance during the visit, or absence to school during some of the consultations. Inclusion criteria were attendance from first to sixth grade; ages 6–12 years; BMI ≥ 85th percentile for age and sex; Hispanic; both parents Hispanics; LSE status; and signed consent from both parents/caregivers and active assent from children. Exclusion criteria were disapproval by the children's physician due to any at-risk medical condition known by the parents. Approvals by the Ethics and Research Committees of the School of Medicine Tecnológico de Monterrey and by the State Education Authorities were obtained. Participants did not receive compensation for participating.

2.2. Clinical Evaluation. Based on the World Health Organization and the American Academy of Pediatrics criteria [14], overweight was considered as BMI ≥ 85th and <95th percentiles and obesity as ≥95th percentile according to age and sex.

Anthropometric measurements were performed in all participants at each school. Standing height was determined to the nearest 0.5 cm (portable Seca stadiometer, North America) and weight to the nearest 0.1 kg while children wore light clothing and no socks or shoes (TANITA TBF 300 scale, Arlington, Illinois). Waist circumference was measured to the nearest 0.1 cm at the level of the umbilicus with a flexible fiberglass tape while the subjects were standing, after gently exhaling, and with no clothing on the area. BMI was calculated by weight (kg) divided by the square of height (m). Measurements were performed by the same three trained registered dietitians (RD) on all children to control the interobserver variability.

2.3. Dietetic Intervention. The principal strategies for the change in energy and food groups consumption were dietary modifications for the children and parental support, as recommended by national associations [1, 13, 14, 19]. Dietetic intervention was given individually by a RD for every child at each school, every three weeks, for a total of 13 visits during the school-year. Each child left the classroom to attend the 45-minute nutrition counseling and was accompanied by a parent or caregiver. Each child and parent or caregiver was seen by the same RD throughout the school-year to favor compliance to the plan and to avoid interexaminer bias. Each session was conducted by the RD in terms that children and parents could understand clearly. Each nutrition counseling session consisted of (1) anthropometric assessment; (2) dietetic assessment by means of 24-hour diet recalls, a standardized food frequency questionnaire that included Mexican foods, and food replicas to aid in estimation of portion sizes; (3) individualized energy restriction and balanced macronutrient dietary planning; (4) provision of structured, tailor-made daily menus and meals for

Table 1: Comparison of anthropometric parameters and nutrient intake at baseline and end of dietetic intervention.

Variable	Sample size $n = 101$				
	Baseline	End of intervention	Mean difference	95% CI*	P value
BMI percentile	96.43 ± 3.32	93.42 ± 8.12	−3.0	(−4.27, −1.75)	0.00
Waist circumference (cm)	83.29 ± 9.17	82.82 ± 9.88	−0.5	(−1.54, 0.61)	0.39
Total energy (kcal/day)	2506.9 ± 700.6	1751 ± 468.2	−755.7	(−907.4, −604.1)	0.00
Carbohydrates					
Energy (kcal/day of carbohydrates)	1366 ± 438.6	1019.1 ± 351.7	−346.8	(−449.2, −244.5)	0.00
Grams (grams)	348.2 ± 149.7	256.3 ± 85.1	−91.9	(−125.0, −58.8)	0.00
Percent calories (%)	54.4 ± 9.132	58.13 ± 9.101	3.7	(1.38, 6.08)	0.00
Protein					
Energy (kcal/day of protein)	400.3 ± 117.9	299.5 ± 87.6	−100.7	(126.9, −74.5)	0.00
Grams (grams)	100.09 ± 29.4	74.39 ± 22.03	−25.7	(−32.47, −18.93)	0.00
Percent calories (%)	16.37 ± 4.14	17.348 ± 3.90	0.99	(0.070, 1.90)	0.03
Fat					
Energy (kcal/day of fat)	713.5 ± 305.0	418.4 ± 184.2	−295.1	(−356.3, −233.9)	0.00
Grams (grams)	79.29 ± 33.88	47.35 ± 19.30	−31.9	(−38.73, −25.13)	0.00
Percent calories (%)	28.032 ± 7.66	24.515 ± 7.96	−3.5	(−5.48, −1.54)	0.00

Data represent mean ± standard deviation. *Confidence interval for the mean difference. The significance level used in paired t-test was 0.05.

the next three weeks for each child; and (5) information given to parents/caregivers about healthy food, eating practices, and portion sizes. Attendance of the parent/caregiver was mandatory to help answer the 24-hour recalls and to assure commitment to follow the dietary recommendations at home. School partnership consisted in giving notification to parents and children one and two days before the visit, letting the child leave the classroom and attend the nutrition program in a room provided by the school. After each visit, the RD recorded the information into the software (NutriKcal VO software, Consinfo, S.C., DF, Mexico), which determined energy intake and diet composition. Entry of data into the software was completed by means of serving/day and days/week including the weekends.

Diet composition (macronutrients) was based on the most recent dietary recommended intake for children ages 6–12 [19]: 25%–35% of total calories from fat, 45%–65% from carbohydrates, and 10%–30% from protein. Additionally, according to the American Heart Association and the National Cholesterol Education Program recommendations for children or adolescents included a variety of foods that are low in saturated fat (<10% kcal), no trans fat, and cholesterol <300 mg/day. The RDs promoted age appropriate serving sizes, including approximately ≥5 servings of fruit and vegetables, ≥3 servings of low fat milk or dairy products, and ≥6 servings of whole-grain products per day; increase of dietary fiber; and reduction of salt intake [20]. As well, children were advised to avoid overconsumption of ED and nutrient-poor foods and beverages [13].

Reduction in calorie intake was approached following the recommendations of the American Heart Association in which children >4 years old with a BMI ≥ 85th percentile may achieve BMI percentile reductions to <85th percentile with weight maintenance during linear growth [1]. As advised [14], progressive restriction of 150–900 calories from actual intake throughout the school-year was recommended so that obese children with BMI > 95th percentile could lose gradually 0.5 kilogram/month and those with BMI > 99th percentile could lose a maximum of 0.9 kilogram/week.

2.4. Statistical Methods. MINITAB version 16 (Minitab Inc., State College, PA, USA) was used to analyze the differences between anthropometric parameters and nutrient intake values at baseline and end of intervention; Microsoft Excel 2007 (Microsoft Corp., Redmond, WA, USA) was used to incorporate the input of data. The results were expressed as mean ± standard deviation (s.d.) and their corresponding 95% confidence intervals (CI). Comparisons between groups for dependent variables were made using paired Student's t-test for means. The mean comparisons between gender groups were determined using t-test for independent samples. All tests were interpreted based on two-tailed hypothesis. The significance level was set at 0.05 in all cases. The statistical power was >0.80 for all statistical tests involved in this study's analysis.

3. Results

Table 1 shows baseline and end of the school-year dietetic intervention values. BMI percentile fell significantly by a mean difference of −3.0 ($P = 0.00$), from 96.43 to 93.42 (−4.27, −1.75; 95% CI). There was a significant decrease of −755.7 calories (−907.4, −604.1; 95% CI; $P = 0.00$) of the total energy intake/day. As well, there was a significant calorie reduction of all macronutrients consumption ($P = 0.00$). Although girls showed greater reduction in anthropometric parameters, total energy consumption/day, and macronutrients intake/day compared to boys, there was no significant gender difference (Table 2). Children maintained the recommended dietary composition of the total energy

TABLE 2: Gender comparison of the mean difference of anthropometric parameters and nutrient intake after dietetic intervention.

Variable	Boys (n = 55)	Girls (n = 46)	95% CI*	P value
BMI percentile	−2.61 ± 4.32	−3.49 ± 8.23	(−1.65, 3.43)	0.49
Waist circumference (cm)	−1.19 ± 4.96	0.4 ± 5.96	(3.74, 0.57)	0.15
Total energy (kcal/day)	−649 ± 693	−883 ± 839	(−69, 536)	0.13
Carbohydrates				
Energy (kcal/day of carbohydrates)	−246 ± 455	−467 ± 566	(20, 423)	0.03
Grams (grams)	−74 ± 188	−114 ± 139	(−26.5, 106.1)	0.24
Percent calories (%)	4.9 ± 12.2	2.4 ± 11.5	(−2.18, 7.24)	0.29
Protein				
Energy (kcal/day of protein)	−92 ± 129	−112 ± 138	(−32.6, 72.9)	0.45
Grams (grams)	−23.8 ± 34.3	−28 ± 34.6	(−9.47, 17.82)	0.55
Percent calories (%)	0.56 ± 4.56	1.49 ± 4.72	(−2.76, 0.906)	0.32
Fat				
Energy (kcal/day of fat)	−291 ± 328	−300 ± 291	(−11.3, 132.8)	0.88
Grams (grams)	−31.6 ± 36.2	−32.4 ± 32.7	(−12.91, 14.53)	0.91
Percent calories (%)	−4.1 ± 10.4	−2.86 ± 9.58	(−5.18, 2.77)	0.55

Data represent mean ± standard deviation. *Confidence interval for the mean difference. The significance level used in t-test was 0.05.

intake/day and by the end of the intervention: fat 25%–35% (mean: 24.52 ± 7.96); carbohydrates 45%–65% (mean: 58.13 ± 9.101); and protein 15%–30% (mean: 17.35 ± 3.90) (Table 1).

Concerning daily servings and servings/week of the different food groups, snacks, fast foods, and beverages, Table 3 shows the baseline and end of the school-year dietetic intervention values. There was a significant increase in servings/day of fruits (1.31 to 1.66) (P = 0.00), and specially of water (2.98 to 4.91) (P = 0.00), while there was a considerable decrease of processed meats (3.13 to 2.19) (P = 0.00), oils (3.76 to 1.39) (P = 0.00), sugar sweetened beverages (2.79 to 1.42) (P = 0.00), saturated fat (1.47 to 0.78) (P = 0.00), desserts and refined-grain bakery products (1.99 to 1.32) (P = 0.00), whole fat milk (1.72 to 1.23) (P = 0.00), sweets (1.85 to 1.35) (P = 0.00), fast food meals (0.96 to 0.63) (P = 0.02), and chips and french fries (1.13 to 0.68) (P = 0.00). There was a significant increase in the number of days/week consumption of fish and poultry (3.76 to 4.54) (P = 0.00) and no difference in whole grains intake.

Regarding the number of days/week intake of foods, there was a significant increase in fruits (3.34 to 4.28) (P = 0.00), fish and poultry (3.76 to 4.54) (P = 0.00), and water consumption (6.62 to 6.87) (P = 0.00), while there was a significant decrease in the intake of processed meats (5.60 to 4.37) (P = 0.00), saturated fat (2.19 to 1.10) (P = 0.00), sweets (3.02 to 2.20) (P = 0.00), sugar sweetened beverages (6.21 to 3.89) (P = 0.00), chips and fries (2.60 to 1.36) (P = 0.00), and desserts and refined-grain bakery products (2.85 to 2.54) (P = 0.00). Although in general girls showed more favorable healthy eating changes in days/week intake compared to boys, there was no significant gender difference, except for oils (Table 4).

4. Discussion

According to the Academy of Nutrition and Dietetics, the number of American children who are overweight has more than tripled among 6- to 11-year-old children, which has major health consequences [13]. It is well recognized that the obesity epidemic in children is due in part to the consumption of unhealthy foods and drinks and low physical activity [1]. This is the first study in Mexico to evaluate the effects of an innovative one school-year, face-to-face, individualized, at school, and parent supported dietetic intervention on eating habits of Hispanic, LSE status, school-aged children. Findings were noteworthy in favor of modification towards healthier eating habits. A significant decrease was found between baseline and end-of-year intervention in BMI percentile by a mean difference of −3.0 (P = 0.00) as well as of energy intake/day, while children maintained their macronutrient consumption within the recommended ranges. Reduction of calorie intake in this population is of impact, as it is well known that the most important factor in obesity development is an imbalance between calorie intake and calorie expenditure.

Diverse studies have found an association between the consumption of ED foods and obesity [8, 21] and higher fat mass [22] in children. On the other hand, a pattern characterized by ND foods was associated with smaller gains in BMI [23]. The findings in this study clearly indicate a significant decline in servings/day and servings/week consumption of processed meats, oils, saturated fat, sweetened beverages, desserts, refined-grain bakery products, whole fat milk, sweets, fast food meals, chips and fries, and all ED foods. On the other hand, children improved further their eating habits by increasing significantly the intake of water and that of fruits, fish, and poultry, which are ND foods. Although the increase in fruits and vegetables is small, it is still significant. These findings produced an impact on the well-being of the children and were in accordance with national recommendations to improve fruit and vegetable consumption and decrease intake of fats and added sugars [20], as well as to favor a low consumption of ED foods and an increased consumption of ND foods [13, 24, 25].

The favorable impact on health habits in this interventional study is even more relevant, considering the fact that our population is from LSE status, and thus, at higher risk, as it is well recognized that downward mobility or

Table 3: Comparison of food groups intake at baseline and end of dietetic intervention.

	Sample size $n = 101$							
	Daily servings				Days/week			
	Baseline	End of intervention	95% CI*	P value	Baseline	End of intervention	95% CI*	P value
Fruits	1.31 ± 0.89	1.66 ± 0.96	(0.087, 0.606)	0.00	3.34 ± 2.24	4.28 ± 2.43	(0.39, 1.48)	0.00
Vegetables	0.98 ± 0.77	1.15 ± 0.81	(−0.027, 0.374)	0.09	3.05 ± 2.65	3.44 ± 2.51	(−0.13, 0.92)	0.14
Whole grains	9.92 ± 3.67	8.35 ± 2.88	(−2.33, −0.797)	0.00	6.95 ± 0.35	6.97 ± 0.22	(−0.06, 0.10)	0.64
Beans and peas	1.97 ± 1.25	1.09 ± 0.40	(−1.12, −0.64)	0.00	5.21 ± 2.15	4.49 ± 2.36	(−1.23, −0.20)	0.00
Meats								
Fish/poultry	2.99 ± 1.62	2.62 ± 1.14	(−0.73, 0.00)	0.05	3.76 ± 2.15	4.54 ± 2.25	(0.25, 1.31)	0.00
Processed meats	3.13 ± 1.43	2.188 ± 1.04	(−1.30, −0.58)	0.00	5.6 ± 1.75	4.37 ± 2.10	(−1.72, −0.73)	0.00
Dairy								
Cheese	1.911 ± 1.23	1.71 ± 1.13	(−0.52, 0.13)	0.24	2.9 ± 2.25	2.6 ± 2.04	(−0.84, 0.24)	0.28
Whole fat milk	1.72 ± 1.15	1.23 ± 0.62	(−0.76, −0.30)	0.00	5.38 ± 2.47	5.23 ± 2.55	(−0.68, 0.38)	0.58
Fats								
Oils	3.76 ± 2.04	1.39 ± 0.74	(−2.78, −1.95)	0.00	6.68 ± 1.33	6.98 ± 0.19	(0.03, 0.56)	0.03
Saturated fat	1.47 ± 1.08	0.777 ± 0.79	(−0.96, −0.42)	0.00	2.19 ± 2.18	1.1 ± 1.36	(−1.61, −0.56)	0.00
Sweets								
Sweets	1.85 ± 1.29	1.35 ± 1.75	(−0.92, −0.06)	0.02	3.02 ± 2.58	2.2 ± 2.86	(−1.58, −0.04)	0.03
Sugar sweetened beverages	2.79 ± 1.99	1.42 ± 1.21	(−1.78, −0.96)	0.00	6.21 ± 1.72	3.89 ± 2.80	(−2.98, −1.67)	0.00
Fast food								
Fast food meals	0.96 ± 1.41	0.629 ± 0.57	(−0.61, −0.05)	0.02	0.613 ± 0.79	0.703 ± 0.70	(−0.09, 0.26)	0.32
Chips, French fries	1.13 ± 1.15	0.68 ± 0.56	(−0.69, −0.20)	0.00	2.69 ± 2.47	1.36 ± 1.62	(−1.87, −0.78)	0.00
Desserts, refined grain bakery	1.99 ± 1.54	1.32 ± 1.59	(−1.07, −0.25)	0.00	2.85 ± 2.54	1.57 ± 2.20	(−1.90, −0.65)	0.00
Water	2.98 ± 2.02	4.91 ± 2.37	(1.43, 2.43)	0.00	6.615 ± 2.03	6.87 ± 0.91	(0.29, 1.12)	0.00

Data represent mean ± standard deviation. *Confidence interval for the mean difference. The significance level used in paired t-test was 0.05.

Table 4: Gender comparison of the mean difference of food groups intake after dietetic intervention.

	Daily servings				Days/week			
	Boys (n = 55)	Girls (n = 46)	95% CI*	P value	Boys (n = 55)	Girls (n = 46)	95% CI*	P value
Fruits	0.73 ± 2.75	1.2 ± 2.78	(−1.56, 0.62)	0.40	0.29 ± 1.51	0.41 ± 1.05	(−0.64, 0.40)	0.65
Vegetables	0.27 ± 2.76	0.54 ± 2.64	(−1.34, 0.80)	0.62	−0.02 ± 1.11	0.40 ± 0.85	(−0.81, −0.02)	0.04
Whole grains	0.00 ± 0.38	0.04 ± 0.46	(−0.21, 0.12)	0.61	−1.55 ± 4.25	−1.59 ± 3.46	(−1.50, 1.59)	0.96
Beans and peas	−0.82 ± 2.55	−0.61 ± 2.71	(−1.25, 0.83)	0.69	−0.88 ± 1.16	−0.89 ± 1.30	(−0.47, 0.49)	0.97
Meats								
Fish/poultry	0.56 ± 2.75	1.04 ± 2.63	(−1.55, 0.59)	0.38	−0.29 ± 2.08	−0.46 ± 1.63	(−0.56, 0.89)	0.66
Processed meats	−0.96 ± 2.61	−1.54 ± 2.34	(−0.40, 1.56)	0.25	−0.93 ± 1.79	−0.95 ± 1.89	(−0.70, 0.74)	0.96
Dairy								
Cheese	−0.11 ± 2.88	−0.52 ± 2.62	(−0.685, 1.51)	0.46	−0.31 ± 1.87	−0.07 ± 1.41	(−0.89, 0.40)	0.46
Whole fat milk	−0.31 ± 2.64	0.04 ± 2.76	(−1.42, 0.71)	0.52	−0.66 ± 1.36	−0.38 ± 0.85	(−0.72, 0.16)	0.21
Fats								
Oils	0.03 ± 0.60	0.61 ± 1.86	(−1.14, 0.00)	0.05	−2.59 ± 1.76	−2.11 ± 2.43	(−1.31, 0.34)	0.25
Saturated fat	−1.06 ± 3.08	−1.12 ± 2.04	(−0.96, 1.07)	0.91	−0.53 ± 1.44	−0.9 ± 1.26	(−0.15, 0.90)	0.17
Sweets								
Sweets	−1.15 ± 4.18	−0.41 ± 3.51	(−2.27, 0.81)	0.35	−0.36 ± 2.28	−0.65 ± 2.06	(−0.57, 1.15)	0.51
Sugar sweetened beverages	−2.13 ± 3.30	−2.57 ± 3.36	(−0.88, 1.75)	0.51	−1.53 ± 2.28	−1.18 ± 1.81	(−1.16, 0.48)	0.41
Fast food								
Fast food meals	0.11 ± 0.79	0.07 ± 1.04	(−0.31, 0.40)	0.81	−0.46 ± 1.54	−0.17 ± 1.25	(−0.85, 0.27)	0.31
Chips, French fries	−1.02 ± 2.59	−1.7 ± 2.92	(−0.41, 1.76)	0.22	−0.44 ± 1.32	−0.47 ± 1.19	(−0.46, 0.53)	0.90
Desserts, refined grain bakery	−1.25 ± 3.01	−1.3 ± 3.37	(−1.21, 1.31)	0.94	−0.23 ± 1.91	−1.18 ± 2.19	(0.14, 1.76)	0.02
Water	0.36 ± 1.75	1.13 ± 2.41	(−1.61, 0.08)	0.08	2.00 ± 2.46	1.85 ± 2.65	(−0.85, 1.16)	0.77

Data represent mean ± standard deviation. *Confidence interval for the mean difference. The significance level used in t-test was 0.05.

stable LSE status has been associated with greater adiposity evaluated by BMI, waist circumference, and triceps skin fold [11]. This link has also been found in cross-sectional studies [10] and in longitudinal ones that even associate LSE status in childhood with adult obesity [26]. Even more, the prevalence of childhood obesity almost doubled across levels of household income [12]. In addition, LSE status has also been associated with poor and unhealthy eating [10, 27] such as low vegetable consumption and high intake of fried foods [9] and consumption of ED fast foods [27]. Thus, the fact that our at-risk population changed their dietary consumption of all food groups in a favorable way is important not only for the reduction in their actual BMI percentiles, but it may also contribute to their health status and in prevention of cardiometabolic chronic diseases such as insulin resistance, diabetes mellitus, dyslipidemias, and the metabolic syndrome in the near future.

Several studies have demonstrated that Hispanic children and adolescents, such as our studied population, have a greater proportion of obesity, visceral fat, and type 2 diabetes [5, 6], as well as greater morbidity and mortality [28]. Besides, research has shown that Hispanic children have a tendency towards nonhealthy eating habits, such as low consumption of fruits, vegetables, and milk and higher intake of saturated fat, fries, fast food, and high ED foods such as refined-grain bakery products [7]. In a study conducted on school-age Mexican children, patterns characterized by high intakes of ED foods were associated with a higher risk of overweight/obesity [8]. These facts highlight the importance of our dietetic intervention, which achieved an improvement towards healthy eating habits in this at-risk Hispanic population.

However, although some school-based interventions in other countries that were directed at curriculum modifications or changing school policies, or the selling or provision of food within the schools have had positive effects on improving healthy eating habits [16], some others have not [17, 18] because they were short-term, they either neglected or poorly addressed what children ate outside of school or the importance of family support [29]. Furthermore, the dietetic interventions have not been carried out on an individualized basis, as ours has been. Our dietetic intervention was carried out at the schools as a partnership. The school administrative personnel and the teachers reminded children of the next nutrition consultation both verbally and by written notification. On the visit day, children were called out of the classroom for their individual consultations with the Rds. This school support facilitated enormously the adherence to the dietetic intervention.

It is also well known that parents influence food preferences and eating behaviors of children, as demonstrated in various studies [7, 15, 29] and as stated by national associations [13, 14]. Previous studies have shown an association between more availability of unhealthy food products, more permissiveness from parents and less healthy food choices among Hispanic children and adolescents [7, 15]. Thus, nutrition education for Hispanic parents of LSE status seems especially important for improving children's diets.

Favorable results of this study might also be due to the fact that parent/caregiver presence was mandatory at the time of the consultations with the RD and they were instructed regarding nutrition education and healthy eating habits for the whole family and how to deal with the food preferences of their particular child participating in the study.

The study had some limitations, though. Voluntary participation in the study and the relatively small sample may have influenced our results and may not be representative of the general population. Not having a control group could have limited the impact of this intervention. The children and their parents/caregivers were likely to be highly motivated and thus the study could be biased in this regard.

Nevertheless, the study had several strengths. Factors contributing to the changes in healthier eating habits and the decrease in BMI percentiles were the parental support, the school partnership, the year-long intervention, the face-to-face consultations with the RDs, and the individualized tailor-made menus that the RDs planned for each child. A long-term follow-up plan is currently being structured to be able to measure the success of the dietary intervention.

5. Conclusions

Our findings in obese, Hispanic, LSE status children demonstrating a change in dietary patterns towards healthier eating habits, contribute to our understanding that maybe the strategy we followed is needed to help overcome obesity and to move towards healthier eating habits. To the best of our knowledge, this is the first initiative of its kind that we found in literature search. Although the solution is complex, intervention strategies that focus on individual children's attitudes and parental behavior should aim at creating individual behavior changes. Having a home and school environment with healthy eating behaviors is recommended to encourage children to maintain these new eating habits in the long term.

Conflict of Interests

The authors declare that there is no conflict of interests regarding the publication of this paper.

Acknowledgments

The authors have no financial interests to declare. The authors would like to thank deeply Lorena Lam, Andrea de la Garza, Daniela Tamargo, Alejandra Ríos-Hernández, Natalia Garza, and Maricel Barbosa, for their invaluable collaboration during the fieldwork, and to Bianca Nieblas for her writting assistance. M.D. Leticia Elizondo-Montemayor affirms that she has listed and obtained written consent from everyone who contributed significantly to the work in this paper.

References

[1] S. R. Daniels, M. S. Jacobson, B. W. McCrindle, H. Robert, and B. M. Sanner, "American heart association childhood obesity research summit report," *Circulation*, vol. 119, no. 15, pp. e489–e517, 2009, Erratum in *Circulation*, vol. 120, pp. e14-e15, 2009.

[2] Food and Agriculture Organization of the United Nations, *The State of Food and Agriculture: Food Systems for Better Nutrition*, FAO, Rome, Italy, 2013, http://www.fao.org/docrep/018/i3300e/i3300e00.htm.

[3] G. Olaiz-Fernández, J. Rivera-Dommarco, T. Shamah-Levy et al., "Encuesta Nacional de Salud y Nutrición 2012: resultados nacionales," Instituto Nacional de Salud Pública (MX), Cuernavaca, México, 2012, http://ensanut.insp.mx/informes/ENSANUT2012ResultadosNacionales.pdf.

[4] L. Elizondo-Montemayor, M. Serrano-González, P. A. Ugalde-Casas, C. Cuello-García, and J. R. Borbolla-Escoboza, "Metabolic syndrome risk factors among a sample of overweight and obese Mexican children," *The Journal of Clinical Hypertension*, vol. 12, no. 5, pp. 380–387, 2010.

[5] S. Cook, M. Weitzman, P. Auinger, M. Nguyen, and W. H. Dietz, "Prevalence of a metabolic syndrome phenotype in adolescents: findings from the Third National Health and Nutrition Examination Survey, 1988–1994," *Archives of Pediatrics and Adolescent Medicine*, vol. 157, no. 8, pp. 821–827, 2003.

[6] E. Fuentes-Afflick and N. A. Hessol, "Overweight in young latino children," *Archives of Medical Research*, vol. 39, no. 5, pp. 511–518, 2008.

[7] R. E. Mazur, G. S. Marquis, and H. H. Jensen, "Diet and food insufficiency among Hispanic youths: acculturation and socioeconomic factors in the Third National Health and Nutrition Examination Survey," *The American Journal of Clinical Nutrition*, vol. 78, no. 6, pp. 1120–1127, 2003.

[8] S. Rodríguez-Ramírez, V. Mundo-Rosas, A. Garcia-Guerra, and T. Shamah-Levy, "Dietary patterns are associated with overweight and obesity in Mexican school-aged children," *Archivos Latinoamericanos de Nutrición*, vol. 61, no. 3, pp. 270–278, 2001.

[9] T. F. Eagle, A. Sheetz, R. Gurm et al., "Understanding childhood obesity in America: linkages between household income, community resources, and children's behaviors," *The American Heart Journal*, vol. 163, no. 5, pp. 836–843, 2012.

[10] Y. Wang and M. A. Beydoun, "The obesity epidemic in the United States—gender, age, socioeconomic, racial/ethnic, and geographic characteristics: a systematic review and meta-regression analysis," *Epidemiologic Reviews*, vol. 29, no. 1, pp. 6–28, 2007.

[11] D. E. Kendzor, M. O. Caughy, and M. T. Owen, "Family income trajectory during childhood is associated with adiposity in adolescence: a latent class growth analysis," *BMC Public Health*, vol. 12, no. 1, article 611, 2012.

[12] C. L. Ogden, M. M. Lamb, M. D. Carroll, and K. M. Flegal, "Obesity and socioeconomic status in children and adolescents: United States, 2005–2008," *National Center for Health Statistics Data Brief*, no. 51, pp. 1–8, 2010.

[13] T. A. Nicklas and D. Hayes, "Position of the American Dietetic Association: nutrition guidance for healthy children ages 2 to 11 years," *Journal of the American Dietetic Association*, vol. 108, no. 6, pp. 1038–1047, 2008.

[14] B. A. Spear, S. E. Barlow, C. Ervin et al., "Recommendations for treatment of child and adolescent overweight and obesity," *Pediatrics*, vol. 120, no. 4, pp. S254–S288, 2007.

[15] C. Vereecken, E. Legiest, I. de Bourdeaudhuij, and L. Maes, "Associations between general parenting styles and specific food-related parenting practices and children's food consumption," *The American Journal of Health Promotion*, vol. 23, no. 4, pp. 233–240, 2009.

[16] J. A. Mendoza, K. Watson, and K. W. Cullen, "Change in dietary energy density after implementation of the Texas Public School Nutrition Policy," *Journal of the American Dietetic Association*, vol. 110, no. 3, pp. 434–440, 2010.

[17] D. L. Katz, M. O'Connell, V. Y. Njike, M.-C. Yeh, and H. Nawaz, "Strategies for the prevention and control of obesity in the school setting: systematic review and meta-analysis," *International Journal of Obesity*, vol. 32, no. 12, pp. 1780–1789, 2008.

[18] M. J. Müller, S. Danielzik, and S. Pust, "School- and family-based interventions to prevent overweight in children," *Proceedings of the Nutrition Society*, vol. 64, no. 2, pp. 249–254, 2005.

[19] Subcommittees on Upper Reference Levels of Nutrients and Interpretation and Uses of Dietary Reference Intakes, and the Standing Committee on the Scientific Evaluation of Dietary Reference Intakes, Food and Nutrition Board, and Institute or Medicine, *Dietary Reference Intakes for Energy, Carbohydrate, Fiber, Fat, Fatty Acids, Cholesterol, Protein, and Amino Acids*, A Report of the Panel on Macronutrients, The National Academies Press, Washington, DC, USA, 2005, http://www.nap.edu/openbook.php?isbn=0309085373.

[20] U. S. Department of Agriculture and U. S. Department of Health and Human Services, *Dietary Guidelines for Americans*, Government Printing Office, Washington, DC, USA, 7th edition, 2010, http://health.gov/dietaryguidelines/dga2010/dietaryguidelines2010.pdf.

[21] S. Lioret, M. Touvier, L. Lafay, J.-L. Volatier, and B. Maire, "Dietary and physical activity patterns in French children are related to overweight and socioeconomic status," *The Journal of Nutrition*, vol. 138, no. 1, pp. 101–107, 2008.

[22] T. A. McCaffrey, K. L. Rennie, M. A. Kerr et al., "Energy density of the diet and change in body fatness from childhood to adolescence; is there a relation?" *The American Journal of Clinical Nutrition*, vol. 87, no. 5, pp. 1230–1237, 2008.

[23] P. K. Newby, D. Muller, J. Hallfrisch, N. Qiao, R. Andres, and K. L. Tucker, "Dietary patterns and changes in body mass index and waist circumference in adults," *The American Journal of Clinical Nutrition*, vol. 77, no. 6, pp. 1417–1425, 2003.

[24] S. E. Barlow, "Expert committee recommendations regarding the prevention, assessment, and treatment of child and adolescent overweight and obesity: summary report," *Pediatrics*, vol. 120, no. 4, pp. 164–192, 2007.

[25] B. J. Rolls, A. Drewnowski, and J. H. Ledikwe, "Changing the energy density of the diet as a strategy for weight management," *Journal of the American Dietetic Association*, vol. 105, no. 5, pp. S98–S103, 2005.

[26] L. C. Senese, N. D. Almeida, A. K. Fath, B. T. Smith, and E. B. Loucks, "Associations between childhood socioeconomic position and adulthood obesity," *Epidemiologic Reviews*, vol. 31, no. 1, pp. 21–51, 2009.

[27] E. A. Jackson, T. Eagle, A. Leidal et al., "Childhood obesity: a comparison of health habits of middle-school students from two communities," *Clinical Epidemiology*, vol. 2009, article 1, pp. 133–139, 2009.

[28] D. R. Thompson, E. Obarzanek, D. L. Franko et al., "Childhood overweight and cardiovascular disease risk factors: the National Heart, Lung, and Blood Institute Growth and Health Study," *The Journal of Pediatrics*, vol. 150, no. 1, pp. 18–25, 2007.

[29] M. D. Hingle, T. M. O'Connor, J. M. Dave, and T. Baranowski, "Parental involvement in interventions to improve child dietary intake: a systematic review," *Preventive Medicine*, vol. 51, no. 2, pp. 103–111, 2010.

20

Effects of Dietary Milled Seed Mixture on Fatty Acid Status and Inflammatory Markers in Patients on Hemodialysis

Danijela Ristic-Medic,[1] Gordana Perunicic-Pekovic,[2] Zorica Rasic-Milutinovic,[3] Marija Takic,[1] Tamara Popovic,[1] Aleksandra Arsic,[1] and Marija Glibetic[1]

[1] *Centre of Research Excellence in Nutrition and Metabolism, Institute for Medical Research, University of Belgrade, P.O. Box 102, 11000 Belgrade, Serbia*
[2] *Department of Nephrology and Dialysis, Clinical Hospital Zemun, University of Belgrade, Belgrade, Serbia*
[3] *Department of Endocrinology, Diabetes and Metabolism, Clinical Hospital Zemun, University of Belgrade, Belgrade, Serbia*

Correspondence should be addressed to Danijela Ristic-Medic; dristicmedic@gmail.com

Academic Editors: E. Kirk and E. van den Heuvel

Background. Plant seeds have gained interest for their health benefits due to their fatty acid content. The objective of this study was to determine the effects of dietary consumption of milled sesame/pumpkin/flax seed mixture on glycemic control, serum lipids, phospholipid fatty acid status, and inflammatory factors in patients on hemodialysis. *Methods.* Thirty patients with well nutrition status (18 male, 12 female) were enrolled in the study. Participants consumed 30 g of milled sesame/pumpkin/flax (6 g/6 g/18 g, resp.) seeds mixture added to their habitual diet. *Results.* Total n-6 and n-3 polyunsaturated fatty acids and levels of linoleic, dihomo-gamma-linolenic (DGLA), arachidonic, alpha-linolenic (ALA), eicosapentaenoic, docosapentaenoic, and docosahexaenoic (DHA) acid were increased after 12 weeks of supplementation. A significant decrease of the serum triglyceride level ($P < 0.001$), glucose, insulin, calculated IR HOMA ($P < 0.05$), and inflammatory markers (TNF-alpha, IL-6, and hs-CRP, $P < 0.001$) was observed after seed mixture treatment. The serum levels of CRP and TNF-alpha negative correlate with ALA, DHA, and DGLA. *Conclusion.* Results of this study indicated that dietary milled sesame/pumpkin/flax seed mixture added to a habitual diet lowered triglyceride and CRP, TNF-alpha, IL-6 levels, affect glycemic control and improved fatty acid profile and pruritus symptoms in hemodialysis patients.

1. Introduction

Fatty acid composition in serum phospholipids can be used not only as a biomarker of dietary fat intake quality, but also as an indicator of disease risk [1, 2]. In observational and intervention studies altered fatty acid composition of phospholipids linked with metabolic and cardiovascular diseases [2–4]. This suggestion implied a continued dietary supply. In our previous studies we showed that patients on hemodialysis have higher level of oleic (18 : 1 n-9) and lower levels of eicosapentaenoic (EPA) and docosahexaenoic (DHA) acids, with low levels of total n-6 and n-3 polyunsaturated fatty acid (PUFA) [5–8]. There are many limitations in the published studies which deal with changes in fatty acid (FA) metabolism and PUFA content in chronic renal failure. However, in general, it can be concluded that patients on hemodialysis need nutritional care programs with an adequate n-6/n-3 PUFA ratio in their diet [9, 10].

The precursor to long-chain n-3 fatty acid is alpha-linolenic acid (ALA), which is elongated to EPA and docosapentaenoic acid (DPA n-3), possibly more in women than in men [11, 12]. According to the available literature, further metabolism of DPA n-3 to DHA is very limited [12, 13]. However, the use of the plant-based n-3 fatty acid to be alternative to consummation of fish may be important for maintaining optimal EPA and DHA status in plasma and cell membranes. It is important to address that serum levels of ALA significantly increased after ingestion of flax oil and milled flaxseed whereas whole flaxseed, did not show the same effect [14, 15]. Flax, pumpkin, and sesame seeds have gained interest for their health benefits due to their fatty acid and lignan contents [16–18]. Flaxseed is also an excellent source of dietary fiber and contains protein and several micronutrients. Sesame and flax seeds are considerably different in the PUFA content, with a high ALA n-3 level (51–55%) in flaxseeds and high linoleic acid (LA) n-6 content in sesame seeds (44%). Since sesame seed is a rich source of n-6 FA and also monounsaturated FA (oleic acid 40%), in addition to diet, increased serum phospholipids LA levels as biomarker of intake are observed [19, 20]. The seeds of pumpkin are rich natural source of LA n-6 (40.4–55.6%), oleic acid, and antioxidant vitamins, such as carotenoids and tocopherol [21, 22]. The ideal ratio of LA n-6 and ALA n-3 in diet is not known, but ratio of 1 : 1-2 has been considered beneficial to health with effects on cell membrane fluidity and membrane function [23]. The balance required in the diet between n-6 and n-3 fatty acid is important due to their competitive nature and their different biological roles [24, 25].

Uremic pruritus is one of common symptoms in patients with end-stage renal disease (ESRD), with approximately 60–90% of patients on hemodialysis suffering from this problem [26, 27]. The pathogenesis of dry, scaly skin, and pruritus is not known but could be related to the abnormal fatty acid profile reported in these patients [10, 28]. It is shown that intervention with fish oil may improve symptoms of pruritus in hemodialysis patients [28].

In the latest prospective cohort study on inflammation and death risk, Noori et al. [29] concluded that a higher dietary n-6/n-3 PUFA ratio appears to be associated with inflammation and a trend toward higher risk of morality in hemodialysis patients. Inflammatory states in ESRD are associated with an elevation of C-reactive protein (CRP) and some proinflammatory cytokines such as interleukin-6 (IL-6) and tumor necrosis factor-alpha (TNF-alpha) [6, 8, 30]. IL-6 is reported to play a central role in the pathophysiology of the adverse effects of inflammation in ESRD patients. The increased activation of inflammatory cytokines such as IL-6 and TNF-alpha may cause muscle breakdown and hypoalbuminemia and may be involved in atherogenesis [31, 32].

The purpose of the present study was prospective evaluation of the effects of milled sesame/pumpkin/flax seed mixture dietary treatments on nutrition status, plasma lipids, phospholipids fatty acid profile, inflammatory markers, and symptoms of pruritus in patients on hemodialysis.

2. Patients and Methods

We cross-sectionally evaluated 65 patients on maintenance hemodialysis from the Department of Nephrology, University Hospital Zemun (Belgrade). For this study we included cohort group of 30 chronic renal failure patients (18 male, 12 female, mean age 55 ± 14 yr; range 42 to 64), who have been selected based on their well nutrition status. All patients had been on maintenance hemodialysis three times a week for at least 6 months and the mean duration of hemodialysis in included patients was 4.76 ± 3.38 yr. The duration of dialysis was defined as the number of months from the initiation of chronic hemodialysis to the time of laboratory data collection. The patients were clinically stable, with adequate nutrition status and with no recorded cardiovascular events (coronary heart disease and cerebrovascular disease). The mean body mass index (BMI) calculated from dry body weight was 22.63±3.44 kg/m^2 (range 19.8 to 27.3). Serum albumin concentration was 46.27 ± 7.22 g/L and serum CRP level was 6.26 ± 4.12 mg/mL. Patients were dialyzed with synthetic membranes and a bicarbonate dialysate with 1.25, 1.5, or 1.75 mmol/L calcium according to the serum calcium phosphate equilibrium and with obligatory use of 1.25-dihydroxy vitamin D3 to control the parathyroid hormone levels. The duration of hemodialysis was individually tailored (4–6 h weekly) to control body fluids and blood chemistries with the aim of achieving Kt/V > 1.2 (1.46 ± 0.13). Patients did not regularly receive epoetin therapy during that time. Antihypertensives were prescribed when it was necessary to obtain predialysis blood pressure < 160/90 mmHg. Patients with a history of nephrotic syndrome, diabetes mellitus, alcohol consummation, systemic illness, or any other disease that might influence lipid metabolism were excluded. None of the patients received lipid lowering drugs, L-carnitine, β-blockersor, vitamin B12 in the 3 months prior to entering the study. Patients received no other medications except multivitamins, calcitriol phosphate binders, and/or iron. Calcium carbonate was used to obtain predialysis serum phosphate level < 2.0 mmol/L. Patients maintained their habitual diets (35 kcal/kg bw, protein intake 1–1.2 g/kg bw, fats < 35% caloric intake) with sodium and potassium restriction. They had low habitual consumption of foods containing soy, fish intake once in two weeks, and no dietary supplementation of oil rich in long-chain fatty acid (fish, sesame, or linseed oil) as determined by diet assessment made at the time of recruitment. All patients were sedentary (<1 h/wk of physical activity), free of alcohol consumption, and nonsmokers. All study participants signed and provided an informed consent document. Study protocol was approved by the ethical review boards of the participating institutions in accordance with the principles of the Declaration of Helsinki.

2.1. Study Design. This study was a cross-sectional and follow-up dietary intervention study. Patients were instructed to mix 30 g per day of milled seed mixture containing 6 g sesame : 6 g pumpkin : 18 g flax (1 : 1 : 3) (company Beyond, Nis, Serbia; seed mixture was made in our laboratory) in 200 mL of fat-free milk (Imlek, Belgrade) in a single evening dose before dinner during the follow-up period of 12 weeks. In the present study, the test milled seed mixture was added to the habitual diet as they have already consumed at least 200 mL of fat-free milk a day at the moment they were recruited for our study. The participants were also instructed to continue to consume a usual amount of milk. Although no modification of the habitual diets for these patients was planned, they were instructed to keep their usual diets and level of physical activity relatively constant throughout the study and to maintain stable body weights. Fatty acid profile of ground seed mixture (analyzed with gas chromatography) was sum of palmitic and stearic fatty acid 18%, oleic acid (OA) 30%, LA 24%, and ALA 28%; polyunsaturated/saturated (PUFA/SFA) fatty acid ratio was 4 : 1 and n-6/n-3 ratio was 1 : 1. Daily fatty acid intake from milled seed mixture was palmitic acid 0.9 g, stearic 0.7 g, OA 3.9 g, LA 2.9 g, and ALA 3.0 g. Specific instructions were given not to take any new supplements or increase the amount of fish in the diet. The patients continued to consume (sunflower oil) n-6 PUFA cooking oils as part of their usual diet. The diet control was done as usual for all study participants by interview during hemodialysis.

For the purpose of this study, uremic pruritus was defined as pruritus appearing in close conjunction with the commencement of dialysis or appearing in conjunction with significant deterioration in renal function [33]. A questionnaire with issues to evaluate subjective feeling of presence and frequency of pruritus was given to patients at baseline and after intervention period. The pruritus questionnaire was used as the short form from Peck et al. [28] for assessment of uremic pruritus in part of the pruritus history. The questions covered the presence of dry skin or itching (yes/no), history of pruritus symptoms (1–4, from never to continuing daily, weekly, fortnightly, or monthly), severity (1–5, from mild to total restlessness), distribution (1–3, single location to generalized), and frequency of symptoms (number of episodes per 24 h).

2.2. Biochemical Determination. Blood samples were taken in the middle of week, after 12–14 h of overnight fasting and immediately prior to dialysis in the beginning of study and after 12 weeks. Serum samples were prepared by 4°C centrifugation of venous blood. Plasma triglyceride, glucose, and total cholesterol concentrations were measured by using standard enzyme color tests (EliTech Diagnostic. Sées, France); HDL cholesterol was determined by the enzyme procedure (EliTech Diagnostic. Sées, France) in supernatant after precipitation by the phosphotungstic acid and LDL cholesterol was estimated by using Friedewald formula. Total phospholipids were determined by the method of Zilversmit and Davis [34]. Insulin level was measured using the radioimmunoassay method (INEP Zemun, Belgrade, Serbia). Fasting insulin and glucose concentrations were used to calculate insulin resistance from the IR-HOMA model (insulin × glucose/22.5) [35].

Serum albumin concentration was determined by using bromcresol green reagent (EliTech Diagnostic. Sées, France). Serum iron was measured by a photometric color test for clinical chemistry analyzers (Olympus System Reagent; Olympus Diagnostica). IL-6 and TNF-alpha concentrations were measured in duplicate by Immunotech IL-6 immunoassays and Immunotech TNF-alpha immunoassays (Beckman Coulter, Fullerton, CA, USA), and hs-CRP was measured by the Olympus (LATEX) assay on the Olympus AU 400 analyzer (Olympus, PA, USA) by methods that have already been reported [7].

2.3. Fatty Acid Determination. Serum lipids were extracted according to method of Sperry and Brand [36] which uses chloroform-methanol mixture (2 : 1, v/v) with 10 mg/100 mL 2.6-di-tert-buthyl-4-methylphenol (BHT) added as an antioxidant. The phospholipids fraction was isolated from the lipid extract using one-dimensional thin-layer chromatography (TLC) in a neutral lipid solvent system hexane-diethyl ether-acetic acid (87 : 12 : 1, v/v/v) using Silica Gel GF plates (C. Merck, Darmstadt, Germany).

Methyl esters of phospholipids FA were prepared by methods that have already been reported [37]. Fatty acid methyl esters derivatives were analyzed by gas chromatography using Varian GC (model 3400, Varian Associates) equipped with SP-2330 (30 m × 0.53 mm i.d., film thickness 0.5 μm; Supelco Inc., Bellefonte, PA) fused silica capillary column. Analysis was performed in duplicate for each sample. Individual FA methyl esters were identified by comparing peak retention times with authentic standards (Sigma Aldrich, Germany) and/or the PUFA-2 standard mixtures (Supelco Inc., Bellefonte, PA). The results were expressed as the relative percentage of total identified FA.

2.4. Statistical Analysis. All the results are expressed as the mean ± SD. Before being statistically analyzed, all data were examined for normality by using the Shapiro-Wilks test. Differences in the absolute changes in fasting plasma triglycerides, total cholesterol, HDL cholesterol, LDL cholesterol, albumin, creatinine, hemoglobin, hs-CRP, TNF-alpha, IL-6, glucose, insulin, iron, calculated IR HOMA, and FA profile of serum phospholipids over the 12-week period of milled seed mixture supplementation were determined using independent-sample t-tests or Mann-Whitney U test for variables with skewed distribution. The Pearson correlation coefficients were computed for examination of the relation between inflammatory factors and fatty acid composition of serum phospholipids. The differences were considered significant at $P \leq 0.05$.

3. Results

3.1. Subject Characteristics. The baseline characteristics of the study participants are presented in Table 1. All participants completed the study and there were no withdrawals. There were no significant differences in the anthropometrical characteristics of hemodialysis patients before and after 12 weeks of milled seed mixture dietary treatments. Most patients (20 participants) had suffered from pruritus for periods ranging from 6 months to 1 year. In most patients (60%), pruritus symptoms were aggravated during the night sleeping period compared to rate of pruritus symptoms during the daytime. Seed mixture added to diet improves the symptoms of pruritus in all patients. The scores for severity, distribution, and frequency of pruritus symptoms on the questionnaire showed a great improvement. Systolic and diastolic blood pressure were significantly decreased after 12 of weeks of treatment ($P < 0.01$). We also found significant decrease of creatinine level ($P < 0.05$) at the end of the study. This seed mixture was well tolerated with no significant side effect in hemodialysis patients.

TABLE 1: The baseline characteristics of study participants and responsiveness to milled seed mixture after twelve weeks.

Variable	Before treatment	After treatment
Age	55 ± 14	
Gender (M/F)	30 (18/12)	
Duration of HD (years)	4.76 ± 3.38	
BMI (kg/m^2)	22.63 ± 3.44	22.81 ± 3.62
SBP (mmHg)	155 ± 14	144 ± 13**
DBP (mmHg)	92 ± 9	86 ± 10**
WBC 10^9/L	6.40 ± 1.46	5.74 ± 1.46
Hematocrit L/L	0.27 ± 0.04	0.26 ± 0.06
Serum creatinine (μmol/L)	785 ± 158	722 ± 156*
Serum urea (μmol/L)	20.56 ± 2.30	19.41 ± 2.34
Serum iron (μmol/L)	13.67 ± 4.77	14.49 ± 4.34*
Serum albumin (g/L)	46.27 ± 7.22	43.74 ± 4.05
Serum glucose (mmol/L)	4.76 ± 1.18	4.28 ± 0.82*
Serum insulin (pg/mL)	23.98 ± 9.42	20.28 ± 6.36*
IR HOMA	5.09 ± 2.82	3.83 ± 1.35*
TNF (mU/L)	1.86 ± 0.90	0.72 ± 0.59***
IL-6 (pg/mL)	2.63 ± 1.45	0.55 ± 0.34***
hs-CRP (mg/L)	6.26 ± 4.12	3.06 ± 1.34***

The values are means ± SD. $^*P \leq 0.05$, $^{**}P \leq 0.01$, and $^{***}P \leq 0.001$ significantly different from baseline.

3.2. Serum Lipids. Effect of milled seed mixture dietary treatments on mean serum lipid values for all participating patients and percentage change are shown in Table 2. After 12 weeks of consuming milled sesame/pumpkin/flax seed mixture in the hemodialysis patients, total and LDL cholesterol concentrations had decreased by 7% and 5% ($P < 0.05$, $P > 0.05$), respectively (Table 2). The Tg/HDL ($P < 0.01$) ratio significantly decreased but TC/HDL and LDL/HDL cholesterol ratios decreases remained non statistic. Serum HDL cholesterol did not differ from baseline values throughout either feeding period. During 12 weeks of seed mixture consumption, serum plasma triglyceride levels decreased by 30% ($P < 0.001$) compared with baseline values (week 0) (Table 2).

3.3. Fatty Acid Profile of Serum Phospholipids. The fatty acid profiles of serum phospholipids before and after treatment are shown in Table 3. Saturated 16 : 0 ($P < 0.01$), 18 : 0 ($P < 0.01$), and total SFA ($P < 0.001$) were significantly decreased and oleic acid ($P < 0.05$) and total MUFA increased ($P < 0.01$) in serum phospholipids after treatments. Percentages of LA ($P < 0.01$), dihomo-γ-linoleic (DGLA; 20 : 3n-6) ($P < 0.01$), AA ($P < 0.05$), ALA ($P < 0.05$), EPA ($P < 0.05$), DPA n-3 ($P < 0.05$), and DHA ($P < 0.01$) in serum phospholipids were significantly higher after 12 weeks of intervention. Consistent with the previous were the increases in n-6 PUFA n-3 PUFA, total PUFA, and PUFA/SFA ratios as well ($P < 0.001$ for all mentioned parameters) (Table 3).

3.4. Glucose Tolerance and Inflammatory Markers. A significant decrease of the glucose, insulin, calculated IR HOMA ($P < 0.05$ for all mentioned variables), and inflammatory markers (TNF-alpha, IL-6, hs-CRP, $P < 0.001$) was observed after dietary intervention (Table 1). The serum levels of CRP negative correlate with ALA, DHA, DGLA, and AA in serum phospholipids (Table 4). There was very strong negative correlation between serum TNF-α and ALA, DHA, LA, and DGLA. The serum levels IL-6 negative correlate with ALA, DPAn-3, DGLA, and AA in serum phospholipids (Table 4).

4. Discussion

The results clearly demonstrate that dietary treatment with milled sesame/pumpkin/flax seeds mixture (30 g; rich in n-6 and n-3 FA) for 12 weeks has the capacity to improve traditional lipid levels, inflammatory markers, and serum fatty acid composition as biomarker of status in hemodialysis patients. We also showed the efficacy of increasing levels of not only EPA, but also DHA in plasma phospholipids by providing its precursor ALA (3.0 g) from seed mixture. That was inconsistent with reports that EPA can limitedly be converted to DHA [12, 38]. Therefore, it is important to emphasize that our patients have low intake of fish, once every two weeks, as poor eating patterns of people in our region [25]. Human clinical studies show that an increase in dietary ALA leads to significant increases in ALA, EPA, and DPAn-3 in the blood [39, 40] and they are carried out using daily intakes of > 5 g ALA. It is well known that fatty acid composition of the serum phospholipids clearly reflects the change of dietary habits [41, 42]. This is proved by analysis of fatty acid status in our hemodialysis patients after dietary treatment. Our findings for changes of LA levels in serum phospholipids, LA being the most represented fatty acid (2.9 g) in our seed mixture beside ALA (3.0 g), are consistent with Okita et al. [42] who reported that the LA levels in serum phospholipids appeared to reflect the dietary LA content.

Table 2: Baseline serum lipids profile responsiveness to milled seed mixture after twelve weeks.

Serum lipids	Baseline (mmol/L)	After treatment (mmol/L)	Change %	Probability
Triglycerides	2.06 ± 1.20	1.44 ± 0.92	−30	$P \leq 0.01$
Total cholesterol	5.47 ± 1.35	5.01 ± 0.81	−7	$P \leq 0.05$
HDL cholesterol	1.30 ± 0.11	1.27 ± 0.14	−2	ns
LDL cholesterol	3.24 ± 1.08	3.08 ± 0.40	−5	ns
TC/HDL ratio	4.26 ± 1.27	4.01 ± 0.75	−6	ns
LDL/HDL ratio	2.53 ± 0.98	2.47 ± 0.47	−2	ns
Tg/HDL ratio	1.61 ± 0.98	1.17 ± 0.76	−27	$P \leq 0.01$
Total phospholipids	2.87 ± 0.74	2.50 ± 0.51	−13	ns

The values are means ± SD.

Table 3: Serum phospholipids fatty acid composition at baseline and changes induced by dietary intervention.

Serum fatty acids	Baseline	After treatment
16:0	25.32 ± 2.39	23.87 ± 2.09**
18:0	16.44 ± 1.74	15.05 ± 1.02**
SFA	41.76 ± 3.22	38.93 ± 2.34***
16:1n-7	0.39 ± 0.16	0.36 ± 0.15
18:1n-9	13.83 ± 1.68	14.92 ± 0.86*
MUFA	14.59 ± 1.66	15.28 ± 0.94**
18:2n-6 LA	24.49 ± 2.62	25.73 ± 1.85**
20:3n-6	2.57 ± 0.79	2.96 ± 0.70**
20:4n-6	11.63 ± 2.31	12.77 ± 2.56*
22:4n-6	0.56 ± 0.14	0.61 ± 0.11
n-6	39.25 ± 3.25	42.06 ± 2.72***
18:3n-3 LNA	0.08 ± 0.03	0.12 ± 0.02*
20:5n-3 EPA	0.18 ± 0.05	0.22 ± 0.08*
22:5n-3	0.46 ± 0.07	0.51 ± 0.10*
22:6n-3 DHA	2.75 ± 0.33	2.99 ± 0.39**
n-3	3.46 ± 0.37	3.84 ± 0.42***
PUFA	42.71 ± 3.39	45.90 ± 2.69***
n-6/n-3 ratio	11.34 ± 1.25	10.91 ± 1.59
PUFA/SFA ratio	1.03 ± 0.15	1.10 ± 0.14***

The values are means ± SD. $^{*}P \leq 0.05$, $^{**}P \leq 0.01$, and $^{***}P \leq 0.001$ significantly different from baseline.

As mentioned above, dietary LA and ALA serve as the precursors for the n-6 and n-3 series of PUFA, respectively, and play an important role in modulation of cardiovascular, inflammatory diseases, immune system, and blood pressure regulation [4, 24, 43]. Their products modulate biosynthesis of potent cellular mediators, eicosanoids. Therefore, increased consumption of food with high n-6/n-3 PUFA ratio leads to thrombosis and inflammatory reactions, while high n-3/n-6 ratio has cardioprotective, antithrombotic, and anti-inflammatory action [4, 44]. However, no reports are available on the effects of plant flax/pumpkin/sesame seed mixture (rich in n-6 and n-3 FA), used as dietary supplement on cardiometabolic risk factors in patients with renal disease compared to many studies with marine n-3 fatty acid. Adding seed mixture to the diets of hemodialysis patients resulted in large drops in blood pressure (BP) of around 11 mmHg systolic and 6 mmHg diastolic after 12 weaks. The evidence for a hypotensive effect of flax or its components is unconvincing [45, 46]. However, dietary supplementation with 8 g/day ALA for 12 weeks used by Paschos et al. [47] lowers both systolic and diastolic BP in dyslipidemic men with magnitude of the hypotensive effect (5 mmHg or 3–6%). Study conducted by Gossell-Williams et al. [48] showed that, in women, receiving pumpkin seed oil (2 g/day) decreased diastolic BP. The antihypertensive effect of seed mixture (rich in n-6 and n-3 FA) may be caused by changes in prostaglandin synthesis, by alteration of membrane fatty acid composition and by subsequent changes in membrane functions [46]. Some investigators have shown that flaxseed supplementation (30 g/day) lowers serum creatinine in healthy subject (32 g/day) [45] and has renoprotective effects in patients with lupus nephritis [49]. In the present study, adding milled sesame/pumpkin/flax seeds mixture (30 g; rich in n-6 and n-3 FA) in the habitual diet is accompanied with reduction of serum creatinine levels. It is well known that there was a strong association of severe pruritus with depression symptoms, poorer sleep, and dry skin in hemodialysis patients [27]. The decrease in frequency symptoms of pruritus in our patients indicated that balanced dietary n-6 and n-3 fatty acid intake improves symptoms of pruritus.

This is the first exploration of the influence of added milled sesame/pumpkin/flax seeds mixture in diet on serum lipids and fatty acid status, so we have a coupled effect of these plant food components. Flaxseed oil (2.4–3.6 g/day) has not shown any hypolipidemic effect in supplementation trials [50]. However, considering the publications, ground flaxseed (30–50 g/day) [16, 17, 51] and sesame seed (50 g/day) [19] have been shown to reduce blood lipids levels. In this regard, meta-analyses on eleven studies examining the effect of whole flaxseed supplementation on lipids levels reported that interventions reduced total and LDL cholesterol by 0.21 mmol/L and 0.16 mmol/L, respectively [52]. It is noteworthy, that the high content of dietary fiber and LA in the sesame seed underlies its capacity to lower serum cholesterol levels [18].

In animal models of diabetes, pumpkin seeds supplementation decreased serum glucose, triglyceride and cholesterol, and CRP levels [53]. It is assumed that the possible potential mechanism of lipid lowering by pumpkin is probably due to fibers effects. It is well known that dietary fiber reduces plasma LDL cholesterol levels, by inhibiting the absorption

TABLE 4: Correlation matrix between inflammatory markers and serum phospholipids fatty acid percentage in dietary intervention treatments.

	CRP	IL-6	TNF	ALA	EPA	DPA	DHA	n-3	LA	DGLA	AA	n-6
CRP	—	0.455**	0.392**	−0.369**	−0.112	−0.224	−0.282*	−0.343**	−0.123	−0.523**	−0.255***	−0.379**
IL-6		—	0.780***	−0.269*	−0.185	−0.286*	−0.213	−0.308*	−0.232	−0.262*	−0.293*	−0.438**
TNF			—	−0.587***	−0.140	−0.197	−0.376**	−0.403**	−0.605***	−0.319**	−0.203	−0.370**

*$P < 0.05$, **$P < 0.01$ and ***$P < 0.001$.

of bile acids and cholesterol, and increases the activity of LDL receptors. Recently, Makni et al. [54] have reported that flax and pumpkin seed mixture supplemented in the diet of diabetic rats has hypoglycemic, hypolipidemic, and nephroprotector effect. In the present study we noticed significant reduction in cholesterol by 8% in hemodialyses patients, after dietary treatment with milled sesame/pumpkin/flax seed mixture. LDL cholesterol is the primary target in cholesterol lowering efforts in patients. In general, 1% increase in the LDL cholesterol level may lead to 2-3% increase in coronary artery disease risk [55]. Results of our study showed that added milled sesame/pumpkin/flax seed mixture in diet decreases slightly but not significantly serum LDL cholesterol by 5%. Meta-analysis [56] based on population prospective studies showed that 1 mmol/L increase in serum triglyceride was associated with a 32% increase in a risk factor for cardiovascular disease (CVD). In the present study, we have 30% (0.6 mmol/L) decreases in serum triglyceride level in hemodialysis patients after dietary treatment with milled sesame/pumpkin/flax seed mixture. However, the data related to the protective role of ALA (3.0 g content of ALA in our flax seed mixture) are less definitive than those of long chain n-3, EPA, and DHA [57, 58]. This reduction in fasting serum triglyceride during our intervention was in contrast with the conclusion that the plant-derived n-3 fatty acid is not equivalent to marine-based fatty acid in terms of lowering triglyceride levels [52]. Our study results indicate that sesame/pumpkin/flax diet treatment in hemodialyzed patients could be beneficial in prevention of CVD as triglyceride level is an important factor that has been implicated in the pathogenesis of cardiovascular complication.

It was suggested that plant-based n-3 fatty acids might influence insulin secretion in vivo and improve glucose use and efficiency [59]. Findings from limited studies suggest that flax meal improves insulin sensitivity, likely because of its soluble fiber content, which may delay postprandial glucose absorption in the gut. However, the trial by McManus et al. [60] revealed no effect of n-3 fatty acids from flaxseed oil on HbA1c, fasting glucose, or insulin levels in patients with well-controlled type 2 diabetes. Dietary milled sesame/pumpkin/flax seed mixture intakes in our study affect glycemic control, significant decreased glucose levels, insulin, and calculated IR HOMA in hemodialysis patients.

CRP plays an important role in atherogenesis [61]. Increased CRP levels exhibit synergy with concurrent hypercholesterolemia to increase CVD risk in both men and women [61]. Several studies have shown that CRP is inversely associated with EPA and DHA levels in both healthy subjects and in patients with stable coronary artery disease [62, 63]. Our results demonstrate that a dietary treatment with milled sesame/pumpkin/flax seeds decreased CRP, IL-6, TNF-alpha levels, and the changes in serum ALA and DHA levels, and ALA+ DPA + EPA + DHA (total n-3 FA) were inversely associated with changes in CRP and TNF-alpha. Therefore, decreasing CRP levels, by dietary interventions, can improve the lipid responses, thereby reducing overall CVD risk. In diseases in which inflammation leads to adverse effects on the progression of clinical parameters, such as renal failure, it is necessary fact that dietary intervention that suppresses the production of proinflammatory markers should be included as part of the prevention. Nonetheless, in a recent systematic review, a possible benefit of dietary ALA consumption in reducing sudden death and nonfatal myocardial infarction was deduced [44]. In line with this and because it has been shown that the levels of serum fatty acids vary according to the choice of different foods in the diet, dietary milled sesame/pumpkin/flax seed mixture supplemented to the habitual diet has beneficial effects on reducing CVD risk in hemodialysis patients. For the interpretation of the results, there should be mentioned that there was no placebo group as a control and that dietary fatty acid intake was not assessed by commonly used dietary assessment methods. Instead, compliance was measured as a change in the serum phospholipid fatty acid composition. Yet, despite these limitations, the status biomarker of dietary fatty acid intake showed the good patients' compliance, which means that the participants adhered to the dietary intervention treatment. In conclusion, milled 6 g sesame/6 g pumpkin/18 g flax seeds mixture per day have possible health-promoting effects due to increased levels of n-3 fatty acids in the serum and decreased inflammatory markers. Further well-designed and controlled studies are needed to determine if using seeds mixture might lead to prevention or regression of atherosclerosis and the resolution of some clinical problems in hemodialyzed patients.

Conflict of Interests

The authors declare that there is no conflict of interests regarding the publication of this paper.

Acknowledgments

This work was supported by Project III41030 financed by the Ministry of Education, Science and Technological Development of the Republic of Serbia. The authors would like to acknowledge the assistance of Vera Blazencić-Mladenović for collecting data and conducting interviews organization.

References

[1] A. Aro, "Fatty acid composition of serum lipids: is this marker of fat intake still relevant for identifying metabolic and cardiovascular disorders?" *Nutrition, Metabolism and Cardiovascular Diseases*, vol. 13, no. 5, pp. 253–255, 2003.

[2] G. Riccardi, R. Giacco, and A. A. Rivellese, "Dietary fat, insulin sensitivity and the metabolic syndrome," *Clinical Nutrition*, vol. 23, no. 4, pp. 447–456, 2004.

[3] B. Vessby, B. Karlström, M. Öhrvall, A. Järvi, A. Andersson, and S. Basu, "Diet, nutrition and diabetes mellitus," *Upsala Journal of Medical Sciences*, vol. 105, no. 2, pp. 151–160, 2000.

[4] D. Ristić-Medić, V. Vučić, M. Takić, I. Karadžić, and M. Glibetić, "Polyunsaturated fatty acid in health and disease," *Journal of the Serbian Chemical Society*, vol. 78, no. 9, pp. 1269–1289, 2013.

[5] V. Ristić, V. Tepšić, D. Ristić-Medić et al., "Plasma and erythrocyte phospholipid fatty acids composition in Serbian hemodialyzed patients," *Renal Failure*, vol. 28, no. 3, pp. 211–216, 2006.

[6] G. B. Perunicic-Pekovic, Z. R. Rasic, S. I. Pljesa et al., "Effect of n-3 fatty acids on nutritional status and inflammatory markers in haemodialysis patients," *Nephrology*, vol. 12, no. 4, pp. 331–336, 2007.

[7] Z. Rasic-Milutinovic, G. Perunicic, S. Pljesa et al., "Effects of N-3 PUFAs supplementation on insulin resistance and inflammatory biomarkers in hemodialysis patients," *Renal Failure*, vol. 29, no. 3, pp. 321–329, 2007.

[8] G. Peruničić-Peković, Z. Rašić-Milutinović, Z. Gluvić, M. Lačković, D. Ristić-Medić, and M. Glibetić, "Inflammation, nutritional status, PUFA profile and outcome in hemodialysis patients," *Archives of Biological Science*, vol. 64, no. 3, pp. 1173–1180, 2012.

[9] B. Baggio, E. Musacchio, and G. Priante, "Polyunsaturated fatty acids and renal fibrosis: pathophysiologic link and potential clinical implications," *Journal of Nephrology*, vol. 18, no. 4, pp. 362–367, 2005.

[10] D. Ristić-Medić, G. Peruničić-Peković, and Z. Rašić-Milutinović, "PUFA status and omega-3 fatty acid supplementation in hemodialysis patients: pathophysiological aspects and clinical outcomes," *Nutritional Therapy and Metabolism*, vol. 29, no. 4, pp. 178–187, 2011.

[11] G. C. Burdge and S. A. Wootton, "Conversion of α-linolenic acid to eicosapentaenoic, docosapentaenoic and docosahexaenoic acids in young women," *British Journal of Nutrition*, vol. 88, no. 4, pp. 411–420, 2002.

[12] G. Burdge, "α-Linolenic acid metabolism in men and women: nutritional and biological implications," *Current Opinion in Clinical Nutrition and Metabolic Care*, vol. 7, no. 2, pp. 137–144, 2004.

[13] G. C. Burdge and P. C. Calder, "α-Linolenic acid metabolism in adult humans: the effects of gender and age on conversion to longer-chain polyunsaturated fatty acids," *European Journal of Lipid Science and Technology*, vol. 107, no. 6, pp. 426–439, 2005.

[14] S. Tarpila, A. Aro, I. Salminen et al., "The effect of flaxseed supplementation in processed foods on serum fatty acids and enterolactone," *European Journal of Clinical Nutrition*, vol. 56, no. 2, pp. 157–165, 2002.

[15] J. A. Austria, M. N. Richard, M. N. Chahine et al., "Bioavailability of alpha-linolenic acid in subjects after ingestion of three different forms of flaxseed," *Journal of the American College of Nutrition*, vol. 27, no. 2, pp. 214–221, 2008.

[16] S. C. Cunnane, S. Ganguli, C. Menard et al., "High α-linolenic acid flaxseed (Linum usitatissimum): some nutritional properties in humans," *British Journal of Nutrition*, vol. 69, no. 2, pp. 443–453, 1993.

[17] S. Sirato-Yasumoto, M. Katsuta, Y. Okuyama, Y. Takahashi, and T. Ide, "Effect of sesame seeds rich in sesamin and sesamolin on fatty acid oxidation in rat liver," *Journal of Agricultural and Food Chemistry*, vol. 49, no. 5, pp. 2647–2651, 2001.

[18] M. Namiki, "Nutraceutical functions of sesame: a review," *Critical Reviews in Food Science and Nutrition*, vol. 47, no. 7, pp. 651–673, 2007.

[19] W.-H. Wu, Y.-P. Kang, N.-H. Wang, H.-J. Jou, and T.-A. Wang, "Sesame ingestion affects sex hormones, antioxidant status, and blood lipids in postmenopausal women," *Journal of Nutrition*, vol. 136, no. 5, pp. 1270–1275, 2006.

[20] M. Lemcke-Norojärvi, A. Kamal-Eldin, L.-Å. Appelqvist, L. H. Dimberg, M. Öhrvall, and B. Vessby, "Corn and sesame oils increase serum γ-tocopherol concentrations in healthy Swedish women," *Journal of Nutrition*, vol. 131, no. 4, pp. 1195–1201, 2001.

[21] W. L. Applequist, B. Avula, B. T. Schaneberg, Y.-H. Wang, and I. A. Khan, "Comparative fatty acid content of seeds of four Cucurbita species grown in a common (shared) garden," *Journal of Food Composition and Analysis*, vol. 19, no. 6-7, pp. 606–611, 2006.

[22] M. N. Xanthopoulou, T. Nomikos, E. Fragopoulou, and S. Antonopoulou, "Antioxidant and lipoxygenase inhibitory activities of pumpkin seed extracts," *Food Research International*, vol. 42, no. 5-6, pp. 641–646, 2009.

[23] A. P. Simopoulos, "Essential fatty acids in health and chronic disease," *American Journal of Clinical Nutrition*, vol. 70, supplement 3, pp. 560S–569S, 1999.

[24] D. Ristic-Medic, G. Ristic, and V. Tepsic, "Alfa linolenic acid and cardiovascular disease," *Medicinski Pregled*, vol. 60, 1, pp. S43–S47, 2007, (Serbian).

[25] D. Medić Ristić, V. Ristić, V. Tepšić et al., "Effect of soybean Leci-Vita product on serum lipids and fatty acid composition in patients with elevated serum cholesterol and triglyceride levels," *Nutrition Research*, vol. 23, no. 4, pp. 465–477, 2003.

[26] M. Stahle-Backdahl, "Uremic pruritus," *Seminars in Dermatology*, vol. 14, no. 4, pp. 297–301, 1995.

[27] G. B. Lopes, F. C. P. Nogueira, M. R. de Souza et al., "Assessment of the psychological burden associated with pruritus in hemodialysis patients using the kidney disease quality of life short form," *Quality of Life Research*, vol. 21, no. 4, pp. 603–612, 2012.

[28] L. W. Peck, E. R. Monsen, and S. Ahmad, "Effect of three sources of long-chain fatty acids on the plasma fatty acid profile, plasma prostaglandin E2 concentrations, and pruritus symptoms in hemodialysis patients," *American Journal of Clinical Nutrition*, vol. 64, no. 2, pp. 210–214, 1996.

[29] N. Noori, R. Dukkipati, C. P. Kovesdy et al., "Dietary omega-3 fatty acid, ratio of omega-6 to omega-3 intake, inflammation, and survival in long-term hemodialysis patients," *American Journal of Kidney Diseases*, vol. 58, no. 2, pp. 248–256, 2011.

[30] R. Ross, "Atherosclerosis—an inflammatory disease," *The New England Journal of Medicine*, vol. 340, no. 2, pp. 115–126, 1999.

[31] A. J. King, J. J. Kehayias, R. Roubenoff, C. H. Schmid, and B. J. G. Pereira, "Cytokine production and nutritional status in hemodialysis patients," *International Journal of Artificial Organs*, vol. 21, no. 1, pp. 4–11, 1998.

[32] P. Stenvinkel, O. Heimbürger, F. Paultre et al., "Strong association between malnutrition, inflammation, and atherosclerosis in chronic renal failure," *Kidney International*, vol. 55, no. 5, pp. 1899–1911, 1999.

[33] G. Yosipovitch, I. Zucker, G. Boner, U. Gafter, Y. Shapira, and M. David, "A questionnaire for the assessment of pruritus: validation in uremic patients," *Acta Dermato-Venereologica*, vol. 81, no. 2, pp. 108–111, 2001.

[34] D. B. Zilversmit and A. K. Davis, "Microdetermination of plasma phospholipids by trichloroacetic acid precipitation," *The Journal of Laboratory and Clinical Medicine*, vol. 35, no. 1, pp. 155–160, 1950.

[35] D. R. Matthews, J. P. Hosker, and A. S. Rudenski, "Homeostasis model assessment: insulin resistance and β-cell function from fasting plasma glucose and insulin concentrations in man," *Diabetologia*, vol. 28, no. 7, pp. 412–419, 1985.

[36] E. J. Matusik Jr., V. B. Reeves, and V. P. Flanagan, "Determination of fatty acid methyl esters. Elimination of tissue-derived contamination and artefacts and preparation of a support-coated acid-modified polyester liquid phase," *Analytica Chimica Acta*, vol. 166, pp. 179–188, 1985.

[37] J. T. Brenna, "Efficiency of conversion of alpha-linolenic acid to long chain n-3 fatty acids in man," *Current Opinion in Clinical Nutrition and Metabolic Care*, vol. 5, no. 2, pp. 127–132, 2002.

[38] D. Ristić-Medić, M. Takić, V. Vučić, D. Kandić, N. Kostić, and M. Glibetić, "Abnormalities in the serum phospholipids fatty acid profile in patients with alcoholic liver cirrhosis—a pilot study," *Journal of Clinical Biochemistry and Nutrition*, vol. 53, no. 1, pp. 49–54, 2013.

[39] G. Zhao, T. D. Etherton, K. R. Martin, S. G. West, P. J. Gillies, and P. M. Kris-Etherton, "Dietary α-linolenic acid reduces inflammatory and lipid cardiovascular risk factors in hypercholesterolemic men and women," *Journal of Nutrition*, vol. 134, no. 11, pp. 2991–2997, 2004.

[40] C. R. Harper, M. J. Edwards, A. P. DeFilipis, and T. A. Jacobson, "Flaxseed oil increases the plasma concentrations of cardioprotective (n-3) fatty acids in humans," *Journal of Nutrition*, vol. 136, no. 1, pp. 83–87, 2006.

[41] K. S. Bjerve, A. M. Brubakk, K. J. Fougner et al., "Omega-3 fatty acids: essential fatty acids with important biological effects, and serum phospholipid fatty acids as markers of dietary ω3-fatty acid intake," *American Journal of Clinical Nutrition*, vol. 57, supplement 5, pp. 801S–806S, 1993.

[42] M. Okita, S. Yoshida, J. Yamamoto et al., "n-3 and n-6 fatty acid intake and serum phospholipid fatty acid composition in middle-aged women living in rural and urban areas in Okayama Prefecture," *Journal of Nutritional Science and Vitaminology*, vol. 41, no. 3, pp. 313–323, 1995.

[43] P. Benatti, G. Peluso, R. Nicolai, and M. Calvani, "Polyunsaturated fatty acids: biochemical, nutritional and epigenetic properties," *Journal of the American College of Nutrition*, vol. 23, no. 4, pp. 281–302, 2004.

[44] C. R. Harper and T. A. Jacobson, "Usefulness of omega-3 fatty acids and the prevention of coronary heart disease," *American Journal of Cardiology*, vol. 96, no. 11, pp. 1521–1529, 2005.

[45] C. Stuglin and K. Prasad, "Effect of flaxseed consumption on blood pressure, serum lipids, hemopoietic system and liver and kidney enzymes in healthy humans," *Journal of Cardiovascular Pharmacology and Therapeutics*, vol. 10, no. 1, pp. 23–27, 2005.

[46] Y. Watanabe, Y.-S. Huang, V. A. Simmons, and D. F. Horrobin, "The effect of dietary n-6 and n-3 polyunsaturated fatty acids on blood pressure and tissue fatty acid composition in spontaneously hypertensive rats," *Lipids*, vol. 24, no. 7, pp. 638–644, 1989.

[47] G. K. Paschos, F. Magkos, D. B. Panagiotakos, V. Votteas, and A. Zampelas, "Dietary supplementation with flaxseed oil lowers blood pressure in dyslipidaemic patients," *European Journal of Clinical Nutrition*, vol. 61, no. 10, pp. 1201–1206, 2007.

[48] M. Gossell-Williams, C. Hyde, T. Hunter et al., "Improvement in HDL cholesterol in postmenopausal women supplemented with pumpkin seed oil: pilot study," *Climacteric*, vol. 14, no. 5, pp. 558–564, 2011.

[49] W. F. Clark, C. Kortas, A. P. Heidenheim, J. Garland, E. Spanner, and A. Parbtani, "Flaxseed in lupus nephritis: a two-year nonplacebo-controlled crossover study," *Journal of the American College of Nutrition*, vol. 20, no. 2, pp. 143–148, 2001.

[50] G. Barceló-Coblijn, E. J. Murphy, R. Othman, M. H. Moghadasian, T. Kashour, and J. K. Friel, "Flaxseed oil and fish-oil capsule consumption alters human red blood cell n-3 fatty acid composition: a multiple-dosing trial comparing 2 sources of n-3 fatty acid," *American Journal of Clinical Nutrition*, vol. 88, no. 3, pp. 801–809, 2008.

[51] S. Dodin, A. Lemay, H. Jacques, F. Légaré, J.-C. Forest, and B. Mâsse, "The effects of flaxseed dietary supplement on lipid profile, bone mineral density, and symptoms in menopausal women: a randomized, double-blind, wheat germ placebo-controlled clinical trial," *The Journal of Clinical Endocrinology and Metabolism*, vol. 90, no. 3, pp. 1390–1397, 2005.

[52] A. Pan, D. Yu, W. Demark-Wahnefried, O. H. Franco, and X. Lin, "Meta-analysis of the effects of flaxseed interventions on blood lipids," *American Journal of Clinical Nutrition*, vol. 90, no. 2, pp. 288–297, 2009.

[53] A. S. Sedigheh, J. Moshtaghian, S. Mahbubeh et al., "Hypoglycaemic and hypolipidemic effects of pumpkin (cucurbita pepo l.) on alloxan-induced diabetic rats," *African Journal of Pharmacy and Pharmacology*, vol. 5, no. 23, pp. 2620–2626, 2011.

[54] M. Makni, H. Fetoui, N. K. Gargouri et al., "Hypolipidemic and hepatoprotective effects of flax and pumpkin seed mixture rich in ω-3 and ω-6 fatty acids in hypercholesterolemic rats," *Food and Chemical Toxicology*, vol. 46, no. 12, pp. 3714–3720, 2008.

[55] "Summary of the second report of the National Cholesterol Education Program (NCEP) expert panel on detection, evaluation, and treatment of high blood cholesterol in adults (adult treatment panel II)," *Journal of the American Medical Association*, vol. 269, no. 23, pp. 3015–3023, 1993.

[56] M. A. Austin, J. E. Hokanson, and K. L. Edwards, "Hypertriglyceridemia as a cardiovascular risk factor," *American Journal of Cardiology*, vol. 81, no. 4, pp. 7B–12B, 1998.

[57] C. Wang, W. S. Harris, M. Chung et al., "n-3 Fatty acids from fish or fish-oil supplements, but not α-linolenic acid, benefit cardiovascular disease outcomes in primary- and secondary-prevention studies: a systematic review," *American Journal of Clinical Nutrition*, vol. 84, no. 1, pp. 5–17, 2006.

[58] E. M. Balk, A. H. Lichtenstein, M. Chung, B. Kupelnick, P. Chew, and J. Lau, "Effects of omega-3 fatty acids on serum markers of cardiovascular disease risk: a systematic review," *Atherosclerosis*, vol. 189, no. 1, pp. 19–30, 2006.

[59] L. Djoussé, S. C. Hunt, W. Tang, J. H. Eckfeldt, M. A. Province, and R. Curtis Ellison, "Dietary linolenic acid and fasting glucose and insulin: the national heart, lung, and blood institute family heart study," *Obesity*, vol. 14, no. 2, pp. 295–300, 2006.

[60] R. M. McManus, J. Jumpson, D. T. Finegood, M. T. Clandinin, and E. A. Ryan, "A comparison of the effects of n-3 fatty acids

from linseed oil and fish oil in well-controlled type II diabetes," *Diabetes Care*, vol. 19, no. 5, pp. 463–467, 1996.

[61] P. Libby, P. M. Ridker, and A. Maseri, "Inflammation and atherosclerosis," *Circulation*, vol. 105, no. 9, pp. 1135–1143, 2002.

[62] T. Pischon, S. E. Hankinson, G. S. Hotamisligil, N. Rifai, W. C. Willett, and E. B. Rimm, "Habitual dietary intake of n-3 and n-6 fatty acids in relation to inflammatory markers among US men and women," *Circulation*, vol. 108, no. 2, pp. 155–160, 2003.

[63] T. Madsen, H. A. Skou, V. E. Hansen et al., "C-reactive protein, dietary n-3 fatty acids, and the extent of coronary artery disease," *American Journal of Cardiology*, vol. 88, no. 10, pp. 1139–1142, 2001.

21

Effect of Probiotics Supplementation on Bone Mineral Content and Bone Mass Density

Kolsoom Parvaneh,[1] Rosita Jamaluddin,[1] Golgis Karimi,[1] and Reza Erfani[2]

[1] *Department of Nutrition and Dietetics, Faculty of Medicine and Health Sciences, University Putra Malaysia, 43400 Serdang, Selangor, Malaysia*
[2] *Department of Orthopaedics and Traumatology, Faculty of Medicine, Universiti Kebengsaan Malaysia, 56000 Kuala Lumpur, Malaysia*

Correspondence should be addressed to Rosita Jamaluddin; rosita@medic.upm.edu.my

Academic Editors: A. Chicco, S. E. Harris, J. Khan, and B. Venn

A few studies in animals and a study in humans showed a positive effect of probiotic on bone metabolism and bone mass density. Most of the investigated bacteria were *Lactobacillus* and *Bifidobacterium*. The positive results of the probiotics were supported by the high content of dietary calcium and the high amounts of supplemented probiotics. Some of the principal mechanisms include (1) increasing mineral solubility due to production of short chain fatty acids; (2) producing phytase enzyme by bacteria to overcome the effect of mineral depressed by phytate; (3) reducing intestinal inflammation followed by increasing bone mass density; (4) hydrolysing glycoside bond food in the intestines by *Lactobacillus* and *Bifidobacteria*. These mechanisms lead to increase bioavailability of the minerals. In conclusion, probiotics showed potential effects on bone metabolism through different mechanisms with outstanding results in the animal model. The results also showed that postmenopausal women who suffered from low bone mass density are potential targets to consume probiotics for increasing mineral bioavailability including calcium and consequently increasing bone mass density.

1. Introduction

Probiotics literally means "for life" and the word is derived from Latin and Greek. However, the definition of probiotics has been varied since it was first coined several years ago [1]. Some of the probiotics are bacterial components comprising of normal human intestinal flora that produce end products of short chain fatty acids and lactate metabolism. These bacterial have potential clinical effects for the treatment or prevention of the intestinal and extra intestinal origin diseases [2, 3]. Most commonly investigated bacteria with health benefit are *Lactobacillus* and *Bifidobacteria*. These effects may be useful for reducing the risk of some diseases [3], such as fatty liver disease, inflammatory bowel disease (IBD), cardiovascular disease (CVD), and diabetes [4–7]. This implies that the intestinal bacteria play an important role in the immune system [8, 9]. Recent researches also indicated the beneficial effects of intestinal microbials on bone health.

One of the main bone diseases which is associated with aging and postmenopausal condition is osteoporosis. Currently, 75 million people in Europe, Japan, and the USA are affected by osteoporosis. In 2020, more than 50 percent of the United States population is estimated to suffer from low bone density [10]. One of the most serious problems among women over 50 years of age is hip fracture due to osteoporosis. The possibility of wrist, hip, or spine fracture is estimated to be parallel to the risk of heart disease (approximately 15%) [11].

Sufficient calcium intake has been reported to support bone growth and prevent bone loss during the aging process. Milk and milk products supply 75% of calcium needed by the body in western countries [12], but the consumption of milk has been failing over the past decade [13]. Some specialists believe that one of the effective treatments for osteoporosis is hormone replacement therapy (HRT). However, because of the side effects of HRT, this treatment is not generally accepted, due to low adhesion, unwillingness, and aversion by many women. Moreover, HRT over long durations of time may lead to increase the risk of some types of cancer [14].

Hence, alternative ways for preventing and treating osteoporosis are being developed and recommended by research scientists worldwide. Exercise, including walking and light running, have been reported to maintain bone mass density (BMD) [15]. Another potential method of fighting osteoporosis is probiotics consumption.

To the best of our knowledge, there is no review paper to determine the effect of probiotic on bone health or metabolism. The following review illustrates recent knowledge on the effects of probiotics on BMD as well as bone mineral content (BMC). The search carried out according to the Google scholar, PubMed, ISI Web of knowledge, Medline, and Cochrane Central Register of Controlled Trials (http://www.cochrane.org/). The terms were used for searching the literature including Probiotics, calcium absorption, BMD, BMC, bone loss, *Lactobacillus*, and *Bifidobacterium*.

2. Probiotics and Bones: Animal Studies

Previous studies indicated that different strains of bacteria such as *Lactobacillus* and *Bifidobacterium* have the potential effect on increasing bone mass density on ovariectomized (OVX) rats and mice which can simulate postmenopausal conditions [16–19].

Chiang and Pan [18] used *Lactobacillus paracasei* (NTU 101) and *Lactobacillus plantarum* (NTU 102) (1×10^8 CFU/ML) in OVX mice. They analyzed the right femur using computed tomography (CT) system, while the left femur was analyzed using scanning electron microscopy (SEM). The results showed that OVX mice fed with NTU 101 and NTU 102 fermented milk had higher trabecular number (Tb.N) compared to OVX and sham-ovariectomized (Sovx) as the control groups. In parallel with previous results, another study on male osteoporosis rats, but using different strain of bacteria, showed that *Lactobacillus helveticus* fermented milk increased BMD and BMC which were measured by using dual-energy X-ray absorptiometry (DEXA) [19].

A study on *Lactobacillus casei, Lactobacillus reuteri,* and *Lactobacillus gasseri* reported higher apparent calcium absorption in growing rats and 35% higher bone weight among the probiotic fed group compared to the control group [20]. Besides, Kim et al. [21] indicated that decreased level of BMD in OVX rats will be significantly improved by administrating *Lactobacillus casei 393* from fermented milk. They assessed the breaking force using a Texture Analyzer. They observed that bone strength of sham-ovariectomy (Sovx) group was higher than the Ovx group. However, after treatment in the Ovx group receiving fermented milk, the bone strength was not different from the Sovx group. No difference in body weight of rats was observed initially, but at the end surprisingly, the Sovx group had lower body weight as compared to the other groups. It was reported that ovariectomy caused an increase in dietary intake of rats and subsequently resulted in weight gain.

A current research showed a significant effect of *L. reuteri* 6475 on bone health via decreasing tumor necrosis factor (TNF) levels and reducing bone resorption. The results showed increasing bone fracture, BMD, BMC, trabecular number and thickness, and decreasing trabecular space in both vertebral and femoral bones. In addition, body weight and fat pad weight showed a decreasing trend in the treated group [16]. Surprisingly, significant effects were observed only in treated healthy male mice not in females. Mutuş et al. [22], also worked on bacillus strain of *licheniformis* and *subtilis* on twenty-five one-year-old broiler chicks which were divided into the control and treatment groups. Diet in treatment group contained *Bacillus licheniformis* and *Bacillus subtilis.* After treatment, no significant difference was observed in the body weight and feed consumption between the two groups, but greater concentration of phosphorus and tibia ash, lateral and medial wall thickness of the tibiotarsi was observed in the group supplemented with probiotics compared to the control group fed with normal diet. While, the normal diet group had greater medullary canal diameter [22].

Bifidobacterium longum from fermented broccoli also showed a significant effect on bone health [17]. Four groups of male rats with different diets including normal diet and high cholesterol (HCD) for control groups and HCD + broccoli, HCD + *Bifidobacterium longum* from fermented broccoli diet for intervention groups were used. Significantly higher serum total cholesterol, higher potential antioxidant (PAO) serum level and 34% higher periodontal GSH/GSSG ratio was observed among intervention groups compared to the control groups. Beside a low number of TRAP-positive osteoclasts was found in the group fed with fermented broccoli compared to the control groups, while no significant differences were observed in body weight of rats between the groups. However, *Bifidobacterium longum* and yacon flour in another study have done by Rodrigues et al. [23] showed contradictory results from other previous studies. They reported no difference between intervention and control groups on femur thickness, length, and strength of fracture. The study involved thirty two male Wistar rats; divided into four groups, with 8 animals in each. Different groups of treatment receiving the following diets: control diet; yacon flour; standard diet + *Bifidobacterium longum*; and yacon flour + *Bifidobacterium longum*. They assessed daily food intake and weekly body weight to determine the efficiency coefficient of food (CEA) by weight gain/total food intake. They observed no differences in body weight, total food intake and feed efficiency after 28 days of treatment, while they showed that mineral content including calcium (Ca), phosphorus (P), and magnesium (Mg) was higher in animals fed with *B. longum* and *B. longum* with yacon flour.

Table 1 summarizes results of some of the animal studies on the effects of probiotics on bones.

3. Probiotics in Human Studies

Based on the knowledge, a study assessed the effects of probiotics on bone in twenty postmenopausal women with a mean

TABLE 1: Animal studies effect of probiotics on bone.

Probiotic strain	Duration	Possible effect on bone	Subject	Method	Author and year
Lactobacillus reuteri 6475	4 weeks	(i) ↑Bone volume fraction (ii) ↑Bone mineral density (iii) ↑Bone mineral content (iv) ↑Trabecular number and thickness of distal femur (v) ↓Trabecular space (vi) ↑Vertebral trabecular bone volume	Healthy male mice	Micro-CT	McCabe et al. 2013 [16]
Bifidobacterium longum, fermented broccoli	12 weeks	↓Number of TRAP-positive osteoclasts	Male Wistar rats	Histologic measurements	Tomofuji et al. 2012 [17]
Bifidobacterium Longum (ATCC 15707)	28 days	(i) Bone weight, thickness, and length/NS (ii) Strength of fracture/NS (iii) ↑Ca, Mg bone content	Male Wistar rats	(i) Stainless-steel caliper (ii) Three-point Texture Analyzer (iii) Plasma emission spectrophotometer	Rodrigues et al. 2012 [23]
Lactobacillus paracasei (NTU 101) and Lactobacillus plantarum (NTU102)	8 weeks	(i) Femur BMD/NS (ii) Tb.Th/NS (iii) ↑Tb.N (iv) ↓Tb.sp	Ovariectomized mice	(i) CT system (ii) SkyScan	Chiang and Pan 2011 [18]
Active Lactobacillus casei 393	6 weeks	(i) Femoral length/NS (ii) ↑Dry weight of femur (iii) ↑Ca and P in dry femur (iv) ↑BMD and BMC (v) ↑Bone strength	Ovariectomized Sprague-Dawley rats	(i) Vernier caliper (ii) Inductively coupled plasma-optical emission (iii) DEXA (iv) Three-point Texture Analyzer	Kim et al. 2009 [21]
Bacillus licheniformis and Bacillus subtilis	6 weeks	(i) ↑Medial and lateral wall thickness of tibiotarsi (ii) ↓Medullary canal diameter	Broiler chicks	(i) Dial caliper (ii) Subtracting the thickness of the medial and lateral walls from the diameter at the diaphysis	Mutuş et al. 2006 [22]
Lactobacillus helveticus LBK-16H	14 weeks	(i) ↑BMD and BMC (ii) ↑Femur weight	Male rats induced-osteoporosis aging	DEXA	Narva et al. 2004 [24]

NS: not significant.
CT: computed tomography.
TRAP: tartrate resistant acid phosphatase.
Ca: calcium.
Mg: magnesium.
BMD: bone mass density.
Tb.Th: trabecular thickness.
Tb.N: trabecular number.
Tb.sp: trabecular separation.
BMC: bone mineral content.
DEXA: dual-energy X-ray absorptiometry.

age of 65 years and mean body mass index (BMI) of 26 [24]. The study was a double-blind randomized crossover study. Subjects comprised of two groups. The group consuming *Lactobacillus helveticus* fermented milk was compared to the control milk consumption group with a six-day washout. A day before starting the study, all subjects were given milk product (600 mg calcium) to avoid different amounts of calcium that may affect urine calcium collected in the morning. The effects of the consumed milk products were assessed by measuring the serum Parathyroid hormone (PTH), ionised calcium (iCa), Ca, P, and carboxyterminal telopeptide of type I collagen (ICTP) at 0, 1, 2, 4, 6, and 8 hours, and urinary calcium (U-Ca) and creatinine (U-Crea) at 0, 2, 4, 6 and 8 hours.

Effect of *Lactobacillus* from fermented milk confirmed the reduction of PTH followed by increased in serum calcium levels. In consequence reduced bone resorption in post-menopausal women. The ionized serum calcium, total calcium, phosphate, and urinary calcium were higher in the group that consumed *L. helveticus* fermented milk compared to the control group [24].

4. In Vitro Studies of Probiotics on Bone

Increasing BMD by *Lactobacillus helveticus* (LBK-16H) was also confirmed by an in vitro study [25]. In this study effects of compounds on osteoblasts and osteoclasts were measured by culturing bone marrow of mice derived from osteoblast and osteoclast precursor [26] with slight modifications [27]. Cells of bone marrow were obtained from the femora and tibia of 8–12-week-old female mice.

The results of calcium accumulation measured in osteoblast cultures found that *Lactobacillus helveticus* (LBK-16H) from fermented milk whey can increase osteoblast activity by 1.3-1.4 times with the 1×10^{-5}, 1×10^{-4}, and 1×10^{-3} solutions. However, no significant effect on bone formation was found in vitro osteoclast cultures [25].

5. Possible Mechanisms

Some possible mechanisms of probiotics on bones exit. One of the potential effects of probiotics on bone possibly occurs via synthesis of vitamins [28]. Vitamins like D, C, K, and folate are involved in metabolism of calcium and are necessarily for bone formation [29, 30]. Moreover, bacteria produce short chain fatty acids which decrease PTH followed by an increase in mineral absorption via their solubilisation [31].

In cereal based food minerals are surrounded by phytate. The availability of minerals such as zinc, iron, copper, and calcium are depressed by phytate [32]. Bacteria produce phytaze enzyme, which can release minerals depressed by phytate, resulting in increased availability of minerals including calcium [33]. Moreover, increasing the bioavailability of minerals also happens in some foods with estrogenic activity due to hydrolysis glycoside bonds of estrogenic food in the intestines by *Lactobacillus* and *Bifidobacteria* [18].

Some probiotics produce peptides that have biological functions on the body. These are called bioactive peptides. Bioactive peptides production varies depending on the kind of bacteria used [34]. *Lactobacillus helveticus* produces the proline-containing peptides isoleucyl-prolyl-proline (IPP) and valyl-prolyl-proline (VPP) which may induce greater availability of minerals. Furthermore, some of the peptides are not absorbed but could support release of minerals from insoluble ion and thus enhance mineral absorption. Another possible mechanism of IPP and VPP is through inhibition preventing the formation of Angiotensin II (Ang II) from Angiotensin I (Ang I) [24]. In in vitro study Ang II stimulated bone resorption [35] and may act as a vasoconstrictor in bone vasculature [36].

Another mechanism of *L. helveticus*-fermented milk could be by reducing PTH and raising calcium levels in the blood serum [24]. Decrease in bone loss by *L. helveticus*-fermented milk was confirmed with casein-o-phosphopeptides (CPP). CPP is produced during digestion of milk in the intestine. In a previous study, dietary CPP has been revealed to prevent osteoporosis in ovariectomized rats by increasing the bioavailability of calcium [21, 37]. Increased calcium absorption by some probiotic bacteria like *Lactobacillus salivarius* (UCC 118) was demonstrated in Caco-2 cells [38].

Oxidative stress stimulates osteoclast differentiation [39] and *Bifidobacterium longum*-fermented broccoli can improve periodontal antioxidant status by decreasing NF-κB gene expression. On the other hand, during the progression of alveolar bone loss iNOS is an important factor for inflammatory response and *Bifidobacterium longum*-fermented broccoli in periodontal tissue downregulates iNOS gene expression. Thus, immune modulatory action and antioxidant effects have a role in the inhibition of osteoclast differentiation of alveolar bone surfaces.

A recent study showed another mechanism in which intake of a probiotic reduces intestinal inflammation and increases bone mass density, meaning that microbes in the gut have a significant effect on bone health [40]. *Lactobacillus reuteri 6475* reduces proinflammatory cytokine levels systemically, which leads to increased bone volume fraction; similarly, it reduces the expression of proinflammatory cytokine in Jejunum and ileum. *Lactobacillus reuteri 6475* affects bone health either through increased calcium uptake by increasing calcium solubility or by reducing epithelial cell inflammation which facilitate the transport or through production and transformation of estrogen like compounds that affect the intestinal epithelium or circulate in the blood and directly affect the bone cells [16].

In addition to metabolic differences, human and laboratory rodents such as rats have physiological, anatomical, and biochemical differences in the gastrointestinal (G.I.) tract. These differences can cause significant variation in nutrients or drug absorption from the oral route. Solubility, dissolution rates and transit times of nutrients or drug molecules can be modified by some physiological factors such as bile, pancreatic juice, and pH. Furthermore, enterohepatic circulation of nutrients and colonic delivery of formulation can be affected by microbial content of the GI tract. On the other hand, the gut microbiota can metabolize a wide range of chemicals which may affect the nutrients absorption. Approximately

Table 2: Possible mechanisms of probiotics on bone.

Possible mechanisms
Produce SCFA → ↑PH → ↑mineral absorption via their solubilisation → ↓bone loss
Produce phytase enzyme → release minerals depressed by phytate → ↑availability of minerals → ↓bone loss
Hydrolysis glycoside bonds of estrogenic food → ↑availability of minerals
Produce IPP and VPP → ↓formation Ang II from Ang I → ↓bone resorption
Produce antioxidant status → ↓osteoclast differentiation → ↓bone loss
Reduces intestinal inflammation → ↓proinflammatory cytokine levels → ↓epithelial cell inflammation → ↑calcium uptake → ↑bone volume fraction

SCFA: short chain fatty acid.
IPP: isoleucyl-prolyl-proline.
VPP: valyl-prolyl-proline.
ANG II: Angiotensin II.
ANG I: Angiotensin II.

400 different microorganisms are found in the GI tract. Although, upper GI tract in human and rabbits contain few organisms, large numbers are found in the stomach and upper intestine of other animals [41].

Previous studies on the effect of probiotics and bone have all confirmed that probiotics can increase BMD and BMC and help reduce osteoporosis by different ways. In the present review, we investigated the possible mechanisms of microbiota on bone health among animal (Table 2). Hence, the exact mechanism of bacteria on bone health among human is still unclear. This question deserves further studies.

Conflict of Interests

The authors declare no conflict of interests regarding the publication of this paper.

Acknowledgments

The authors would like to thank the editors and reviewers for their comments and suggestions to improve the paper and have undertaken the revision taking into account all the points suggested by the reviewers.

References

[1] J. M. T. Hamilton-Miller, "Probiotics and prebiotics in the elderly," *Postgraduate Medical Journal*, vol. 80, no. 946, pp. 447–451, 2004.

[2] A. C. Ouwehand, S. Salminen, and E. Isolauri, "Probiotics: an overview of beneficial effects," *Antonie van Leeuwenhoek*, vol. 82, no. 1-4, pp. 279–289, 2002.

[3] M. B. Roberfroid, "Prebiotics and probiotics: are they functional foods?" *American Journal of Clinical Nutrition*, vol. 71, no. 6, pp. 1682s–1687s, 2000.

[4] P. Harsh, M. R. Hogarehalli, K. B. Virender, and G. Sunita, "Probiotics as potential biotherapeutics in the management of type 2 diabetes-prospects and perspectives," *Diabetes/Metabolism Research and Reviews*, vol. 29, no. 2, pp. 103–112, 2013.

[5] V. Pietro, M. Claudia, V. Claudio, and M. Ida, "Probiotics: a possible role in treatment of adult and pediatric non alcoholic fatty liver disease," *Annals of Hepatology*, vol. 12, no. 1, pp. 161–163, 2012.

[6] Z. Wang, E. Klipfell, B. J. Bennett et al., "Gut flora metabolism of phosphatidylcholine promotes cardiovascular disease," *Nature*, vol. 472, no. 7341, pp. 57–65, 2011.

[7] W. Kevin and Q. Eamonn, "Probiotics in the management of irritable bowel syndrome and inflammatory bowel disease," *Current Opinion in Gastroenterology*, vol. 29, no. 2, pp. 184–189, 2013.

[8] H. Chung, S. J. Pamp, J. A. Hill, N. K. Surana, S. M. Edelman, and E. B. Troy, "Gut immune maturation depends on colonization with a host-specific microbiota," *Cell*, vol. 149, no. 7, pp. 1578–1593, 2012.

[9] E. Jirillo, F. Jirillo, and T. Magrone, "Healthy effects exerted by prebiotics, probiotics, and symbiotics with special reference to their impact on the immune system," *International Journal for Vitamin and Nutrition Research*, vol. 82, no. 3, pp. 200–208, 2012.

[10] National Osteoporosis Foundation, 2012.

[11] K. M. Chan, M. Anderson, and E. M. C. Lau, "Exercise interventions: defusing the world's osteoporosis time bomb," *Bulletin of the World Health Organization*, vol. 81, no. 11, pp. 827–830, 2003.

[12] M. Osler, B. L. Heitmann, and M. Schroll, "Ten year trends in the dietary habits of Danish men and women. Cohort and cross-sectional data," *European Journal of Clinical Nutrition*, vol. 51, no. 8, pp. 535–541, 1997.

[13] R. E. Black, S. M. Williams, L. E. Jones, and A. Goulding, "Children who avoid drinking cow milk have low dietary calcium intakes and poor bone health," *American Journal of Clinical Nutrition*, vol. 76, no. 3, pp. 675–680, 2002.

[14] C. Picherit, V. Coxam, C. Bennetau-Pelissero et al., "Daidzein is more efficient than genistein in preventing ovariectomy-induced bone loss in rats," *Journal of Nutrition*, vol. 130, no. 7, pp. 1675–1681, 2000.

[15] P. A. Downey and M. I. Siegel, "Bone biology and the clinical implications for osteoporosis," *Physical Therapy*, vol. 86, no. 1, pp. 77–91, 2006.

[16] L. R. McCabe, R. Irwin, L. Schaefer, and R. A. Britton, "Probiotic use decreases intestinal inflammation and increases bone density in healthy male but not female mice," *Journal of Cellular Physiology*, vol. 228, no. 8, pp. 1793–1798, 2013.

[17] T. Tomofuji, D. Ekuni, T. Azuma et al., "Supplementation of broccoli or *Bifidobacterium longum*-fermented broccoli suppresses serum lipid peroxidation and osteoclast differentiation

on alveolar bone surface in rats fed a high-cholesterol diet," *Nutrition Research*, vol. 32, no. 4, pp. 301–307, 2012.

[18] S.-S. Chiang and T.-M. Pan, "Antiosteoporotic effects of *Lactobacillus*-fermented soy skim milk on bone mineral density and the microstructure of femoral bone in ovariectomized mice," *Journal of Agricultural and Food Chemistry*, vol. 59, no. 14, pp. 7734–7742, 2011.

[19] M. Narva, M. Collin, C. Lamberg-Allardt et al., "Effects of long-term intervention with *Lactobacillus helveticus*-fermented milk on bone mineral density and bone mineral content in growing rats," *Annals of Nutrition and Metabolism*, vol. 48, no. 4, pp. 228–234, 2004.

[20] K. Z. Ghanem, I. H. Badawy, and A. M. Abdel-Salam, "Influence of yoghurt and probiotic yoghurt on the absorption of calcium, magnesium, iron and bone mineralization in rats," *Milchwissenschaft*, vol. 59, no. 9-10, pp. 472–475, 2004.

[21] J. G. Kim, E. Lee, S. H. Kim, K. Y. Whang, S. Oh, and J.-Y. Imm, "Effects of a *Lactobacillus casei* 393 fermented milk product on bone metabolism in ovariectomised rats," *International Dairy Journal*, vol. 19, no. 11, pp. 690–695, 2009.

[22] R. Mutuş, N. Kocabağli, M. Alp, N. Acar, M. Eren, and S. S. Gezen, "The effect of dietary probiotic supplementation on tibial bone characteristics and strength in broilers," *Poultry Science*, vol. 85, no. 9, pp. 1621–1625, 2006.

[23] F. C. Rodrigues, A. S. B. Castro, C. V. Rodrigues, S. A. Fernandes, E. A. F. Fontes, and T. T. Oliveira, "Yacon flour and *Bifidobacterium longum* modulate bone health in rats," *Journal of Medicinal Food*, vol. 15, no. 7, pp. 664–670, 2012.

[24] M. Narva, R. Nevala, T. Poussa, and R. Korpela, "The effect of *Lactobacillus helveticus* fermented milk on acute changes in calcium metabolism in postmenopausal women," *European Journal of Nutrition*, vol. 43, no. 2, pp. 61–68, 2004.

[25] M. Narva, J. Halleen, K. Väänänen, and R. Korpela, "Effects of *Lactobacillus helveticus* fermented milk on bone cells in vitro," *Life Sciences*, vol. 75, no. 14, pp. 1727–1734, 2004.

[26] Q. Qu, M. Perälä-Heape, A. Kapanen et al., "Estrogen enhances differentiation of osteoblasts in mouse bone marrow culture," *Bone*, vol. 22, no. 3, pp. 201–209, 1998.

[27] N. Takahashi, H. Yamana, S. Yoshiki et al., "Osteoclast-like cell formation and its regulation by osteotropic hormones in mouse bone marrow cultures," *Endocrinology*, vol. 122, no. 4, pp. 1373–1382, 1988.

[28] R. D. Hancock and R. Viola, "The use of micro-organisms for L-ascorbic acid production: current status and future perspectives," *Applied Microbiology and Biotechnology*, vol. 56, no. 5-6, pp. 567–576, 2001.

[29] M. L. Villa, R. Marcus, R. R. Delay, and J. L. Kelsey, "Factors contributing to skeletal health of postmenopausal Mexican-American women," *Journal of Bone and Mineral Research*, vol. 10, no. 8, pp. 1233–1242, 1995.

[30] P. Weber, "The role of vitamins in the prevention of osteoporosis—a brief status report," *International Journal for Vitamin and Nutrition Research*, vol. 69, no. 3, pp. 194–197, 1999.

[31] J. M. Campbell, G. C. Fahey Jr., and B. W. Wolf, "Selected indigestible oligosaccharides affect large bowel mass, cecal and fecal short-chain fatty acids, pH and microflora in rats," *Journal of Nutrition*, vol. 127, no. 1, pp. 130–136, 1997.

[32] H. W. Lopez, C. Coudray, M.-A. Levrat-Verny, C. Feillet-Coudray, C. Demigné, and C. Rémésy, "Fructooligosaccharides enhance mineral apparent absorption and counteract the deleterious effects of phytic acid on mineral homeostasis in rats," *Journal of Nutritional Biochemistry*, vol. 11, no. 10, pp. 500–508, 2000.

[33] G. Q. Lan, N. Abdullah, S. Jalaludin, and Y. W. Ho, "Efficacy of supplementation of a phytase-producing bacterial culture on the performance and nutrient use of broiler chickens fed corn-soybean meal diets," *Poultry Science*, vol. 81, no. 10, pp. 1522–1532, 2002.

[34] C. Matar, J. Amiot, L. Savoie, and J. Goulet, "The effect of milk fermentation by *Lactobacillus helveticus* on the release of peptides during in vitro digestion," *Journal of Dairy Science*, vol. 79, no. 6, pp. 971–979, 1996.

[35] H. Hagiwara, Y. Hiruma, A. Inoue, A. Yamaguchi, and S. Hirose, "Deceleration by angiotensin II of the differentiation and bone formation of rat calvarial osteoblastic cells," *Journal of Endocrinology*, vol. 156, no. 3, pp. 543–550, 1998.

[36] Y. F. Ma, M. Stimpel, H. Liang, S. Pun, and W. S. S. Jee, "Impact of antihypertensive therapy on the skeleton: effects of moexipril and hydrochlorothiazide on osteopenia in spontaneously hypertensive ovariectomized rats," *Journal of Endocrinology*, vol. 154, no. 3, pp. 467–474, 1997.

[37] T. Bennett, A. Desmond, M. Harrington et al., "The effect of high intakes of casein and casein phosphopeptide on calcium absorption in the rat," *British Journal of Nutrition*, vol. 83, no. 6, pp. 673–680, 2000.

[38] J. Gilman and K. D. Cashman, "The effect of probiotic bacteria on transepithelial calcium transport and calcium uptake in human intestinal-like caco-2 cells," *Current Issues in Intestinal Microbiology*, vol. 7, no. 1, pp. 1–6, 2006.

[39] K. H. Baek, K. W. Oh, W. Y. Lee et al., "Association of oxidative stress with postmenopausal osteoporosis and the effects of hydrogen peroxide on osteoclast formation in human bone marrow cell cultures," *Calcified Tissue International*, vol. 87, no. 3, pp. 226–235, 2010.

[40] K. Sjögren, C. Engdahl, P. Henning, U. H. Lerner, V. Tremaroli, and M. K. Lagerquist, "The gut microbiota regulates bone mass in mice," *Journal of Bone and Mineral Research*, vol. 27, no. 6, pp. 1357–1367, 2012.

[41] T. T. Kararli, "Comparison of the gastrointestinal anatomy, physiology, and biochemistry of humans and commonly used laboratory animals," *Biopharmaceutics and Drug Disposition*, vol. 16, no. 5, pp. 351–380, 1995.

Skeletal Muscle Mass Indices in Healthy Young Mexican Adults Aged 20–40 Years: Implications for Diagnoses of Sarcopenia in the Elderly Population

H. Alemán-Mateo and Roxana E. Ruiz Valenzuela

Coordinación de Nutrición, Centro de Investigación en Alimentación y Desarrollo (CIAD), A.C. Carretera a La Victoria Km. 0.6, 83304 Hermosillo, Sonora, Mexico

Correspondence should be addressed to H. Alemán-Mateo; helio@ciad.mx

Academic Editors: S. Hirsch and M. A. Kamimura

Background and Objectives. Skeletal muscle and skeletal muscle indices in young adults from developing countries are sparse. Indices and the corresponding cut-off points can be a reference for diagnoses of sarcopenia. This study assessed skeletal muscle using dual-energy X-ray absorptiometry (DXA) in healthy male and female subjects aged 20–40 years and compared their appendicular skeletal muscle mass (ASM) and total-body skeletal muscle (TBSM) indices using certain cut-off points published in the literature. *Methods.* A sample of 216 healthy adults men and women from northwest Mexico was included. Body composition was assessed by DXA and several published DXA-derived skeletal muscle indices were compared. *Results.* Both, ASM and TBSM were higher in men compared to the women group (23.0 ± 3.4 versus 15.9 ± 1.6 kg; $P < 0.05$ and 26.5 ± 4.1 versus 16.9 ± 1.9 kg; $P < 0.05$, resp.). These differences were also valid for both indices. When derived cut-off points were compared with the most reported indices, significant differences were found. *Interpretation and Conclusion.* Published cut-off points from Caucasians are higher than cut-off point derived in this sample of Mexican subjects. The new DXA-derived cut-off points for ASM proposed herein may improve diagnoses of sarcopenia in the geriatric Mexican population.

1. Introduction

Skeletal muscle (SM) plays a central role in many biological functions, such as movement and metabolism, so disruptions in this component of body composition can have a marketed influence on health and disease [1]. Also, we cannot ignore the influence of this factor on nutritional status and functionality at older ages. Skeletal muscle in both men and women subjects remains relatively constant during the third and fourth decades of life but begins to decline noticeably at ~45 years of age [2–4]. It has been suggested that the maintaining muscle mass in old age is a key factor for conserving physical capacity and enabling independent lifestyles in old age. Human skeletal muscle mass depends basically on stature, weight, age, and gender. In a published study these factors explained >80% between-individual within-ethnic group (African-Americans and Caucasians) differences in SM mass [3].

The loss of SM is a common problem in older adults from around the world that reaches a prevalence ranging from 7% to over 50% [5]. At one time, the age-related loss of skeletal muscle was called sarcopenia, but now its definition is not limited only to the loss of muscle mass. Sarcopenia comprised the loss both muscle mass and strength with a risk of adverse outcomes such as physical disability, poor quality of life, and even death [5]. In terms of diagnoses, sarcopenia is characterized by low muscle mass plus low muscle strength or low physical performance. To establish "low muscle mass", some researchers have assessed the total or appendicular skeletal muscle in young adults (the age range in which muscle reaches a plateau and then remains relatively constant). It is important to highlight that the absolute skeletal muscle mass (kg) is normally converted to skeletal muscle indices. Baumgartner et al. [6] summed the muscle mass of the four limbs assessed by DXA and used the term appendicular skeletal muscle mass (ASM) to refer to this sum. They then defined the appendicular skeletal muscle mass index (ASMI) as ASM/height^2 (kg/m^2). ASMI two-standard deviations below the mean ASMI of healthy young male and female reference groups were defined as the gender-specific cut-off points for sarcopenia (original term used).

Several cut-off points based on the ASMI or total-body SM mass index (TBSMI) have been derived [6–13]; however, these cut-off points depend on several factors: the measurement technique used, age range, sex, ethnicity, and the availability suitable references studies. For the Mexican case, unfortunately, no such reference SM data exist, so the few published studies on sarcopenia have used a cut-off point based on an ASMI derived from a young Caucasian population [14]; even though could well bias the prevalence of the loss of skeletal muscle or sarcopenia. In addition, several studies have shown significant differences in the prevalence of sarcopenia when different indices are used interchangeably or are applied to populations distinct from the original sex-specific group of subjects [15]. Due to these issues, the recommendation is that these indices would ideally refer to sex-specific ethnic group populations [5]. Therefore, this study assessed skeletal muscle using dual-energy X-ray absorptiometry in healthy male and female subjects aged 20–40 years and compared their ASM and TBSM indices using certain cut-off points published in the literature.

2. Materials and Methods

2.1. Study Design and Subjects. This is a cross-sectional, non-probability study that included 216 apparently healthy adult men and women from northwest Mexico. All volunteers were selected on the bases of inclusion and exclusion criteria. All men and (nonpregnant) female subjects were between 20 and 40 years of age, were apparently healthy by self-report, and were either born in the state of Sonora, Mexico or had lived there for at least five years. Subjects were excluded if their body weight or height was outside the DXA bed dimensions. Subjects who reported changes in body weight in the last six months due primary to caloric restriction or increased physical activity were not included. For safety reason, pregnant women were not invited to participate and those who were positive on a pregnancy test (DIAGMEX commercial test) were not included for the DXA measurements. Also, volunteers who were taking medications that affect body composition and those with protein supplementation were excluded. Most volunteers had lifestyles that involved only light occupational and leisure time activities. Finally, trained technicians took all anthropometric and body composition measurements of subjects under fasting conditions or at least two hours after subject's most recent meal or drink.

2.2. Anthropometry

2.2.1. Body Weight. This variable was measured with subjects dressed in light clothing and shoes less (avoiding extra weight such as wallets, money, and phones). The Digital Electronic Scale (PV-150 K DNA, Japan) used was calibrated before taking measurements.

2.2.2. Height. This was measured without shoes and according to our standardized protocol, using a calibrated Holtain stadiometer (Holtain Ltd, Dyfed, UK).

2.2.3. Body Mass Index. BMI was calculated on the basis of body weight and height measurements and classified according to WHO's 1997 cut-off points [16].

2.3. Body Composition. The evaluation of body composition including the lean tissue was carried out under fasting conditions or at least two hours after the most recent light meal or drinks, following established guidelines and using a DXA (DPX-MD+; GE Lunar Madison, WI, USA). Regional body composition components were determined from the DXA scans, following the recommended anatomical landmarks. The sum of nonfat plus nonbone tissue in both arms and legs was used to represent ASM [17]. Limb skeletal muscle mass represents 75% of total body skeletal muscle [18]. Other body composition components, such as total body lean tissue and fat mass, were also assessed. From DXA-derived ASM, total-body skeletal muscle mass was predicted using Kim's equation [19].

2.4. Skeletal Muscle Mass Indices and Cut-Off Points. Two indices were calculated: ASMI as ASM/height^2 (kg/m^2) and TBSMI as TBSM/height^2 (kg/m^2). Two cut-off points were established considering two standard deviations below the mean of both indices derived from the SM assessed in a sample of healthy young man and women from northwest Mexico.

2.5. Skeletal Muscle Mass Indices and Cut-Off Points Derived from the Other Populations. For this study, Baumgartner et al., Sanada et al., Lau et al., Wen et al., and Kim et al.'s sex-specific cut-off points for ASMI [6–10] and Lau et al., Tichet et al., Chien et al., and Masanes et al. [8, 11–13] sex-specific cut-off points for TBSMI were used for purposes of comparison.

2.6. Statistical Analyses. Results are presented as mean standard deviations by sex, while significant differences between man and women were tested by a two-sample t-test. A one-sample t-test was also used to test the significant differences between our sex-specific cut-off points compared to the different published ASMI and TBSMI cut-off points derived from a young adult ethnic group populations.

3. Results

This study included 216 subjects, 63% were men and the rest women. Average was 27.6 ± 5.2 years, with a range of 18 to 40 years. The mean BMI was 24.7 kg/m^2 which falls into the "normal" range according to the WHO's classification. Regarding the anthropometric data collected, a significant

TABLE 1: Anthropometry and body composition components of healthy young Mexican adults.

Variables	Men (n = 136)	Women (n = 80)	Both men and women
Age, (years)	27.3 ± 5.0	28.2 ± 5.6	27.6 ± 5.2
Weight, (kg)	77.9 ± 13.0	60.4 ± 8.5*	71.5 ± 14.3
Height, (m)	1.74 ± 0.1	1.61 ± 0.04*	1.69 ± 0.08
BMI, (kg/m^2)	25.7 ± 3.6	23.2 ± 3.1*	24.7 ± 3.6
ASM, (kg)	23.0 ± 3.4	15.9 ± 1.6*	20.1 ± 4.7
ASMI, (kg/m^2)	7.5 ± 0.8	5.8 ± 0.5*	6.6 ± 1.1
TBSM, (kg)	26.5 ± 4.1	16.9 ± 1.9*	22.9 ± 5.7
TBSMI, (kg/m^2)	8.6 ± 1.0	6.5 ± 0.6*	7.8 ± 1.3
FFM, (kg)	52.9 ± 7.1	34.2 ± 3.2*	46.0 ± 10.8
Fat mass, (kg)	20.5 ± 8.5	22.2 ± 6.6**	21.2 ± 4.9
Truncal fat, (kg)	13.1 ± 5.4	11.3 ± 3.8**	12.4 ± 7.9

BMI: body mass index; ASM: appendicular skeletal muscle mass; ASMI: appendicular skeletal muscle mass index; TBSM: total-body skeletal muscle mass; TBSMI: total-body skeletal muscle mass index; FFM: fat-free mass (total lean tissue plus total bone mineral content); $^*P < 0.001$; $^{**}P < 0.05$.

TABLE 2: Sex-effect on the proposed cut-off points based on two standard deviations below the mean value of the ASMI and TBSMI derived from healthy young Mexican adults.

Variables	Men (n = 136)	Women (n = 80)	P value
ASMI, (kg/m^2)	5.86	4.72	0.0001
TBSMI, (kg/m^2)	6.63	5.22	0.0001

ASMI: appendicular skeletal muscle mass index; TBSMI: total-body skeletal muscle mass index.

gender effect was found. As expected, the male group weighed 18 kg more than the female group ($P < 0.001$), and height in former was higher than in the latter by an average 13 cm ($P < 0.001$). These differences were reflected significantly in the BMI measurements, and similar results were found for the body composition components assessed. Both, ASM and TBSM were higher in men compared to the mean value for the women's group. These differences were also valid for both indices. However, total and truncal fat were significantly higher in the women group (Table 1).

Table 2 shows the effect of gender on the new proposed cut-off points based on two standard deviations below the mean value of both indices, derived from the sample included. Both indices were significantly higher in the men's group. When these cut-off points were compared to the most often reported indices in the literature, significant differences were found for all indices derived from other sex-specific ethnic groups, except those from a sample of Chinese and Hong Kong men and a sample of Chinese women (Table 3).

TABLE 3: Comparison between the proposed sex-specific cut-off points against some published indices from around the world.

Indices by authors	Sex-specific cut-off points	
	Men	Women
ASMI, (kg/m^2)		
Alemán and Ruiz, 2014	5.86	4.72
Baumgartner et al., 1988	7.26*	5.45*
Sanada et al., 2010 [7]	6.87*	5.46*
Lau et al., 2005 [8]	5.72*	4.82
Wen et al., 2011 [9]	5.80	4.30*
Kim et al., 2009 [10]	7.40*	5.10*
TBSMI, (kg/m^2)		
Alemán and Ruiz, 2014	6.71	5.22
Lau et al., 2005 [8]	7.66*	6.40*
Tichet et al., 2008 [11]	8.60*	6.20*
Chien et al., 2008 [12]	8.90*	6.50*
Mesanes et al., 2012	8.31*	6.68*

ASMI: appendicular skeletal muscle mass index; TBSMI: total-body skeletal muscle mass index.
$^*P < 0.001$.

4. Discussion

This is the first study to use DXA with a sample of young Latin American adults to determine indices based on our skeletal muscle estimates. The cut-off points derived from this sample of male and female Mexican subjects may improve diagnoses of sarcopenia in the Mexican geriatric population or among Latin American people with similar characteristics to those in the sample assessed herein. Overall results confirm the effect of gender on most of the anthropometric and body composition components and DXA-derived indices. In addition, our results showed significant differences with most of the sex-specific population indices published. These results emphasize that these published indices cannot be used interchangeably.

The expected results on the differences between the derived indices from this sample and those published previously can be related to the determinants of differences in body composition, especially skeletal muscle. It is well recognized that skeletal muscle depends on age, gender, ethnicity, body weight, height, and longer extremities [3, 20, 21]; therefore skeletal muscle indices could depend on the same factors. In order to assess the clinical impact of those indices physical performance test should be assess in order to look the association between the sex-specific cut-off points and physical disabilities in different ethnic groups, but we cannot ignore the effect of the techniques used to measure muscle mass since its highly likely that all these determinants may influence the indices.

The indices derived from some Caucasian populations are higher (i.e., Baumgarnert et al.'s cut-off points of 7.26 and 5.45 for young man and women adults, resp., [6]) because, in general, Caucasian people are taller than Latina American or Asian populations, while in the case of the African-American people we find significantly greater skeletal muscle mass [20] and it has been reported longer appendicular bone lengths [22, 23] compared to Caucasian subjects. If we compared the African-Americans with other ethnic groups, the results would probably not change. For all these reasons, plus the high prevalence of loss of skeletal muscle and sarcopenia around the world, and the clinical impact of these conditions, more research is needed to obtain good reference studies that will establish valid SM cut-off points for populations worldwide and to translate this information to the clinical practice in order to detect patients with low muscle mass or sarcopenia.

The clinical implication of the results of this study is that the interchangeably use of these cut-off points may under- or overestimate real prevalence of loss of skeletal muscle mass or sarcopenia in older people in Mexico or other Latin American countries. Specifically, if we were to use the cut-off points reported by Baumgartner et al., a significant underestimation of the prevalence of the loss of skeletal muscle mass or sarcopenia would be reported for older people, characterized by low skeletal muscle mass or ASMI [20]. Similarly, after applying the ASMI criteria for sarcopenia in a study of an elderly Chinese population Wen et al. [9] concluded that this method may not be appropriate for diagnosing sarcopenia in that group because no older adults in the study were diagnosed with this condition. The criteria based on the skeletal muscle index proposed by Janssen et al. [24] showed greater discriminating power in identifying persons with low handgrip strength. Considering the findings from Wen et al. [9] in addition to having sex-specific cut-off points for different populations or ethnic groups it is clear that the use of other criteria for sarcopenia and clinical assessments of functionality is required for target population.

With respect to clinical implications of the results of this study mentioned before, it is important to consider that skeletal muscle is a required component for diagnoses of sarcopenia [5]. Therefore, the cut-off points for muscle strength in the young reference population or low physical performance in elderly participant in addition to the sex-specific cut-off points for skeletal muscle may improve diagnosis of sarcopenia in the target elderly population.

4.1. Strengths and Limitations. The strength of this study rests on the use of DXA to assess lean tissue, since this technique accurately measures ASM. The comparison with other cut-off points based on DXA-derived ASM is another strength, although the use of a nonrandom sampling method and the nonpopulation-based nature of this work limit the ability to generalize results. For these reasons, future population-based studies are needed to obtain better reference cut-off points for ASM and other body composition components in the young Mexican adult population. Also, we are aware that the reported cut-off points based on ASM or TBSM derived from a young adults population adjusted to the dimensions of the DXA bed could be another important limitation, as individuals taller than 1.96 meters could not be assessed by DXA. The estimates of TBSMI using a published DXA-equation derived from a Caucasian population and the absence of a gold standard method to assess TBSM could be an additional limitation.

5. Conclusion

In conclusion, this study confirms an effect of sex on several body composition components and DXA-derived indices such as ASMI and TBSMI in the sample of young adult assessed. Published cut-off points from Caucasians are higher than those derived in this sample of men and women Mexican subjects so the use of those published indices interchangeably could underestimate the prevalence of the loss of skeletal muscle mass or sarcopenia in older people characterized by low skeletal muscle mass or ASMI. The new DXA-derived cut-off points for ASM proposed herein may improve diagnoses of sarcopenia in the geriatric Mexican population or that of other Latin American countries with similar characteristics to those assessed in our study sample.

Conflict of Interests

The authors declare that they have no conflict of interests regarding the publication of this paper.

Authors' Contributions

H. Alemán-Mateo was the main author of the paper and project director and participated in concept, design, data collection, data analysis, data interpretation, and writing and Roxana E. Ruiz Valenzuela participated in data collection, data analysis, and data interpretation.

Acknowledgments

The authors thank Centro de Investigación en Alimentación y Desarrollo, and CONACYT (S0008-2010-1-140157) for the funding provided for this phase of the study. The authors are especially grateful to the volunteers for their unconditional participation in the project and also Ana Cristina Gallegos for her technical assistance.

References

[1] I. Janssen and R. Ross, "Linking age-related changes in skeletal muscle mass and composition with metabolism and disease," *Journal of Nutrition, Health and Aging*, vol. 9, no. 6, pp. 408–419, 2005.

[2] S. P. Tzankoff and A. H. Norris, "Effect of muscle mass decrease on age-related BMR changes," *Journal of Applied Physiology Respiratory Environmental and Exercise Physiology*, vol. 43, no. 6, pp. 1001–1006, 1977.

[3] D. Gallagher, M. Visser, R. E. De Meersman et al., "Appendicular skeletal muscle mass: effects of age, gender, and ethnicity," *Journal of Applied Physiology*, vol. 83, no. 1, pp. 229–239, 1997.

[4] I. Janssen, S. B. Heymsfield, Z. Wang, and R. Ross, "Skeletal muscle mass and distribution in 468 men and women aged 18–88 yr," *Journal of Applied Physiology*, vol. 89, no. 1, pp. 81–88, 2000.

[5] A. J. Cruz-Jentoft, J. P. Baeyens, J. M. Bauer et al., "Sarcopenia: European consensus on definition and diagnosis," *Age and Ageing*, vol. 39, no. 4, pp. 412–423, 2010.

[6] R. N. Baumgartner, K. M. Koehler, D. Gallagher et al., "Epidemiology of sarcopenia among the elderly in New Mexico," *American Journal of Epidemiology*, vol. 147, no. 8, pp. 755–763, 1998.

[7] K. Sanada, M. Miyachi, M. Tanimoto et al., "A cross-sectional study of sarcopenia in Japanese men and women: reference values and association with cardiovascular risk factors," *European Journal of Applied Physiology*, vol. 110, no. 1, pp. 57–65, 2010.

[8] E. M. C. Lau, H. S. H. Lynn, J. W. Woo, T. C. Y. Kwok, and L. J. Melton III, "Prevalence of and risk factors for sarcopenia in elderly Chinese men and women," *Journals of Gerontology A*, vol. 60, no. 2, pp. 213–216, 2005.

[9] X. Wen, M. Wang, C.-M. Jiang, and Y.-M. Zhang, "Are current definitions of sarcopenia applicable for older Chinese adults?" *Journal of Nutrition, Health and Aging*, vol. 15, no. 10, pp. 847–851, 2011.

[10] T. N. Kim, S. J. Yang, H. J. Yoo et al., "Prevalence of sarcopenia and sarcopenic obesity in Korean adults: the Korean sarcopenic obesity study," *International Journal of Obesity*, vol. 33, no. 8, pp. 885–892, 2009.

[11] J. Tichet, S. Vol, D. Goxe, A. Salle, G. Berrut, and P. Ritz, "Prevalence of sarcopenia in the French senior population," *Journal of Nutrition, Health and Aging*, vol. 12, no. 3, pp. 202–206, 2008.

[12] M.-Y. Chien, T.-Y. Huang, and Y.-T. Wu, "Prevalence of sarcopenia estimated using a bioelectrical impedance analysis prediction equation in community-dwelling elderly people in Taiwan," *Journal of the American Geriatrics Society*, vol. 56, no. 9, pp. 1710–1715, 2008.

[13] F. Masanes Toran, A. Culla, M. Navarro-Gonzalez et al., "Prevalence of sarcopenia in healthy community-dwelling elderly in an urban area of Barcelona (Spain)," *Journal of Nutrition, Health and Aging*, vol. 16, no. 2, pp. 184–187, 2012.

[14] M. C. Velázquez Alva, M. E. Irigoyen Camacho, J. Delgadillo Velázquez, and I. Lazarevich, "The relationship between sarcopenia, undernutrition, physical mobility and basic activities of daily living in a group of elderly women of Mexico city," *Nutrición Hospitalaria*, vol. 28, no. 2, pp. 514–521, 2013.

[15] A. Y. Bijlsma, C. G. M. Meskers, C. H. Y. Ling et al., "Defining sarcopenia: the impact of different diagnostic criteria on the prevalence of sarcopenia in a large middle aged cohort," *Age*, vol. 35, no. 3, pp. 871–881, 2013.

[16] World Health Organisation, *Obesity: Preventing and Managing the Global Epidemic: Report of the WHO Consultation of Obesity*, World Health Organization, Geneva, Switzerland, 1997.

[17] S. B. Heymsfield, R. Smith, M. Aulet et al., "Appendicular skeletal muscle mass: measurement by dual-photon absorptiometry," *American Journal of Clinical Nutrition*, vol. 52, no. 2, pp. 214–218, 1990.

[18] R. D. Hansen, C. Raja, A. Aslani, R. C. Smith, and B. J. Allen, "Determination of skeletal muscle and fat-free mass by nuclear and dual- energy X-ray absorptiometry methods in men and women aged 51–84 y," *American Journal of Clinical Nutrition*, vol. 70, no. 2, pp. 228–233, 1999.

[19] J. Kim, Z. Wang, S. B. Heymsfield, R. N. Baumgartner, and D. Gallagher, "Total-body skeletal muscle mass: estimation by a new dual-energy X-ray absorptiometry method," *American Journal of Clinical Nutrition*, vol. 76, no. 2, pp. 378–383, 2002.

[20] H. Aleman-Mateo, S. Y. Lee, F. Javed et al., "Elderly Mexicans have less muscle and greater total and truncal fat compared to African-Americans and Caucasians with the same BMI," *Journal of Nutrition, Health and Aging*, vol. 13, no. 10, pp. 919–923, 2009.

[21] A. M. Silva, W. Shen, M. Heo et al., "Ethnicity-related skeletal muscle differences across the lifespan," *American Journal of Human Biology*, vol. 22, no. 1, pp. 76–82, 2010.

[22] L. Gerace, A. Aliprantis, M. Russell et al., "Skeletal differences between black and white men and their relevance to body composition estimates," *American Journal of Human Biology*, vol. 6, no. 2, pp. 255–262, 2005.

[23] R. M. Malina, "Regional body composition: age, sex, and ethnic variation," in *Human Body Composition*, A. F. Roche, S. B. Heymsfield, and T. G. Lohman, Eds., pp. 217–255, Human Kinetics, Champaign, Ill, USA, 1996.

[24] I. Janssen, S. B. Heymsfield, and R. Ross, "Low relative skeletal muscle mass (sarcopenia) in older persons is associated with functional impairment and physical disability," *Journal of the American Geriatrics Society*, vol. 50, no. 5, pp. 889–896, 2002.

23

Changes in Iron Metabolism and Oxidative Status in STZ-Induced Diabetic Rats Treated with Bis(maltolato) Oxovanadium (IV) as an Antidiabetic Agent

Cristina Sánchez-González,[1] Carlos López-Chaves,[1] Cristina E. Trenzado,[2] Pilar Aranda,[1] María López-Jurado,[1] Jorge Gómez-Aracena,[3] María Montes-Bayón,[4] Alfredo Sanz-Medel,[4] and Juan Llopis[1]

[1] *Department of Physiology, Faculty of Pharmacy, University of Granada, 18071 Granada, Spain*
[2] *Department of Cellular Biology, Faculty of Sciences, University of Granada, 18071 Granada, Spain*
[3] *Department of Analytical Chemistry, Faculty of Chemistry, University of Oviedo, 33007 Oviedo, Spain*
[4] *Department of Preventive Medicine and Public Health, Faculty of Medicine, University of Málaga, 29071 Málaga, Spain*

Correspondence should be addressed to Juan Llopis; jllopis@ugr.es

Academic Editors: A. Chicco and T. Strand

The role of vanadium as a micronutrient and hypoglycaemic agent has yet to be fully clarified. The present study was undertaken to investigate changes in the metabolism of iron and in antioxidant defences of diabetic STZ rats following treatment with vanadium. Four groups were examined: control; diabetic; diabetic treated with 1 mgV/day; and Diabetic treated with 3 mgV/day. The vanadium was supplied in drinking water as bis(maltolato) oxovanadium (IV) (BMOV). The experiment had a duration of five weeks. Iron was measured in food, faeces, urine, serum, muscle, kidney, liver, spleen, and femur. Superoxide dismutase, catalase, NAD(P)H: quinone-oxidoreductase-1 (NQO1) activity, and protein carbonyl group levels in the liver were determined. In the diabetic rats, higher levels of Fe absorbed, Fe content in kidney, muscle, and femur, and NQO1 activity were recorded, together with decreased catalase activity, in comparison with the control rats. In the rats treated with 3 mgV/day, there was a significant decrease in fasting glycaemia, Fe content in the liver, spleen, and heart, catalase activity, and levels of protein carbonyl groups in comparison with the diabetic group. In conclusion BMOV was a dose-dependent hypoglycaemic agent. Treatment with 3 mgV/day provoked increased Fe deposits in the tissues, which promoted a protein oxidative damage in the liver.

1. Background

Diabetes is a pathological state that affects many metabolic processes and is associated with alterations to antioxidant defences and the metabolism of trace elements, which may contribute to the development of the disease.

The role of vanadium (V) as a micronutrient for humans, its essentiality, distribution, and toxicology, as well as its biological and pharmacological activity, are still not fully understood [1]. Rising levels of V in the environment, together with growing interest in the pharmacological effects of some of its compounds, have led to the study of V metabolism becoming an important area of current research.

In plasma, V is bound mainly to transferrin and to a lesser degree to other molecules, such as albumin [2–4]. Elsewhere, it is distributed primarily in the bone, kidney, and liver [1, 2, 4]. However, its interactions with other elements are not well understood.

Some V complexes have been shown to possess hypoglycaemic or insulin-mimetic properties [5–8], but many aspects remain to be determined, such as the interactions with other elements involved in antioxidant defence. Moreover, weight training athletes are reported to use it to improve performance [9]. According to some authors, V improves glucose metabolism and prevents the oxidant damage caused by diabetes [10].

Table 1: Digestive and metabolic utilization of Fe on days 28–35 of study.

	C	DM	DMV	DMVH	P_{test}
Food intake (g/day)	15 ± 2	33 ± 2.4[a]	26.9 ± 2[a,b]	13.8 ± 1.1[b,c]	$P < 0.001$
Water intake (mL/day)	17 ± 4	324 ± 36[a]	191 ± 41[a,b]	14 ± 7[b,c]	$P < 0.001$
V intake (μg/day)	1 ± 0.1	1.9 ± 0.1[a]	965 ± 104[a,b]	3228 ± 350[a,b,c]	$P < 0.001$
Fe intake (I) (μg/day)	668 ± 88	1472 ± 105[a]	1197 ± 89[a,b]	614 ± 50[b,c]	$P < 0.001$
Faecal excretion (F) (μg/day)	497 ± 75	1219 ± 106[a]	888 ± 50[a,b]	430 ± 78[b,c]	$P < 0.001$
Urinary excretion (U) (μg/day)	29 ± 8	118 ± 95[a]	103 ± 22[a]	47 ± 17[a,b,c]	$P < 0.001$
Absorbed (A); $A = (I - F)$ (μg/day)	171 ± 78	253 ± 56[a]	308 ± 68[a]	184 ± 59[b,c]	$P < 0.01$
Retained (R); $R = [I - (F + U)]$ (μg/day)	142 ± 79	134 ± 52	205 ± 66[b]	137 ± 64[c]	NS

Values shown are means ± SD, C: control rats; DM: diabetic STZ rats; DMV: diabetic STZ rats treated with 1 mgV/day; DMVH: diabetic STZ rats treated with 3 mgV/day. [a]Different from group C; [b]different from group DM; [c]different from group DMV. $P < 0.05$. NS: not significant.

However, other authors have related V with prooxidant effects [11, 12], because it does not normalize alterations in the metabolism of various elements that are associated with diabetes [12]. Therefore, the widespread use of V as a potential insulin-mimetic agent is subject to evaluation of the toxicity associated with its prooxidant effect.

Diabetes has been associated with alterations in iron (Fe) homeostasis both in humans and in animal models [13]. The generation of reactive oxygen species by prooxidant metals such as Fe may be a mechanism which aggravates this disease. Previous studies have reported that diabetes produces an accumulation of Fe in the tissues together with increased excretion of this metal [14]. Concerning the effect of diabetes on Fe content in the liver, opinions are mixed; some authors have observed increased Fe [15], while others have found no changes [11]. Little is known about the effects of exposure to V on Fe metabolism in diabetes [11] and therefore we consider it important to study whether V-treated diabetic rats experience alterations in the metabolism of Fe and in the activity of liver enzymes related to antioxidant defence. The results obtained will clarify the role of V as a micronutrient and the level of its biological activity as an antidiabetic agent.

2. Materials and Methods

2.1. Animals and Diets. The experiment was carried out over a period of five weeks. Male *Wistar* rats (Charles River Laboratories, L' Arbresle, France) weighing 190–220 g at the beginning of the experimental period were randomly distributed into four groups: control group (C): 9 healthy rats; diabetic group (DM): 8 STZ-induced diabetic rats; diabetic treated group (DMV): 8 STZ-induced diabetic rats treated with 1 mg V/d (administered as 6.2 mg BMOV/d); and high-dose diabetic group (DMVH): 8 STZ-induced diabetic rats treated with 3 mg V/d (administered as 18.7 mg BMOV/d).

All groups were fed with the semisynthetic AIN-93 diet (which provided 44.5 mg Fe and 60 μg V/kg food) and were allowed free access to drinking water (Milli-Q quality) throughout the experimental period. In the DM, DMV, and DMVH groups, type I diabetes was induced by single intraperitoneal administration of streptozotocin (STZ) (Sigma-Aldrich, St. Louis, MO, USA) at a dose of 60 mg/kg body weight, as a diabetogenic agent. Seven days later, the induction of diabetes was confirmed by measuring blood glucose levels on three occasions (9 a.m., 2 p.m., and 7 p.m.). Animals with a glucose concentration (random glycaemia) >13.8 mmol/L and with polyuria, polydipsia, and hyperphagia were considered diabetic [16].

In all cases, the BMOV solution was prepared and administered daily in the drinking water for 35 days, a sufficient time for the effects of V to become apparent [11, 17, 18]. BMOV was synthesised according to published procedures [19]. During the experimental period, the animals' weight gain and intake of food and water were monitored. Every day at 9 a.m., the surplus water from the previous day was removed and the amount consumed was calculated. Table 1 shows the water and V intake.

On day 35, after overnight fasting, the rats were anaesthetised by intraperitoneal injection of 5 mg sodium pentobarbital/100 g body weight (Sigma-Aldrich, St. Louis, MO, USA) and exsanguinated by cannulating the posterior aorta. Blood was collected and centrifuged at 1200 ×g for 15 minutes to separate the serum. The gastrocnemius muscle, kidney, liver, spleen, heart, and femur were removed, weighed, placed in preweighed polyethylene vials, and stored at −80°C. During the last seven days of the experimental period, the faeces and urine were collected every 24 h and stored at −80°C in polyethylene bottles for subsequent analysis. All animals were housed from day 0 of the experiment in individual metabolic cages designed for the separate collection of faeces and urine. The cages were located in a well-ventilated, temperature-controlled room (21 ± 2°C) with relative humidity of 40–60% and a 12-hour light:dark period.

The following biological indices were calculated: absorbed as [I − F] and retained as [I − (F + U)], where I = intake, F = faecal excretion, and U = urinary excretion.

All experiments were carried out in accordance with Directional Guides Related to Animal Housing and Care (European Community Council, 1986) and all procedures were approved by the Animal Experimentation Ethics Committee of the University of Granada.

2.2. Analytical Methods. V and Fe in the diet, serum, and tissues were determined by ICP-MS (Agilent 7500, Tokyo, Japan) after digestion of the corresponding material using a microwave oven (Milestone, Sorisole, Italy). All the plastic containers used in the analysis were previously cleaned with superpure nitric acid and ultrapure water (18.2 Ω) obtained using a Milli-Q system (Millipore, Bedford, MA, USA). For Fe determination, 0.2 g of the corresponding samples was taken and 6 mL of a mixture (1 : 1) of nitric acid (65%) and hydrogen peroxide (30%), both of Suprapur quality (Merck, Darmstadt, Germany), was introduced directly into the microwaved vessels. The samples were then digested by applying the following programme: power 1000 W, 2 min ramp to 85°C, 4 min ramp to 135°C, 5 min ramp to 230°C held for 15 min. After digestion, the extracts were collected and made up to a final volume of 30 mL with Milli-Q water for subsequent analysis. Further dilutions of samples were prepared when necessary. Similarly, for the analysis of V, 0.5 g of each serum sample was treated with 8 mL of a mixture of nitric acid, hydrogen peroxide, and water in a 1 : 1 : 6 ratio in the microwave digester. After digestion, the extracts were collected and made up to a final volume of 10 mL with Milli-Q water for subsequent analysis. Calibration curves for Fe and V were prepared using stock solutions of 1000 mg/L of each element (Merck), using Ga as an internal standard. The internal standard was added to each sample in the same conditions. Calibration curves were prepared using 5 points with ranges of 0-1 mg/L and 0-0.1 mg/L for Fe and V, respectively. The total metal content in the tissues was obtained by interpolation in the corresponding graphs; for this purpose, each sample was measured three times. The accuracy of the method used was evaluated by comparison with certified reference materials such as Seronorm (Billingstad, Norway) and NIST 8414 (Gaithersburg, MD, USA) obtaining results of 68.9 ± 2.4 mg/kg for Fe and 0.00391 ± 0.00087 mg/kg for V, these values being in agreement with the certified ones (estimated in the case of V) of 71.2 ± 9.2 mg/kg and 0.0050 mg/kg, respectively. Additionally, spiking experiments were conducted: the concentration of Fe was analysed in three aliquots of the same sample, two of which had previously been enriched with different concentrations of Fe: 0.25 and 1 mg/L. The same procedure was carried out for V, using in this case concentrations of 0.06 and 0.1 mg/L. The recoveries calculated were 92–98% in all cases.

Glycaemia levels were determined using the sensor ACCU-CHEK AVIVA (Roche, Mannheim, Germany). Liver samples were homogenised in an ice-cold buffer (100 mM Tris-HCl, 0.1 mM EDTA, and 0.1% triton X-100 (v/v), pH 7.8) at a ratio of 1 : 9 (w/v). Homogenates were centrifuged at 30,000 rpm for 30 min in a Centrikon H-401 (Germany) centrifuge. After centrifugation, the supernatant was collected and frozen at −80°C until analysed. All enzymatic assays were carried out at 25 ± 0.5°C using a Power Wavex microplate scanning spectrophotometer (Bio-Tek Instruments, USA) in duplicate in 96-well microplates (UVStar, Greiner Bio-One, Germany). The enzymatic reactions were started by the addition of the tissue extract. The specific assay conditions were as follows.

Superoxide dismutase (SOD; EC 1.15.1.1) activity was measured spectrophotochemically by the ferricytochrome C method using xanthine/xanthine oxidase as the source of superoxide radicals [20]. The method was adapted according to Trenzado et al. [21]. The reaction mixture consisted of 50 mM potassium phosphate buffer (pH 7.8), 0.1 mM EDTA, 0.1 mM xanthine, 0.013 mM cytochrome C, and 0.024 IU mL^{-1} xanthine oxidase. One activity unit was defined as the amount of enzyme necessary to produce a 50% inhibition of the ferricytochrome C reduction rate measured at 550 nm.

Catalase (CAT; EC 1.11.1.6) activity was determined by measuring the decrease in H_2O_2 concentration at 240 nm [22]. The reaction mixture contained freshly prepared 10.6 mM H_2O_2 in 50 mM potassium phosphate buffer (pH 7.0).

NAD(P)H:quinone-oxidoreductase-1 (NQO1; EC 1.6.99.2) activity was determined by measuring DCPIP reduction at 600 nm [23]. The reaction mixture contained 50 mM Tris-HCl (pH 7.6), 50 μM 2,6-dichlorophenol indophenol (DCPIP), and 0.5 mM NADH. A control reaction with distilled water (three measures average) was assayed and subtracted from each sample reaction. For these enzymes, one unit of activity is defined as the amount of enzyme required to transform 1 μmol of substrate/min under the above assay conditions. The levels of protein carbonyl groups were assessed using Protein Carbonyl Kit (Cayman Chemical Company, MI, USA). The protein content of the supernatant solutions was determined by the Bradford method [24], using bovine serum albumin as the standard.

All biochemicals, including substrates, coenzymes, and purified enzymes, were obtained from Roche (Mannheim, Germany) or Sigma Chemical Co. (St. Louis, MO, USA). All other chemicals came from Merck (Darmstadt, Germany) and were of reagent grade.

2.3. Statistical Analysis. Descriptive statistical parameters (means and standard deviations) were obtained for each of the variables studied. Statistical comparisons among the four groups were performed by the analysis of the variance (ANOVA) test. For the bivariate analysis, Pearson's coefficient of correlation was calculated. All analyses were performed using the Statistical Package for Social Science 15.0 (SPSS, Chicago, IL, USA). Differences were considered statistically significant at a probability level <5%.

3. Results

Table 1 shows the food, water, and V intake and the digestive and metabolic utilisation of Fe. The diabetic rats showed an increase in food and water intake, in Fe excreted in faeces and urine, and in Fe absorbed, but no changes were found in Fe retained, compared to the nondiabetic control rats. Treatment with 1 mg V/d decreased the intake of food and water and the faecal excretion of Fe and increased Fe retained compared to those in the untreated diabetic rats. Treatment with 3 mg V/d decreased the intake of food and water, the faecal and urinary excretion of Fe, and Fe absorbed and retained compared to those in the diabetic untreated rats and to those in the diabetic rats treated with 1 mg V/d. The rats treated with 3 mg V/d had values of food and water intake, faecal excretion of Fe, and Fe absorbed and retained similar to those of the controls.

TABLE 2: Iron content in kidney, liver, spleen, muscle, heart, and femur (mg/kg dry tissue) on day 35.

	C	DM	DMV	DMVH	P_{test}
Kidney	255 ± 43	359 ± 74[a]	299 ± 51	290 ± 53	$P < 0.05$
Liver	404 ± 54	428 ± 65	505 ± 82[a,b]	530 ± 73[a,b]	$P < 0.05$
Spleen	3043 ± 646	1849 ± 718[a]	2410 ± 670	3918 ± 671[a,b,c]	$P < 0.001$
Muscle	50 ± 14	68 ± 19[a]	70 ± 14[a]	46 ± 5[b,c]	$P < 0.01$
Heart	340 ± 26	353 ± 56	356 ± 44	420 ± 46[a,b,c]	$P < 0.05$
Femur	40 ± 4	61 ± 4[a]	69 ± 6[a,b]	64 ± 19[a]	$P < 0.001$

Values shown are means ± SD, C: control rats; DM: diabetic STZ rats; DMV: diabetic STZ rats treated with 1 mgV/day; DMVH: diabetic STZ rats treated with 3 mgV/day. [a]Different from group C; [b]different from group DM; [c]different from group DMV. $P < 0.05$.

TABLE 3: Activity of superoxide dismutase (SOD), catalase (CAT), NAD(P)H: quinone-oxidoreductase-1 (NQO1), and protein carbonyl group levels in the liver on day 35.

	C	DM	DMV	DMVH	P_{test}
SOD (U/mg protein)	685 ± 81	672 ± 83	743 ± 74	718 ± 70	NS
CAT (U/mg protein)	389 ± 97	295 ± 29[a]	402 ± 76[b]	733 ± 73[a,b,c]	$P < 0.001$
NQO1 (mU/mg protein)	173 ± 72	269 ± 87[a]	242 ± 59	155 ± 57[b,c]	$P < 0.05$
Protein carbonyl groups (pm/mg protein)	134 ± 33	130 ± 38	196 ± 40[a,b]	186 ± 21[a,b]	$P < 0.01$

Values shown are means ± SD. C: control rats; DM: diabetic STZ rats; DMV: diabetic STZ rats treated with 1 mgV/day; DMVH: diabetic STZ rats treated with 3 mgV/day. [a]Different from group C; [b]different from group DM; [c]different from group DMV. $P < 0.05$. NS: not significant.

However, treatment with 3 mg V/d provoked urinary losses of Fe greater than those recorded for the controls.

Table 2 shows the Fe content in the tissues studied. Diabetes provokes increased Fe levels in kidney, skeletal muscle, and femur and decreased Fe content in the spleen. Treatment with 1 mg V/d increased Fe levels in liver and femur, in comparison with those in the untreated diabetic rats. Treatment with 3 mg V/d restored Fe in the muscle to levels similar to those of the control group but increased the content of Fe in the liver, spleen, and heart versus that in the controls and untreated diabetic rats. Moreover, this dose increased Fe in spleen and heart, in comparison to that in the group treated with 1 mg V/d.

Table 3 shows the activities of SOD, CAT, NQO1, and protein carbonyl group levels. There was a decrease in CAT and an increase in NQO1 activity in the untreated diabetic rats. The two doses of V tested reduced the activity of NQO1 and increased that of CAT and protein carbonyl groups versus that in the controls and untreated diabetic rats.

The bivariate study revealed the existence of significant relations, among which the following are particularly important. V intake correlated negatively with Fe content in liver ($r = 0.46$; $P < 0.01$), heart ($r = 0.43$; $P < 0.05$), and femur ($r = 0.55$; $P < 0.01$). The intake of V also correlated positively with the activity of CAT ($r = 0.61$; $P < 0.01$) and protein carbonyl group levels ($r = 0.46$; $P < 0.05$).

4. Discussion

The doses of V used in the present study (1 mg V/d, approximately 5 mg V/kg body weight/d, and 3 mg V/d, approximately 15 mg V/kg body weight/d) are low in comparison with those administered in many other studies and much lower than LD50 (lethal dose 50) (41–90 mg V/kg body weight) [10, 11, 25]. The sample size has been designed according to most of the studies performed in this field [2, 10, 11, 13, 14].

The hyperphagia associated with diabetes leads to increased food (Fe) intake, which accounts for the increased net absorption of Fe observed in the untreated diabetic group [26]. Despite the high Fe absorption and high urinary losses of Fe, the polyuria that accompanies diabetes meant that the total amount of Fe retained in the untreated diabetic rats was similar to that of the controls (Table 1).

The treatment of diabetic rats with 1 mg V/d decreased food intake (Fe intake) in comparison with that in the untreated diabetic rats. It has been suggested that the decrease in food intake could be because V heightens the effects of leptin, thus reducing food intake [27]. Other authors have suggested that the reduction in food and water intake could be due to the fact that V reduces the increased production of neuropeptide Y (NPY) that occurs in diabetes [28]. However, in the treated animals the net quantity of Fe retained increased (Table 1). In this group, there was a reduction in faecal losses of the cation, which would account for the increased amount of Fe retained, in comparison with that in the untreated diabetic rats.

The dose of 3 mg V/d administered to the diabetic rats had a clear antidiabetic effect, normalizing glycaemia [12] and reducing the hyperphagia (Fe intake) and polydipsia that accompany diabetes; food and water intake approached the levels found in the controls (Table 1). The reduced food consumption was the main reason why the rats in this group presented values of Fe absorbed similar to those of the controls and significantly lower than those of the other groups of diabetic rats.

In the group of untreated diabetic rats, the Fe content increased in various tissues. Previous studies have also described increased Fe content in various organs, and in this respect there is a high degree of agreement in the case of the kidney [14, 15]. One study showed that renal transferrin receptor expression increased in STZ-induced diabetic rats [13], which could explain the accumulation of Fe observed in the kidney (Table 2). Treatment with 3 mg V/d produced a significant increase in Fe content in the liver, heart, and spleen (Table 2), possibly due to the erythropoietic suppression and the greater uptake of Fe by hepatocytes, macrophages, and cardiac myocytes. The increased Fe content in the heart reveals the existence of Fe overload, because the heart is an organ where Fe is deposited when the storage organs become saturated. This overhead indicates a worsening of the situation, which could cause malfunctions in the organs affected.

The presence of metal ions (especially Fe) and the activation of macrophages by cytokines and/or abnormal metabolites are known to lead to an overproduction of reactive oxygen species (ROS). To determine whether the increased Fe in the liver affects the oxidative status of this organ, we designed a study of the activity of enzymes (SOD, CAT) directly related to the control of the iron-induced ROS production (Table 3). In addition, NQO1 activity was studied (Table 3). The activity of NQO1 increases in response to xenobiotics, oxidants, heavy metals, and carcinogens, which has led to the suggestion that the enzyme may offer protection against the toxic effects of these agents [29]. In order to determine whether the generationof ROS caused protein oxidative damage, we examined protein carbonyl group levels. These abnormal metabolites, too, favor the production of ROS. The liver was chosen for this study due to its importance in Fe metabolism and because the treatment produced significant Fe deposits in this organ.

Our results showed that in the untreated diabetic rats there were no changes in the activity of SOD, while CAT decreased and NQO1 increased. These findings are consistent with those of previous studies concerning SOD [30, 31] and CAT [32]. The increased NQO1 activity in diabetic rats may favor a decrease in the formation of reactive oxygen species, which would explain why no changes in SOD appear, together with the decreased CAT activity in this group. Treatment with 1 mg V/d increased the hepatic content of Fe, which was accompanied by nonsignificant increases in SOD, increased hepatic CAT, and raised levels of protein carbonyl groups. Treatment with 3 mg V/d caused an increase in Fe content in the tissues. Fe was deposited mainly in the kidney, liver, spleen, and heart. This situation was accompanied by an increase in CAT activity and a decrease in that of NQO1 in the liver. Recent *in vitro* studies with HepG2 cells [33] have shown that exposure to V (ammonium metavanadate) at low concentrations does not modify the activity of NQO1 but that the latter decreases when the dose is increased. These authors suggested that V inhibits the gene expression of NQO1.

Although our study used a different V compound and our results were obtained *in vivo*, they corroborated those mentioned above; with a dose of 1 mg V/d, no significant changes were observed, whereas enzyme activity decreased when the dose of 3 mg V/d was used, in relation to that in the untreated diabetic rats. Previous studies have shown that V decreases GPx activity and increases malondialdehyde levels in the livers of healthy rats [34] and of diabetic rats treated with V [12]. The decrease in NQO1 and GPx activity, together with the enlarged pool of liver Fe, may have increased the production of hydroxyl radicals. The strong CAT activity response appears to be insufficient to prevent the increased formation of protein carbonyl groups, which would suggest that the treatment provoked oxidative damage to the liver proteins.

5. Conclusion

Our results showed that treatment with 3 mV/d (administered as 18.7 mg BMOV/d) caused an iron overload in tissues that impaired antioxidant defences and produced protein oxidative damage in the liver. However, further studies are needed to better determine the effects arising from these interactions in order to determine optimum levels for pharmacological use, thus reducing or preventing toxic effects.

Conflict of Interests

There is no conflict of interests related to the authors or consortium members, since the project was funded by public funds. This project is dedicated to basic research and there are no commercial interests.

Acknowledgments

The authors are grateful for support received from the Consejería de Innovación, Ciencia y Empresa, Andalusian Regional Government (Project P06-CTS-01435).

References

[1] F. H. Nielsen, "Other trace elements," in *Present Knowledge in Nutrition*, E. E. Ziegler and L. J. Filder, Eds., pp. 364–370, ILSI Press, Washington, DC, USA, 7th edition, 1996.

[2] K. De Cremer, M. Van Hulle, C. Chéry et al., "Fractionation of vanadium complexes in serum, packed cells and tissues of Wistar rats by means of gel filtration and anion-exchange chromatography," *Journal of Biological Inorganic Chemistry*, vol. 7, no. 7-8, pp. 884–890, 2002.

[3] B. D. Liboiron, K. H. Thompson, G. R. Hanson, E. Lam, N. Aebischer, and C. Orvig, "New insights into the interactions of serum proteins with bis(maltolato)oxovanadium(IV): transport and biotransformation of insulin-enhancing vanadium pharmaceuticals," *Journal of the American Chemical Society*, vol. 127, no. 14, pp. 5104–5115, 2005.

[4] T. Iglesias-González, C. Sánchez-González, M. Montes-Bayón, J. Llopis-González, and A. Sanz-Medel, "Absorption, transport and insulin-mimetic properties of bis(maltolato)oxovanadium (IV) in streptozotocin-induced hyperglycemic rats by integrated mass spectrometric techniques," *Analytical and Bioanalytical Chemistry*, vol. 402, no. 1, pp. 277–285, 2012.

[5] C. Orvig, K. H. Thompson, M. Battell, and J. H. McNeill, "Vanadium compounds as insulin mimics," *Metal ions in Biological Systems*, vol. 31, pp. 575–594, 1995.

[6] K. H. Thompson and C. Orvig, "Vanadium in diabetes: 100 years from Phase 0 to Phase I," *Journal of Inorganic Biochemistry*, vol. 100, no. 12, pp. 1925–1935, 2006.

[7] K. Kawabe, Y. Yoshikawa, Y. Adachi, and H. Sakurai, "Possible mode of action for insulinomimetic activity of vanadyl(IV) compounds in adipocytes," *Life Sciences*, vol. 78, no. 24, pp. 2860–2866, 2006.

[8] K. H. Thompson, J. Lichter, C. LeBel, M. C. Scaife, J. H. McNeill, and C. Orvig, "Vanadium treatment of type 2 diabetes: a view to the future," *Journal of Inorganic Biochemistry*, vol. 103, no. 4, pp. 554–558, 2009.

[9] D. G. Barceloux, "Vanadium," *Journal of Toxicology*, vol. 37, no. 2, pp. 265–278, 1999.

[10] R. Yanardag and S. Tunali, "Vanadyl sulfate administration protects the streptozotocin-induced oxidative damage to brain tissue in rats," *Molecular and Cellular Biochemistry*, vol. 286, no. 1-2, pp. 153–159, 2006.

[11] M. H. Oster, J. M. Llobet, J. L. Domingo, J. B. German, and C. L. Keen, "Vanadium treatment of diabetic Sprague-Dawley rats results in tissue vanadium accumulation and pro-oxidant effects," *Toxicology*, vol. 83, no. 1–3, pp. 115–130, 1993.

[12] C. Sanchez-Gonzalez, C. Bermudez-Peña, F. Guerrero-Romero et al., "Effect of bis(maltolato)oxovanadium (IV) (BMOV) on Se nutritional status in diabetic STZ rats," *British Journal of Nutrition*, vol. 108, pp. 893–899, 2012.

[13] D. T. Ward, K. Hamilton, R. Burnand, C. P. Smith, D. R. Tomlinson, and D. Riccardi, "Altered expression of iron transport proteins in streptozotocin-induced diabetic rat kidney," *Biochimica et Biophysica Acta*, vol. 1740, no. 1, pp. 79–84, 2005.

[14] L. Cai, S. Chen, T. Evans, M. G. Cherian, and S. Chakrabarti, "Endothelial-1-mediated alteration of metallothionein and trace metals in the liver and kidneys of chronically diabetic rats," *International Journal of Experimental Diabetes Research*, vol. 3, no. 3, pp. 193–198, 2002.

[15] A. Dogukan, N. Sahin, M. Tuzcu et al., "The effects of chromium histidinate on mineral status of serum and tissue in fat-fed and streptozotocin-treated type II diabetic rats," *Biological Trace Element Research*, vol. 131, no. 2, pp. 124–132, 2009.

[16] American Diabetes Association, "Standards of medical care in diabetes—2013," *Diabetes Care*, vol. 36, supplement 1, pp. S11–S66, 2013.

[17] J. B. Majithiya, R. Balaraman, R. Giridhar, and M. R. Yadav, "Effect of bis[curcumino]oxovanadium complex on non-diabetic and streptozotocin-induced diabetic rats," *Journal of Trace Elements in Medicine and Biology*, vol. 18, no. 3, pp. 211–217, 2005.

[18] S. Tas, E. Sarandol, S. Z. Ayvalik, Z. Serdar, and M. Dirican, "Vanadyl sulfate, taurine, and combined vanadyl sulfate and taurine treatments in diabetic rats: effects on the oxidative and antioxidative systems," *Archives of Medical Research*, vol. 38, no. 3, pp. 276–283, 2007.

[19] J. H. McNeill, V. G. Yuen, H. R. Hoveyda, and C. Orvig, "Bis(maltolato)oxovanadium(IV) is a potent insulin mimic," *Journal of Medicinal Chemistry*, vol. 35, no. 8, pp. 1489–1491, 1992.

[20] J. M. McCord and I. Fridovich, "Superoxide dismutase. An enzymic function for erythrocuprein (hemocuprein)," *Journal of Biological Chemistry*, vol. 244, no. 22, pp. 6049–6055, 1969.

[21] C. Trenzado, M. C. Hidalgo, M. García-Gallego et al., "Antioxidant enzymes and lipid peroxidation in sturgeon Acipenser naccarii and trout Oncorhynchus mykiss. A comparative study," *Aquaculture*, vol. 254, no. 1–4, pp. 758–767, 2006.

[22] H. Aebi, "[13] Catalase in vitro," *Methods in Enzymology*, vol. 105, pp. 121–126, 1984.

[23] J. Sturve, E. Stephensen, and L. Förlin, "Effects of redox cycling compounds on DT diaphorase activity in the liver of rainbow trout (Oncorhynchus mykiss)," *Comparative Hepatology*, vol. 4, article 4, 2005.

[24] M. M. Bradford, "A rapid and sensitive method for the quantitation of microgram quantities of protein utilizing the principle of protein dye binding," *Analytical Biochemistry*, vol. 72, no. 1-2, pp. 248–254, 1976.

[25] EFSA, "Opinion of the scientific panel on dietetic products, nutrition and allergies on a request from the commission related to the tolerable upper intake level of vanadium (Request no EFSA-Q-2003-018)," *The EFSA Journal*, vol. 33, pp. 1–22, 2004, http://www.efsa.eu.int/ .

[26] A. L. Lau and M. L. Failla, "Urinary excretion of zinc, copper and iron in the streptozotocin-diabetic rat," *Journal of Nutrition*, vol. 114, no. 1, pp. 224–233, 1984.

[27] J. Wilsey, M. K. Matheny, and P. J. Scarpace, "Oral vanadium enhances the catabolic effects of central leptin in young adult rats," *Endocrinology*, vol. 147, no. 1, pp. 493–501, 2006.

[28] I. M. Liu, T. C. Chi, and J. T. Cheng, "Decrease of hypothalamic neuropeptide Y gene expression by vanadyl sulfate in streptozotocin-induced diabetic rats," *Hormone and Metabolic Research*, vol. 33, no. 2, pp. 96–100, 2001.

[29] C. Foppolia, F. Marcob, C. Blarzinoc, M. Perluigib, C. Cinib, and R. Cocciab, "Biological response of human diploid keratinocytes to quinone producing compounds: role of NAD(P)H:quinone oxidoreductase 1," *The International Journal of Biochemistry & Cell Biology*, vol. 37, pp. 852–863, 2005.

[30] Y. Y. Jang, J. H. Song, Y. K. Shin, E. S. Han, and C. S. Lee, "Protective effect of boldine on oxidative mitochondrial damage in streptozotocin-induced diabetic rats," *Pharmacological Research*, vol. 42, no. 4, pp. 361–371, 2000.

[31] G. Sadi and T. Güray, "Gene expressions of Mn-SOD and GPx-1 in streptozotocin-induced diabetes: effect of antioxidants," *Molecular and Cellular Biochemistry*, vol. 327, no. 1-2, pp. 127–134, 2009.

[32] M. A. Abou-Seif and A.-A. Youssef, "Evaluation of some biochemical changes in diabetic patients," *Clinica Chimica Acta*, vol. 346, no. 2, pp. 161–170, 2004.

[33] G. Abdelhamid, A. Anwar-Mohamed, M. M. Elmazar, and A. O. S. El-Kadi, "Modulation of NAD(P)H: Quinone oxidoreductase by vanadium in human hepatoma HepG2 cells," *Toxicology in Vitro*, vol. 24, no. 6, pp. 1554–1561, 2010.

[34] C. Sanchez-Gonzalez, C. Bermudez-Peña, C. E. Trenzado et al., "Changes in the antioxidant defence and in selenium concentration in tissues of vanadium exposed rats," *Metallomics*, vol. 4, pp. 814–819, 2012.

Antioxidant Activity and Phenolic Content of Microwave-Assisted *Solanum melongena* Extracts

Loredana Salerno, Maria N. Modica, Valeria Pittalà, Giuseppe Romeo, Maria A. Siracusa, Claudia Di Giacomo, Valeria Sorrenti, and Rosaria Acquaviva

Dipartimento di Scienze del Farmaco, Università degli Studi di Catania, Viale A. Doria 6, 95125 Catania, Italy

Correspondence should be addressed to Maria N. Modica; mmodica@unict.it

Academic Editors: Y.-C. Huang, N. Parletta, and U. Uusitalo

Eggplant fruit is a very rich source of polyphenol compounds endowed with antioxidant properties. The aim of this study was to extract polyphenols from eggplant entire fruit, pulp, or skin, both fresh and dry, and compare results between conventional extraction and microwave-assisted extraction (MAE). The effects of time exposure (15, 30, 60, and 90 min) and solvent (water 100% or ethanol/water 50%) were also evaluated. The highest amount of polyphenols was found in the extract obtained from dry peeled skin treated with 50% aqueous ethanol, irradiated with microwave; this extract contained also high quantity of flavonoids and showed good antioxidant activity expressed by its capacity to scavenge superoxide anion and to inhibit lipid peroxidation.

1. Introduction

Polyphenols have received a great deal of attention in recent years due to their powerful antioxidant properties. Polyphenols are present at high concentrations in a variety of fruits and vegetables. Many studies have demonstrated that consumption of fruits and vegetables rich of polyphenols is related to a reduced risk of coronary heart diseases, neurodegenerative diseases, and certain forms of cancer [1–3].

With the aim of studying vegetables with antioxidant properties, we focused our interest on eggplant (*Solanum melongena* L.). Eggplant is a worldwide diffused vegetable and a common food; the whole eggplant fruit possesses antioxidant activity and is ranked among the top ten vegetables in terms of oxygen radical absorbance capacity [4]. Antioxidant activity of eggplant was tested by different assays [5]. There are several research publications describing phenolic compounds extracted from eggplant and the health benefits associated with their use. Besides antioxidant activity of entire fruit [6], pulp [7], or skin [8, 9], a number of pharmacological properties were reported: hepatoprotective [10], anti-inflammatory [11], hypolipidemic [12], antiallergic [13], and anticancer [14]. Usually, observed activities well correlated with the total phenolic content of the eggplant fruit.

The quantity and quality of phenols present in fruit and vegetables may be significantly influenced by cultivar, environment, soil type, growing, storage conditions, and cooking. Luthria et al. [15] did not observe significant difference in the total phenolic content of eggplant samples grown with organic and conventional farming practices. Scalzo et al. [16] studied changes in antioxidant activity of aqueous eggplant extracts before or after grilling and boiling, concluding that thermal treatment commonly used before consumption of this vegetable can increase the content and biological activity of antioxidant compounds present in eggplants. Moreover, quantity and quality of phenols may depend on extraction procedures. Usually traditional methods, such as solvent extraction, were employed to study the phenolic composition of eggplant [17, 18].

In the recent years, faster and more efficient novel techniques including ultrasound-assisted extraction, microwave-assisted extraction (MAE), supercritical fluid extraction, and accelerated solvent extraction have been developed for the extraction of nutraceuticals from plants and foods [19]. These techniques often shorten the extraction time, decrease the solvent consumption, increase the extraction yields, and enhance the quality of extracts because of reduced risk of degradation of thermolabile constituents. A number of recent reports suggested that extraction of phenolic compounds from various sources and antioxidant capacity could be enhanced via MAE [20–23]. To the best of our knowledge there are no reports on MAE of phenolic compounds from eggplant; the present study was designed to investigate the utility of MAE to extract phenolic antioxidant compounds from eggplant entire fruit, pulp, or skin, both fresh and dry; a comparison was made between conventional extraction and MAE. The effects of time exposure (15, 30, 60, and 90 min) and solvent (water 100% or ethanol/water 50%) were also evaluated. Water and ethanol were chosen as solvents for environmental reasons and possible food application. The extract containing the higher quantity of polyphenols was further analyzed to determine the flavonoid content and antioxidant activity. To this purpose, the ability of this extract to scavenge superoxide anion, to quench a stable radical, and to inhibit *in vitro* lipid peroxidation was evaluated.

2. Materials and Methods

2.1. Materials. Eggplant was purchased from a local distributor. Gallic acid, Folin-Ciocalteu reagent, and nicotinamide-adenine dinucleotide reduced form (NADH), catechin, 1-diphenyl-2-picrylhydrazyl (DPPH), and xylenol orange were purchased from Sigma-Aldrich Co. (St. Louis, MO, USA). All reagents and solvents used were of reagent grade unless otherwise specified.

2.2. Sample Preparation and Extraction Procedures. The fruit was cut into pieces and homogenized (entire eggplant). The peeled skin and pulp were homogenized separately. All the fresh samples were kept at −20°C until use. A number of homogenates were lyophilized to obtain dry samples, which were kept at −20°C until use.

Polyphenolic compounds were extracted from eggplant entire fruit, skin, or pulp (fresh or dry) using a conventional method or a microwave instrument (Focused Microwave Synthesis System CEM Discovery). The extraction variables evaluated were irradiation time (15, 30, 60, and 90 min) and solvent (deionized water 100% and 50% aqueous ethanol). A constant temperature (100°C) and a constant solvent volume of 50 mL for 1.5 g of fresh or dry entire eggplant, pulp, or skin were chosen for the current study. Dry entire eggplant, pulp and skin were obtained by lyophilization from 24, 25, and 20 g of fresh samples, respectively.

2.2.1. Microwave-Assisted Extraction. Microwave irradiation was accomplished with a CEM Discovery instrument and took place in 80 mL closed reactor vessels containing accurately weighed samples. A stir bar was placed in each reactor vessel, which was then inserted into the microwave oven. Conditions within the reaction vessel were power 150 W, pressure 150 Psi, temperature 100°C, run time 2 min, and then the time selected for each experiment (15, 30, 60, and 90 min). After microwave treatment, samples were allowed to cool and then an amount of mixture was transferred to a test tube for centrifugation; the supernatant was used for the total phenols determination.

2.2.2. Conventional Extraction. Fresh or dry entire eggplant, pulp, or skin were suspended in solvent, agitated with stir bar, and then heated in an oil bath with a temperature control system (Heidolph EKT 3001) performed at 100°C for the chosen time. Following treatment, the mixture was cooled and then an amount of mixture was transferred to a test tube for centrifugation; the supernatant was used for determination of total phenols.

2.3. Total Phenols Determination. The concentration of total phenolic content was determined spectrophotometrically, using the Folin-Ciocalteu total phenols procedure, described by Ballard et al. [20], with slight modifications. Gallic acid standard solutions were prepared at 0.0, 0.0125, 0.025, 0.050, 0.100, and 0.150 mg/mL. Test extracts (0.1 mL) appropriately diluted or the gallic acid standards (0.1 mL) were transferred to 15 mL test tubes. Folin-Ciocalteu reagent (0.2 N, 3.0 mL) was added to each test tube and mixed using a vortex mixer. After 1 min, 2.0 mL of 9.0% (w/v) Na_2CO_3 in water was added and the obtained solution was mixed and left at room temperature. After 2 h, absorbance was determined at λ = 765 nm, using a PriXma UV 1200 spectrophotometer. The concentration of total phenolic compounds in the extracts was determined comparing the absorbance of the extract samples to that of the gallic acid standard solutions. All samples were analyzed in triplicate. Total phenolic content (TPC) was expressed as gallic acid equivalents (GAE) in mg per 1.5 g fresh or dry eggplant.

2.4. Total Flavonoid Content. The total flavonoid concentration was measured using a colorimetric assay described by Zhishen et al. [24], with slight modifications. Catechin standard solutions were prepared at 0.0, 0.004, 0.008, 0.016, 0.032, and 0.064 mg/mL. Briefly, 25 μL of the eggplant extract and/or catechin standard solutions was added to a 100 μL of water. At time zero, 7.5 μL of 5% $NaNO_2$ was added; at 5 min, 7.5 μL of 10% $AlCl_3$ was added; at 6 min, 50 μL of 1 M NaOH was added. Each reaction mixture was then immediately diluted with 60 μL of water and mixed. Absorbances of the mixtures upon the development of pink color were determined at λ = 510 nm relative to a prepared blank. The total flavonoid content of the samples is expressed as catechin equivalents (CE) in mg per 1.5 g extract. All samples were determined in triplicate.

2.5. Antioxidant Activities. Based on results regarding polyphenolic and flavonoid content, the extract obtained from dry peeled skin treated with 50% aqueous ethanol solution under microwave-assisted extraction (EPS50MAE) was selected to evaluate antioxidant activities. EPS50MAE was dried on Rotavapor and the dry mass was dissolved in phosphate buffered saline (PBS).

Table 1: Phenolic content of water extracts and 50% aqueous ethanol extracts of fresh and dry entire eggplant, pulp, and skin at 100°C for 15 min, with conventional method or microwave-assisted extraction (MAE). Values are reported in mg gallic acid equivalents ± SD ($n = 3$) on 1.5 g of eggplant.

	Fresh (water)	Fresh (water/ethanol)	Dry (water)	Dry (water/ethanol)
Entire fruit*	0.84 ± 0.03	0.76 ± 0.07	3.51 ± 0.04	6.98 ± 0.01
Entire fruit**	1.07 ± 0.05	1.18 ± 0.08	5.95 ± 0.04	8.04 ± 0.02
Pulp*	0.99 ± 0.07	1.63 ± 0.17	6.74 ± 0.07	8.23 ± 0.16
Pulp**	0.97 ± 0.14	0.84 ± 0.05	7.20 ± 0.06	10.26 ± 0.04
Skin*	2.75 ± 0.02	2.93 ± 0.06	10.17 ± 0.07	14.25 ± 0.06
Skin**	2.82 ± 0.02	2.94 ± 0.03	9.18 ± 0.04	15.05 ± 0.15

*Conventional method. **MAE.

Table 2: Comparison of phenolic content of water extracts and 50% aqueous ethanol extracts of dry entire eggplant and skin at 100°C at variable heating times, with conventional method or microwave-assisted extraction (MAE). Values are reported in mg gallic acid equivalents ± SD ($n = 3$) on 1.5 g of eggplant.

	15 min (water)	30 min (water)	60 min (water)	90 min (water)	90 min (water/ethanol)
Entire fruit*	3.51 ± 0.04	6.66 ± 0.03	10.19 ± 0.06	14.63 ± 1.35	15.35 ± 0.19
Entire fruit**	5.95 ± 0.04	8.38 ± 0.06	21.33 ± 0.05	36.81 ± 0.04	15.19 ± 0.25
Skin*	10.17 ± 0.07	11.85 ± 0.04	21.97 ± 0.50	34.02 ± 0.16	36.13 ± 0.09
Skin**	9.18 ± 0.04	10.82 ± 0.04	18.99 ± 0.14	35.02 ± 0.16	47.09 ± 0.62

*Conventional method. **MAE.

2.5.1. Quenching of DPPH. The free radical scavenging capacity of eggplant extract was tested by its ability to bleach the stable DPPH radical. The reaction mixture contained 86 μM DPPH and different amounts of EPS50MAE in a total volume of 1 mL of ethanol to obtain concentrations of EPS50MAE ranging from 8.75 to 875 μg/mL. After 10 min at room temperature the absorbance at $\lambda = 517$ nm was recorded. Results are expressed as percentage decrease in absorbance with respect to control. Trolox (30 μM), a water-soluble derivative of vitamin E, was used as standard; it had a quenching activity of 100%.

2.5.2. Scavenger Effect on Superoxide Anion. Superoxide anion was generated *in vitro* as reported by Acquaviva et al. [25]. The assay mixture contained in a total volume of 1 mL : 100 mM triethanolamine-diethanolamine buffer, pH 7.4, 3 mM NADH, 25 mM/12.5 mM ethylene diamine tetra-acetic acid (EDTA)/$MnCl_2$, and 10 mM β-mercaptoethanol; some samples contained EPS50MAE at different concentrations of (875–8.75 μg/mL). After 20 min incubation at 25°C, the decrease in absorbance was measured at $\lambda = 340$ nm. Results are expressed as percentage of inhibition of NADH oxidation with respect to control. Superoxide dismutase (SOD) 80 mU/mL was used as standard; it had a scavenging activity of 100%.

2.5.3. Determination of Lipid Hydroperoxide Levels in the Plasma of a Healthy Donor. Plasmatic lipid hydroperoxide levels were evaluated by oxidation of Fe^{2+} to Fe^{3+} in the presence of xylenol orange (FOX assay) at $\lambda = 560$ nm [26]. Heparinized venous blood was collected after overnight fasting; plasma was separated by centrifugation at 800 g for 20 min. Plasma aliquots (500 μL) were diluted 1 : 1 with oxygenated PBS and incubated at 37°C for 2 h with or without different concentrations of EPS50MAE (875–8.75 μg/mL) in a total volume of 1 mL. Calibration was obtained using hydrogen peroxide (0.2–20 μM). Results are expressed as percentage of inhibition with respect to control (plasma incubated in absence of test compounds).

2.5.4. Statistical Analyses. The data are presented as means ± SD for 4 experiments in triplicate. One-way variance analysis and Student's t-test were used where appropriate; $P < 0.05$ was regarded as significant.

3. Results and Discussion

3.1. Polyphenolic and Flavonoid Content. It is known that numerous fruits and vegetables contain high amount of polyphenols which can be beneficial for human health [27]. Eggplant is listed among the top ten vegetables in terms of oxygen radical absorbance capacity [4]. In addition, this plant is consumed throughout the world and it is endowed with many potential pharmacological properties [7, 9–14]. As first aim, in this research we wanted to determine the amount of polyphenolic compounds in various parts of the vegetable (skin, pulp, or entire fruit) and to compare the effect of MAE with a conventional method. Results are summarized in Tables 1 and 2 and are expressed as mg gallic acid equivalents on 1.5 g of eggplant. Firstly we determined the content of polyphenolic compounds on samples of both fresh and dry entire fruit, pulp, and skin, using both water and 50% aqueous ethanol as solvents, at 100°C for a fixed time of 15 min (Table 1). Methanol or other organic extraction solvents, instead of ethanol, often used for the extraction of polyphenols from plants and food [10], were avoided for their

TABLE 3: DPPH radical, superoxide anion scavenging activity, and inhibition of lipid peroxidation by different concentrations of EPS50MAE. Each value represents the mean ± SD of 4 experiments in triplicate.

	DPPH radical scavenging activity	Superoxide anion scavenging activity	Inhibition of lipid peroxidation
875 μg/mL	30%	100%	40%
435 μg/mL	12%	100%	20%
175 μg/mL	8%	100%	10%
87.5 μg/mL	0%	84%	0%
43.5 μg/mL	0%	80%	0%
17.5 μg/mL	0%	52%	0%
8.75 μg/mL	0%	30%	0%
IC_{50} (μg/mL)	>875 μg/mL	17 ± 0.3 μg/mL*	>875 μg/mL

Values had a standard deviation of ≤10%. $^*P < 0.001$ versus the other tests we evaluated.

toxicity that would not allow the use of these data for food application. Among the various parts of eggplant examined, peeled skin contains the major amount of polyphenolic compounds with respect to entire fruit and pulp, both in fresh and dry samples. These results suggest the use of skin, waste production of eggplants, as source of polyphenols for nutraceutical extraction; in addition, content of polyphenols in dry samples is greater than that in fresh, but not proportional to the amount of starting fresh materials used. This is probably due to the matrix of the dry samples that does not permit an extraction similar to that of the fresh. However, comparison of the results in fresh and dry eggplant suggests consumption of entire fresh fruit for beneficial salutary effects since the quantity of polyphenols present is sufficient to contribute to the daily intake of bioflavonoids [28]. The effects of various investigated parameters (microwave irradiation and solvents), were different if we compare fresh with dry materials. Usually, microwave irradiation with respect to conventional method and solvent composition (50% aqueous ethanol with respect to 100% water), significantly increase the polyphenol extraction for dry materials in all examined samples, entire fruit, pulp and skin. On the contrary, generally both parameters do not influence polyphenols extraction for fresh materials. In a next step we compared the content of polyphenolic compounds in samples of dry entire fruit or skin at different heating times (15, 30, 60 and 90 min) using 100% water. Results, showed in Table 2, demonstrate that heating time increases the yield of polyphenolic compounds and microwave irradiation positively affects this yield on entire plant, but not on skin. Finally, we tested the effect of the employment of the use of 50% aqueous ethanol solution to determine the quantity of polyphenols in dry entire fruits and skin maintained at 100 °C for 90 min, with conventional and microwave irradiation; water/ethanol showed to be very effective solvent particularly on skin treated with microwave irradiation. Consequently, the extract obtained from dry peeled skin treated with 50% aqueous ethanol solution under microwave-assisted extraction for 90 min (EPS50MAE) was selected for further analyses. In this extract the content of flavonoid compounds was also determined. Results demonstrate that EPS50MAE contained 13.5 mg CE/1.5 g extract which well correlated with the amount of total phenolic compounds.

3.2. Antioxidant Activities. Antioxidant activity of EPS50MAE in this study was assessed by the use of three tests: (i) *in vitro* quenching of DPPH radical, (ii) *in vitro* scavenger effect on superoxide anion, and (iii) "*ex vivo cell-free system*" to evaluate lipid peroxidation inhibitory activity.

Free radical species such as superoxide and hydrogen peroxide have both been implicated in several diseases such as atherosclerosis, chronic inflammation, and cancer. In particular, it is now recognized that the extremely reactive hydroxyl radical ($^{\bullet}OH$) derived from O_2^{-} and H_2O_2 causes DNA strand scission in cellular damage [29]. The importance of removing active oxygen species from living organisms is becoming clear, while there is growing interest in the protective mechanisms whereby antioxidants that scavenge reactive oxygen species (ROS) may have a potential therapeutic use [30].

The free radical scavenging activity of EPS50MAE was tested by its ability to bleach the stable DPPH radical [25]. This assay provides information on the reactivity of test sample with a stable free radical. Because of its odd electron, DPPH gives a strong absorption band at 517 nm in visible spectroscopy (deep violet color). As this electron becomes paired off in the presence of a free radical scavenger, the absorption vanishes, and the resulting decolorization is stoichiometric with respect to the number of electrons taken up. In this assay, this extract did not show a significant DPPH quenching capacity, probably due to the large size and high stability of this radical. In addition it was not possible to test higher concentrations because the reaction mixture became opalescent.

Since the antioxidant effects of polyphenols could be due both to their free radical scavenging and/or chelating activities, to investigate the superoxide anion scavenging capacity of the extract, we used a method which excludes the Fenton-type reaction and the xanthine/xanthine oxidase system. Results reported in Table 3 are expressed as IC_{50} (μg/mL) which represents the concentration of EPS50MAE required to scavenge 50% superoxide anion formation. EPS50MAE inhibited superoxide anion formation in a dose-dependent manner with IC_{50} value of 17 ± 0.3 μg/mL; this last result would suggest that components of the extract are able to scavenge the small free radical superoxide anion and then contribute to antioxidant activity of EPS50MAE.

There is growing evidence that oxidative stress may represent one of the agents involved in the initiation and/or progression of many human diseases including atherosclerosis, postischemic reperfusion injury, inflammation, aging, and neurodegenerative pathologies (Parkinson's and Alzheimer's diseases). In addition, several experimental results link the overproduction of ROS to biological damage. ROS, in fact, are able to chemically alter virtually all the major classes of biomolecules (proteins, nucleic acids, and lipids). Like other aerobic organisms, humans have evolved a variety of mechanisms to protect themselves from the potentially deleterious effects of ROS; nevertheless, oxidative stress occurs when the generation of free radicals exceeds the capacity of a cell to defend or repair itself.

Since *in vitro* studies have shown that phenolic compounds may prevent lipid peroxidation and formation of atherosclerotic plaques [31, 32], in this study the antioxidant activity of EPS50MAE was also evaluated by measuring antilipoperoxidative capacity in human plasma incubated with or without extract for 2 h at 37°C. Results of this study showed that the addition of EPS50MAE determined an inhibition of lipid peroxidation (Table 3) even though this effect was moderate with respect to superoxide anion scavenging activity. The ability of EPS50MAE to counteract *in vitro* plasmatic lipid peroxidation may contribute to prevention of the formation of atherosclerotic plaques and subsequent cardiovascular diseases.

4. Conclusions

Antioxidant activity of polyphenols may have health-promoting and disease-preventing effects. Consequently, consumption of eggplant, which contains polyphenols, or extracts of polyphenols from eggplant, may have a potential therapeutic use. Our study confirms that polyphenols are present in various parts of eggplant, in particular skin, suggesting the use of the entire vegetable as food; MAE may be an attractive alternative to conventional method to improve the amount of polyphenols extracted, in particular for nutraceutical application. Extraction of skin with 50% aqueous ethanol with microwave irradiation was particularly effective. In addition, our study provides evidence that EPS50MAE exhibits interesting antioxidant properties, expressed by its capacity to scavenge superoxide anion and to inhibit lipid peroxidation.

Conflict of Interests

The authors declare that there is no conflict of interests regarding the publication of this paper.

Acknowledgments

This work was supported by grants from the Italian MIUR and the University of Catania.

References

[1] B. Halliwell, "Free radicals, antioxidants, and human disease: curiosity, cause, or consequence?" *The Lancet*, vol. 344, no. 8924, pp. 721–724, 1994.

[2] M. T. Huang and T. Ferraro, "Phenolic compounds in food and cancer prevention," in *Phenolic Compounds in Food and their Effects on Health. II. Antioxidants and Cancer Prevention*, pp. 8–34, American Chemical Society, Washington, DC, USA, 1992.

[3] H.-C. Hung, K. J. Joshipura, R. Jiang et al., "Fruit and vegetable intake and risk of major chronic disease," *Journal of the National Cancer Institute*, vol. 96, no. 21, pp. 1577–1584, 2004.

[4] G. Cao, E. Sofic, and R. L. Prior, "Antioxidant capacity of tea and common vegetables," *Journal of Agricultural and Food Chemistry*, vol. 44, no. 11, pp. 3426–3431, 1996.

[5] H.-Y. Huang, C.-K. Chang, T. K. Tso, J.-J. Huang, W.-W. Chang, and Y.-C. Tsai, "Antioxidant activities of various fruits and vegetables produced in Taiwan," *International Journal of Food Sciences and Nutrition*, vol. 55, no. 5, pp. 423–429, 2004.

[6] P. M. Hanson, R.-Y. Yang, S. C. S. Tsou, D. Ledesma, L. Engle, and T.-C. Lee, "Diversity in eggplant (*Solanum melongena*) for superoxide scavenging activity, total phenolics, and ascorbic acid," *Journal of Food Composition and Analysis*, vol. 19, no. 6-7, pp. 594–600, 2006.

[7] A. P. Singh, D. Luthria, T. Wilson et al., "Polyphenols content and antioxidant capacity of eggplant pulp," *Food Chemistry*, vol. 114, no. 3, pp. 955–961, 2009.

[8] Y. Noda, T. Kneyuki, K. Igarashi, A. Mori, and L. Packer, "Antioxidant activity of nasunin, an anthocyanin in eggplant peels," *Toxicology*, vol. 148, no. 2-3, pp. 119–123, 2000.

[9] L. Azevedo, P. L. A. de Lima, J. C. Gomes, P. C. Stringheta, D. A. Ribeiro, and D. M. F. Salvadori, "Differential response related to genotoxicity between eggplant (*Solanum melanogena*) skin aqueous extract and its main purified anthocyanin (delphinidin) *in vivo*," *Food and Chemical Toxicology*, vol. 45, no. 5, pp. 852–858, 2007.

[10] P. Akanitapichat, K. Phraibung, K. Nuchklang, and S. Prompitakkul, "Antioxidant and hepatoprotective activities of five eggplant varieties," *Food and Chemical Toxicology*, vol. 48, no. 10, pp. 3017–3021, 2010.

[11] S.-W. Han, J. Tae, J.-A. Kim et al., "The aqueous extract of *Solanum melongena* inhibits PAR2 agonist-induced inflammation," *Clinica Chimica Acta*, vol. 328, no. 1-2, pp. 39–44, 2003.

[12] S. Sudheesh, G. Presannakumar, S. Vijayakumar, and N. R. Vijayalakshmi, "Hypolipidemic effect of flavonoids from *Solanum melongena*," *Plant Foods for Human Nutrition*, vol. 51, no. 4, pp. 321–330, 1997.

[13] Y.-M. Lee, H.-J. Jeong, H.-J. Na et al., "Inhibition of immunologic and nonimmunologic stimulation-mediated anaphylactic reactions by water extract of white eggplant (*Solanum melongena*)," *Pharmacological Research*, vol. 43, no. 4, pp. 405–409, 2001.

[14] K. Matsubara, T. Kaneyuki, T. Miyake, and M. Mori, "Antiangiogenic activity of nasunin, an antioxidant anthocyanin, in eggplant peels," *Journal of Agricultural and Food Chemistry*, vol. 53, no. 16, pp. 6272–6275, 2005.

[15] D. Luthria, A. P. Singh, T. Wilson, N. Vorsa, G. S. Banuelos, and B. T. Vinyard, "Influence of conventional and organic agricultural practices on the phenolic content in eggplant pulp: plant-to-plant variation," *Food Chemistry*, vol. 121, no. 2, pp. 406–411, 2010.

[16] R. L. Scalzo, M. Fibiani, G. Mennella et al., "Thermal treatment of eggplant (*Solanum melongena* L.) increases the antioxidant content and the inhibitory effect on human neutrophil burst," *Journal of Agricultural and Food Chemistry*, vol. 58, no. 6, pp. 3371–3379, 2010.

[17] T. Ichiyanagi, Y. Kashiwada, Y. Shida, Y. Ikeshiro, T. Kaneyuki, and T. Konishi, "Nasunin from eggplant consists of cis-trans isomers of delphinidin 3-[4-(*p*-coumaroyl)-L-rhamnosyl (1 → 6)glucopyranoside]-5-glucopyranoside," *Journal of Agricultural and Food Chemistry*, vol. 53, no. 24, pp. 9472–9477, 2005.

[18] K. Helmja, M. Vaher, T. Püssa, and M. Kaljurand, "Analysis of the stable free radical scavenging capability of artificial polyphenol mixtures and plant extracts by capillary electrophoresis and liquid chromatography-diode array detection-tandem mass spectrometry," *Journal of Chromatography A*, vol. 1216, no. 12, pp. 2417–2423, 2009.

[19] L. Wang and C. L. Weller, "Recent advances in extraction of nutraceuticals from plants," *Trends in Food Science and Technology*, vol. 17, no. 6, pp. 300–312, 2006.

[20] T. S. Ballard, P. Mallikarjunan, K. Zhou, and S. O'Keefe, "Microwave-assisted extraction of phenolic antioxidant compounds from peanut skins," *Food Chemistry*, vol. 120, no. 4, pp. 1185–1192, 2010.

[21] G. E. Inglett, D. J. Rose, D. Chen, D. G. Stevenson, and A. Biswas, "Phenolic content and antioxidant activity of extracts from whole buckwheat (*Fagopyrum esculentum* Möench) with or without microwave irradiation," *Food Chemistry*, vol. 119, no. 3, pp. 1216–1219, 2010.

[22] N. Sutivisedsak, H. N. Cheng, J. L. Willett, W. C. Lesch, R. R. Tangsrud, and A. Biswas, "Microwave-assisted extraction of phenolics from bean (*Phaseolus vulgaris* L.)," *Food Research International*, vol. 43, no. 2, pp. 516–519, 2010.

[23] E. Nkhili, V. Tomao, H. El Hajji, E.-S. El Boustani, F. Chemat, and O. Dangles, "Microwave-assisted water extraction of green tea polyphenols," *Phytochemical Analysis*, vol. 20, no. 5, pp. 408–415, 2009.

[24] J. Zhishen, T. Mengcheng, and W. Jianming, "The determination of flavonoid contents in mulberry and their scavenging effects on superoxide radicals," *Food Chemistry*, vol. 64, no. 4, pp. 555–559, 1999.

[25] R. Acquaviva, A. Russo, A. Campisi et al., "Antioxidant activity and protective effect on DNA cleavage of resveratrol," *Journal of Food Science*, vol. 67, no. 1, pp. 137–141, 2002.

[26] L. Salerno, M. N. Modica, G. Romeo et al., "Novel inhibitors of nitric oxide synthase with antioxidant properties," *European Journal of Medicinal Chemistry*, vol. 49, pp. 118–126, 2012.

[27] C. S. Yang, J. M. Landau, M.-T. Huang, and H. L. Newmark, "Inhibition of carcinogenesis by dietary polyphenolic compounds," *Annual Review of Nutrition*, vol. 21, pp. 381–406, 2001.

[28] M. Yoshizumi, K. Tsuchiya, K. Kirima, M. Kyaw, Y. Suzaki, and T. Tamaki, "Quercetin inhibits Shc- and phosphatidylinositol 3-kinase-mediated c-Jun N-terminal kinase activation by angiotensin II in cultured rat aortic smooth muscle cells," *Molecular Pharmacology*, vol. 60, no. 4, pp. 656–665, 2001.

[29] B. Halliwell and J. M. C. Gutteridge, "Role of free radicals and catalytic metal ions in human disease: an overview," *Methods in Enzymology*, vol. 186, pp. 1–85, 1990.

[30] C. A. Rice-Evans, N. J. Miller, and G. Paganga, "Structure-antioxidant activity relationships of flavonoids and phenolic acids," *Free Radical Biology and Medicine*, vol. 20, no. 7, pp. 933–956, 1996.

[31] T. Tsuda, F. Horio, J. Kitoh, and T. Osawa, "Protective effects of dietary cyanidin 3-*O*-β-D-glucoside on liver ischemia-reperfusion injury in rats," *Archives of Biochemistry and Biophysics*, vol. 368, no. 2, pp. 361–366, 1999.

[32] P. C. Hollman, M. N. Bijsman, Y. van Gameren, E. P. Cnossen, J. H. de Vries, and M. B. Katan, "The sugar moiety is a major determinant of the absorption of dietary flavonoid glycosides in man," *Free Radical Research*, vol. 31, no. 6, pp. 569–573, 1999.

25

Effect of Storage on the Physicochemical and Flavour Attributes of Two Cultivars of Strawberry Cultivated in Northern India

Rachna Mishra and Abhijit Kar

Division of Post Harvest Technology, Indian Agricultural Research Institute, Pusa Campus, New Delhi 110 012, India

Correspondence should be addressed to Abhijit Kar; abhijit8366@gmail.com

Academic Editors: K. Ebihara, A. Ferrante, and A. Turrini

An attempt was made to understand the changes in physicochemical quality (total soluble solids, titratable acidity, ascorbic acid, total sugars, total phenolics, anthocyanin content, and cupric reducing antioxidant capacity assay) and total volatile/aroma compounds of two cultivars of strawberry (Camarosa and Chandler) during storage at 5°C for 9 days at an interval of three days. Observations indicated a significant quantitative difference both in the physicochemical and in total volatile content among the cultivars indicating the importance of cultivar for determining the postharvest quality and shelf life. At the end of 9 days of storage significant changes in the physicochemical and total volatile/aroma compounds were observed. Total antioxidants and total phenols were found to increase significantly, whereas total soluble solids and total sugars decreased with the advent of storage period for both cultivars. Total anthocyanin contents however remained almost constant throughout the storage period. Titratable acidity in Camarosa reduced with the increase in the storage period whereas it remained almost constant in Chandler. Ascorbic acid increased in Camarosa whereas the same decreased significantly in Chandler. Significantly higher contents of esters and terpenoids in Camarosa indicated a better retention of the typical fruits flavour of strawberry compared to that of Chandler.

1. Introduction

Intake of fresh fruits and vegetables helps in preventing a number of chronic diseases like cancer and cardiovascular diseases [1]. Increased consumer demand for high quality fruit having attractive appearance, high nutritional value, and good taste combined with the reported health benefits from biologically active components like antioxidants and phenolics [2] has enabled enhanced attention among the researchers for the retention of the quality (both physicochemical and flavour) of the fresh fruits.

Strawberry (*Fragaria x ananassa* Duch.) is one of the most popular, nutritious fruits among all the berries and is cultivated in almost all countries of the world. It has a delicious taste and unique flavor widely accepted and consumed in fresh or processed form. Aroma in strawberry mainly constitutes a complex mixture of esters, aldehydes, alcohols, and sulfur compounds. Among the hundreds of volatiles identified in strawberry, esters are known to be the most important contributors to its typical fruity flavor. Differences in strawberry aroma compounds among cultivars have been reported by several authors [3, 4]. In addition to its attractive flavour strawberry has an extremely attractive bright red appearance because of anthocyanins. The anthocyanin found predominantly constitutes pelargonidin 3-glucoside. The other minor ones include cyanidin 3-glucoside and pelargonidin 3-rutinoside [5]. In addition to its flavouring compounds and anthocyanins, strawberry is also found to be rich in antioxidant [6, 7], flavonols [6], phenolic compounds [8], and ascorbic acid [9].

Strawberries are highly perishable having a very limited shelf life [10]. Low temperature storage helps in extending the shelf life to some extent [11]. In fact several studies have been aimed in the past toward the extension of the shelf life of strawberry [3, 5]. Most of the biochemical constituents such as anthocyanins, vitamin C, antioxidant, total phenolics, and flavour are greatly affected by the cultivar, stage of harvest, and the postharvest storage conditions.

Strawberry is an important fruit with respect to its nutritional content as well as its flavour. Flavor of strawberry is considered to be an important aspect of its quality. Although difficult to define, qualify, and quantify, this elusive and complex trait is important to consumers and deserves adequate attention. Flavor quality of strawberry is an important factor in an increasingly competitive global market. Flavor maintenance becomes a challenge to maintain as shelf life and marketing distances increase due to new storage, handling, and transport technologies.

Flavor and aroma are perhaps the most elusive and subjective quality traits. Flavor mainly constitutes a combination of sweetness and sourness, whereas aroma represents the mixture of sugars, acids, and volatiles. Volatile biosynthesis and its contribution to fruit eating quality are very complex, and are influenced by many factors, such as cultivar, harvest maturity, postharvest handling, and storage [12, 13].

Measurement of aroma compounds is difficult and time consuming. The disadvantage of classical flavor isolation procedures of steam distillation and/or solvent extraction is that it could qualitatively and quantitatively modify the flavor profile of a sample. Static headspace methods have replaced the traditional technique as it is said to more closely reflect the true flavor profile, but compounds which are present at low levels may not be detected at all. Therefore, solid phase microextraction (SPME) which is a rapid sampling technique, where volatiles interact with a fiber-coated probe inserted into the sample headspace, has been developed and widely adopted.

Hence, an attempt was made to study a quantitative analysis of physicochemical parameters (total soluble solids, titratable acidity, ascorbic acid, total sugars, total phenolics, anthocyanin content, and cupric reducing antioxidant capacity assay) and total volatile/aroma compounds of two predominantly grown cultivars of strawberries (Camarosa and Chandler) in order to understand the qualitative changes during its storage at 5°C. These two varieties were selected since they are predominately cultivated in India.

2. Materials and Methods

2.1. Material. About 30 kg of strawberries fruits of each of the varieties (Cv. Camarosa and Chandler) of uniform size and colour were freshly harvested from a private farmer's field, washed thoroughly to remove any extraneous material, surface-dried using blotting paper, divided into three lots per variety, and were stored at 5 ± 1°C and 85 ± 5% relative humidity. Fruits were evaluated for physicochemical and volatile content at the beginning and subsequently at three-day intervals up to the 9th day. All analyses were performed in triplicate and results were expressed as fresh weight (f.w.) basis.

2.2. Total Soluble Solids (TSS) and Titratable Acidity (TA) Determinations. TSS was analyzed with the help of a hand held digital refractometer whereas TA was determined by titration method using 0.1 N NaOH and phenolphthalein as an indicator [14].

2.3. Ascorbic Acid (AA) and Total Sugar Determination. 2 g of crushed sample was extracted with metaphosphoric acid (3%) and the total AA was determined by titrating a known weight of sample against 2,6-dichlorophenol-indophenol dye [14]. Result was expressed in mg/100 g of fresh fruit. Total sugar was determined by using Lane and Eynon method [14].

2.4. Determination of Total Phenols. Total phenols were quantified using 1 g homogenate (pulp homogenized in a blender) using the method described by Singleton et al. [15]. Total phenol was extracted in methanol (80%) and left for 2 hrs. The extract was centrifuged at 10,000 rpm for 15 min. About 0.1 mL of the supernatant was mixed with 2 mL of saturated sodium carbonate, 0.5 mL of Folin-Ciocalteu reagent, and 2.9 mL of distilled water and incubated at 27°C for 1 hr and the absorbance read at 765 nm using a spectrophotometer. Total phenolic content was expressed as gallic acid equivalents in mg/100 g fresh weight.

2.5. Total Anthocyanins Content. Total anthocyanin contents were determined using pH differential spectrophotometric (absorbance at 520 and 700 nm) method [16] and expressed as milligram pelargonidin-3-glucoside (molar extinction coefficient of 22,400 and molecular weight of 433.2 g/mol) per 100 g fresh weight.

2.6. Cupric Reducing Antioxidant Capacity (CUPRAC) Assay. CUPRAC assay was done by the method developed by Apak et al. [17]. To 100 μL of sample aliquot, 1 mL each of copper (II) chloride solution (10^{-2} M), neocuproine solution (7.5×10^{-3} M), and ammonium acetate buffer solution (pH 7) solution were mixed. The tubes were stoppered and, after 1 h, absorbance at 450 nm was recorded against a reagent blank. Results were expressed as μmol TE/g.

2.7. Analysis of Aroma Compounds/Volatiles. Headspace sampling method was adopted using a 100 μm fused-silica fibre coated with polydimethylsiloxane (PDMS) (Supelco, Bellefonte, PA, USA). 5 g of the homogenized fruit pulp was taken in a 20 mL vial and subjected to GC-MS analysis. Sample was first equilibrated for 10 min at 38°C and maintained at 38°C throughout the 30 min assay. After 30 min of extraction the SPME syringe was introduced into the injector port at a temperature of 240°C using splitless injection for further analysis. Volatile compounds were analysed using a Varian 450-GC/240-MS apparatus equipped with a VF-5 ms (30 m $\times$ 0.25 mm $\times$ 0.25 μm) fused-silica capillary column. Helium (1 mL/min) was used as a carrier gas. The oven operated at the following ramp rates: 40°C–120°C at 6°C/min; 70°C–170°C at 4°C/min; and 180°C–240°C at 6°C/min. Thermal desorption was subsequently allowed for 15 min. The transfer line and ion source temperatures were maintained at 280°C and 180°C, respectively. The energy of electron was 70 eV and ion mass/charge ratio 20–450 m/z under full scan mode. The components were identified by comparison of mass spectra and retention time data with Wiley and NIST library and authentic standards. Quantification was achieved by using 3-chlorophenol as an internal standard.

2.8. Statistical Analysis. Experiments were performed according to completely randomized design having three replications. Two factor Analysis of Variance (ANOVA) with cultivar and time as factors was performed using PROC GLM

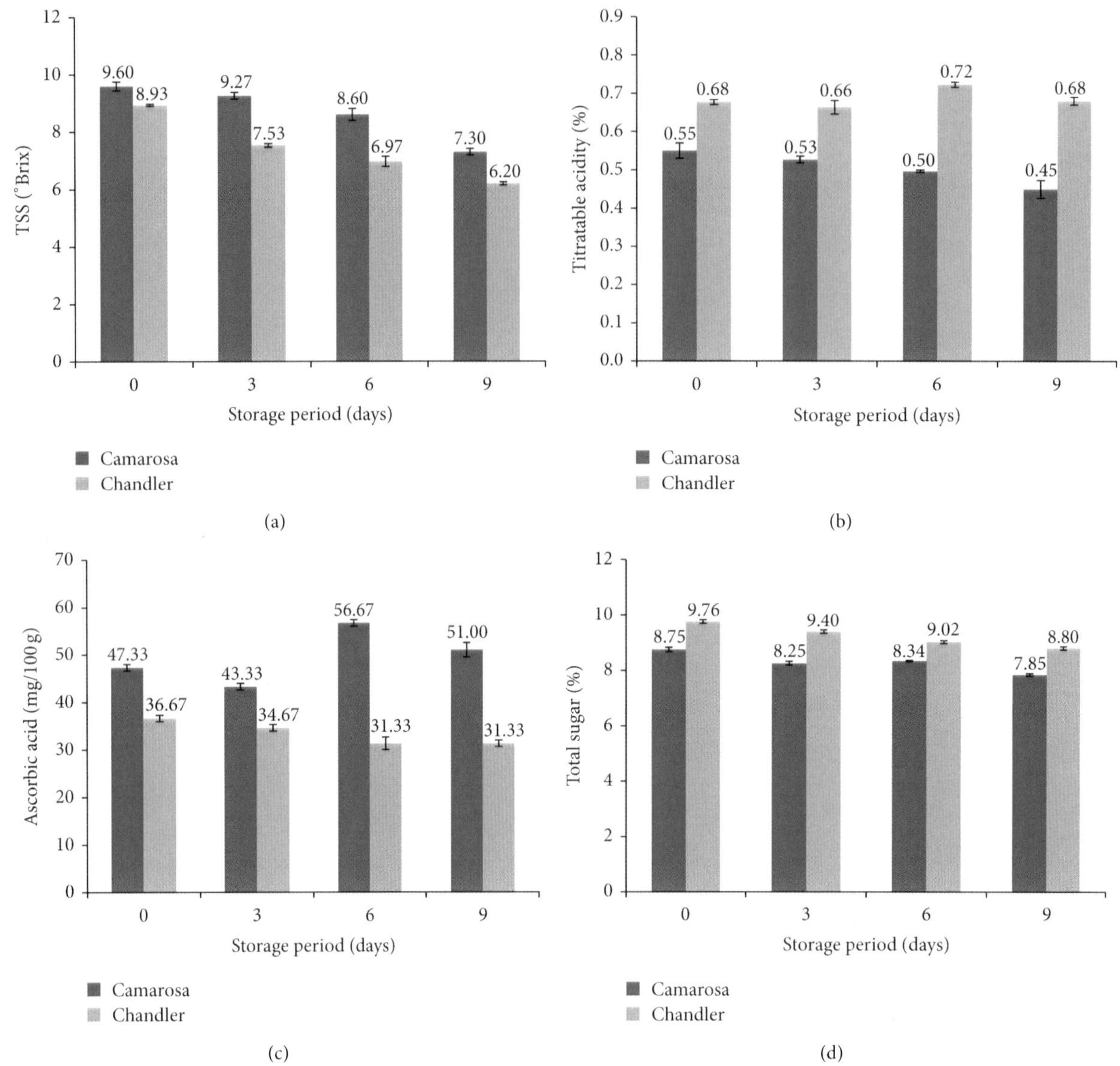

FIGURE 1: Changes in physicochemical parameters of strawberries during storage at 5°C (a) TSS, (b) titratable acidity, (c) ascorbic acid, and (d) total sugar.

of SAS to understand the effect of time period and variety on the fruit quality (TSS, Titratable Acidity, Ascorbic Acid, Total Sugar, Total Phenolics, Total Anthocyanin, Antioxidant Capacity, and Volatiles).

3. Results and Discussion

3.1. TSS, TA, AA, and Total Sugar. TSS for both cultivars decreased with the increase in the storage period (Figure 1(a)). Both varieties were found to be significantly different in their TSS contents. For both varieties, storage period was found to have a significant effect on the TSS content. The decrease in the TSS content after nine days of storage was more for Chandler (about 30%) in comparison to Camarosa (about 24%). The significant loss suggests decrease in total sugars and may be attributed to the enhanced respiration rate of the fruits during storage. Similar results have been reported by Gil et al. [5] and Pelayo et al. [3].

TA has been expressed in terms of percentage citric acid since citric acid constitutes a major chunk of the acids in strawberry [3, 18]. TA in case of Camarosa decreased with the advent of the storage period (Figure 1(b)). Pelayo et al. [3] also reported similar results in three different strawberry cultivars. However, it remained almost constant even at the end of 9th day of storage in case of Chandler. TA of both cultivars was found to be significantly different from each other. Chandler variety showed a significantly higher TA content compared to Camarosa throughout the storage period.

Ascorbic acid, a predominant form of vitamin C, is known to be highly unstable. Temperature is reported to have a significant effect on the ascorbic acid retention. The AA content reduced with the increase in the storage period for Chandler

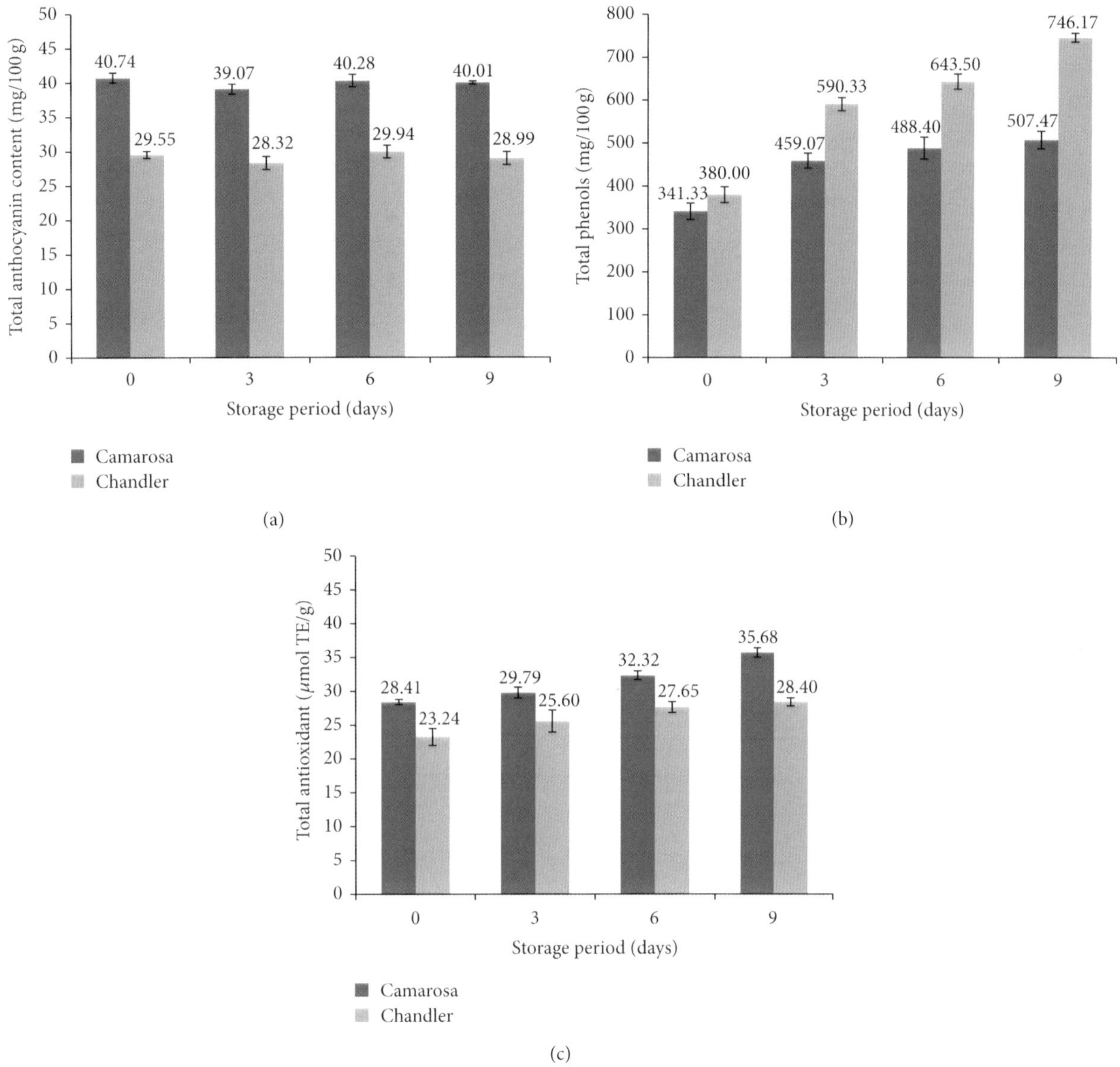

FIGURE 2: Changes in (a) total anthocyanin content, (b) total phenols, and (c) Total antioxidants of strawberry (Camarosa and Chandler) during storage at 5°C.

which could be attributed to the activity of ascorbate oxidase which promotes ascorbic acid to dehydroascorbic acid [19]. The decrease was about 15% (Figure 1(c)). On the other hand, the AA content fluctuated quite a bit with the storage period in case of Camarosa. However, the total AA content increased at the end of 9 days of storage indicating synthesis of ascorbic acid during storage as reported by Cordenunsi et al. [20].

High sugar and high acid content are the known precursors of good strawberry flavor. Total sugar content also followed a trend similar to that of TSS. However, at the end of the nine-day storage period, both cultivars have almost similar total sugar loss (Figure 1(d)). In this case also ANOVA indicated a significant effect of both storage period and variety. The loss in sugars can be mostly explained by the hydrolysis of sucrose and the utilization of the corresponding reducing sugars in the fruit respiration since strawberry does not have much starch to support total sugar synthesis after harvest. Castro et al. [21] also reported loss of total sugar in strawberries during storage.

3.2. Total Anthocyanin, Total Phenols, and CUPRAC Assay. Pelargonidin-3-glucoside is the most prevalent anthocyanin pigment which is responsible for red color of strawberry. Camarosa and Chandler were found to have significantly different total anthocyanin contents (Figure 2(a)) which can be mainly attributed to the varietal characteristics. ANOVA indicated a nonsignificant effect of storage period on the total anthocyanin content for both cultivars which indicates that the colour of fruits of both varieties was retained at the end of 9 days of storage. Kalt and McDonald [22] have reported an increase in the anthocyanin content of strawberry during storage whereas Ayala-Zavala et al. [23] reported a decrease in anthocyanin content when the strawberries were stored at 5°C. The biosynthetic pathway for the anthocyanin is

Table 1: Identified aroma compounds by SPME method in both cultivars of strawberry stored at 5°C.

Compound	Relative concentration of aroma volatiles (%)							
	Camarosa				Chandler			
	Days of storage				Days of storage			
	0	3	6	9	0	3	6	9
Esters								
Methyl butanoate	0.070	0.079	0.079	0.089	0.039	0.036	0.034	0.031
Ethyl butanoate	0.060	0.159	0.256	0.327	0.075	0.098	0.289	0.292
Hexyl butanoate	0.350	0.328	0.292	0.246	0.270	0.301	0.376	0.375
Methyl hexanoate	9.360	8.276	5.432	4.488	0.007	0.189	0.400	0.505
Ethyl hexanoate	2.701	2.692	2.802	3.658	0.024	0.021	0.179	0.272
Hexyl hexanoate	0.157	0.181	0.196	0.162	1.050	1.053	0.848	0.898
Propyl hexanoate	0.222	0.202	0.238	0.246	1.042	0.876	0.645	nd
Methyl octanoate	0.232	0.243	0.230	0.247	0.033	1.761	5.238	8.254
Benzyl acetate	0.380	0.321	0.142	0.061	0.055	0.796	0.621	0.898
n-Octyl acetate	0.926	0.869	0.421	0.559	0.100	0.098	0.231	0.243
n-Octyl butyrate	0.480	0.431	0.334	0.392	1.143	1.013	0.901	0.915
(2Z)-2-Hexenyl butyrate	0.410	0.376	0.319	0.208	0.190	0.178	0.191	0.170
Terpenoids								
Linalool	0.611	0.602	0.592	0.569	0.426	0.536	0.839	1.704
α-Terpineol	0.197	0.182	0.170	0.132	nd	nd	nd	nd
α-Terpinene	0.024	0.029	0.041	0.062	0.029	0.023	0.017	0.025
Nerolidol	19.836	19.129	17.281	11.717	1.653	1.532	0.989	1.173
Alcohols and aldehydes								
1-Nonanol	0.403	0.482	0.768	1.050	0.029	0.018	0.023	0.187
2-Hexen-1-ol, (z)	2.006	2.004	2.121	2.836	1.042	1.041	1.079	1.488
2-Hexenal, (E)	0.031	0.025	0.032	0.036	0.021	0.019	0.017	0.020
2-Hexyl-1-octanol	0.145	0.018	0.075	0.082	0.170	0.009	nd	nd
Furanones								
2,5-Dimethyl-4-hydroxy-3(2H)-furanone	0.278	0.243	0.412	0.267	0.013	0.013	0.06	nd
Mesifurane	0.232	0.232	0.208	0.222	nd	nd	nd	nd
Others								
α-Farnesene	0.470	0.462	0.436	0.530	0.018	0.111	0.271	0.363
Dodecalactone	0.530	0.531	0.438	0.506	nd	nd	nd	nd

known to be uninhibited by storage at low temperatures [22]. However, in the varieties under consideration in this study the pathway seems to have been sufficiently inhibited so as not to inflict any changes in the total anthocyanin content even after 9 days of storage.

The initial total phenol content of both varieties was slightly different from each other but was not found to be significantly different from each other (Figure 2(b)). However, the difference becomes statistically significant all the subsequent period of storage under consideration. A remarkable increase in the total phenols was observed in both cultivars which may be attributed to the hydrolysis of the tannins which are reported to be dominant in strawberries [24].

Antioxidant activity of fruit can be estimated using ferric reducing antioxidant power (FRAP), oxygen radical absorbance capacity (ORAC), or cupric reducing antioxidant capacity (CUPRAC) assay. CUPRAC assay for the estimation of antioxidant capacity was adopted for this study because of its distinctive documented advantages like simplicity, clarity of endpoint, readily available instrumentation, good intra- and interassay reproducibility, and high throughout for routine analysis by Prior et al. [25]. Variety as well as storage period had a significant effect on the antioxidant activity exhibited by CUPRAC assay. The antioxidant activity increased with the increase in the storage period for both varieties. However, the increase was higher in Camarosa for each difference in time periods than that of Chandler (Figure 2(c)). The results are in agreement with the ORAC values reported by Ayala-Zavala et al. [23].

Kalt and McDonald [22] also reported changes in phenolic composition, anthocyanin, and antioxidant capacities in strawberry, raspberry, and highbush and lowbush blueberries during postharvest storage treatments. They also reported correlation of antioxidant capacity with phenolic and anthocyanin content.

3.3. Aroma Compound. Typical aroma of strawberries comes from not only one or a few impact aroma compounds, but also from numerous volatiles present at certain concentrations and in a particular balance among them. Thus, strawberry aroma is a result of a combined perception of many aromatic constituents [26].

The aroma profile did not vary qualitatively but only quantitatively among genotypes in their aroma profile (Table 1). Both produced the same major aroma compounds (esters, terpenoids, and furanones) with the exceptions of mesifurane which was not found in Chandler and nerolidol which was found in significantly higher quantity in Camarosa compared to Chandler.

Esters are one of the most important volatile compounds in fruit flavour. Fruity, green grass and other flavour notes of strawberries are emanated by a complex mixture of esters [26]. Esters accounted for the majority of the aroma compounds in both cultivars. Prominent among the esters were methyl hexanoate, ethyl hexanoate, hexyl hexanoate, propyl hexanoate, n-octyl butyrate, and n-octyl acetate. The total esters content of Camarosa reduced with the advent of the storage period, whereas that of Chandler increased significantly with the increase in the storage period. The increase in Chandler is mainly due to the enhanced production of methyl octanoate which can be attributed to the activity of fermentative and volatile biosynthesis related enzymes and isoenzyme in response to senescence and stress conditions [3].

The terpenoid profile of both varieties was dominated by nerolidol and linalool which are considered to be an important contributor to the fresh aroma of strawberry. Nerolidol was found to be significantly higher in Camarosa than in Chandler. However, the same significantly decreased with the increase in the storage period.

Many short-chain alcohols and acids have been found in strawberries [27]; however, since most of short-chain alcohols and acids have very high sensory thresholds, they contribute very little to the overall aroma of strawberry and thus their concentrations were not quantified. Concentrations of alcohols were found to be higher in Camarosa compared to those of Chandler. Hexanal, the only aldehyde identified and associated with the green and cut grass odour characteristics in fruits, was found in higher concentration (almost 50% more) in Camarosa compared to that in Chandler.

Furanones are also the main contributors to the aroma of fresh strawberries other than esters. 2,5-Dimethyl-4-hydroxy-3(2H)-furanone (furaneol) and mesifurane were the two furanones which were found in Camarosa. Both furaneol and mesifurane have strong, sweet, and pleasant odors. Furaneol imparts caramel burnt sugar notes at high concentrations and becomes fruity at lower concentrations [28]. Chandler, however, did not have any detectable mesifuran. Mesifurane is described as having a more sherry-like aroma [29]. Recently, Larsen and Poll [30] found that a mixture of furaneol and ethyl butanoate presented a strawberry-like odor. Total furanone content was retained over the period of storage in Camarosa while in case of Chandler it was totally lost by the end of the 9 days of storage.

Among other compounds, α-farnesene and dodecalactone were found in Camarosa. However, dodecalactone was found only in Camarosa. α-Farnesene was found to increase with the storage period for both varieties, whereas dodecalactone remained constant over the entire storage period.

4. Conclusions

The present study revealed that storage of strawberry has a significant effect on the physicochemical parameters and aroma volatiles of strawberry. Total antioxidants and total phenols were found to increase significantly for both varieties with the increase in the storage period. Similarly, total soluble solids and total sugars decreased with the increase in the storage period for both cultivars. Total anthocyanin content of both varieties remained almost constant throughout the storage period. Titratable acidity in Camarosa reduced with the increase in the storage period whereas it remained almost constant in Chandler. In case of ascorbic acid there was an increase in case of Camarosa whereas the same decreased significantly in Chandler. Significantly higher contents of esters and terpenoids in Camarosa indicated a better retention of the typical fruits flavour of strawberry compared to that of Chandler.

Conflict of Interests

The authors declare that there is no conflict of interests regarding the publication of this paper.

References

[1] L. Reddivari, J. Vanamala, S. Chintharlapalli, S. H. Safe, and J. C. Miller Jr., "Anthocyanin fraction from potato extracts is cytotoxic to prostate cancer cells through activation of caspase-dependent and caspase-independent pathways," *Carcinogenesis*, vol. 28, no. 10, pp. 2227–2235, 2007.

[2] J. He and M. M. Giusti, "Anthocyanins: natural colorants with health-promoting properties," *Annual Review of Food Science and Technology*, vol. 1, pp. 163–187, 2010.

[3] C. Pelayo, S. E. Ebeler, and A. A. Kader, "Postharvest life and flavor quality of three strawberry cultivars kept at 5°C in air or air + 20 kPa CO_2," *Postharvest Biology and Technology*, vol. 27, no. 2, pp. 171–183, 2003.

[4] E. Kafkas and S. Paydas, "Evaluation and Identification of volatile Compounds of Some Promising Strawberry Genotypes Using HS-SPME Technique by GC/MS," *World Journal of Agricultural Sciences*, vol. 3, no. 2, pp. 191–195, 2007.

[5] M. I. Gil, D. M. Holcroft, and A. A. Kader, "Changes is strawberry anthocyanins and other polyphenols in response to carbon dioxide treatments," *Journal of Agricultural and Food Chemistry*, vol. 45, no. 5, pp. 1662–1667, 1997.

[6] H. Wang, G. Cao, and R. L. Prior, "Total antioxidant capacity of fruits," *Journal of Agricultural and Food Chemistry*, vol. 44, no. 3, pp. 701–705, 1996.

[7] I. M. Heinonen, A. S. Meyer, and E. N. Frankel, "Antioxidant activity of berry phenolics on human low-density lipoprotein and liposome oxidation," *Journal of Agricultural and Food Chemistry*, vol. 46, no. 10, pp. 4107–4112, 1998.

[8] K. Robards, P. D. Prenzler, G. Tucker, P. Swatsitang, and W. Glover, "Phenolic compounds and their role in oxidative processes in fruits," *Food Chemistry*, vol. 66, no. 4, pp. 401–436, 1999.

[9] B. R. Cordenunsi, J. R. Oliveira do Nascimento, M. I. Genovese, and F. M. Lajolo, "Influence of cultivar on quality parameters and chemical composition of strawberry fruits grown in Brazil," *Journal of Agricultural and Food Chemistry*, vol. 50, no. 9, pp. 2581–2586, 2002.

[10] C. Han, C. Lederer, M. McDaniel, and Y. Zhao, "Sensory evaluation of fresh strawberries (*Fragaria ananassa*) coated with chitosan-based edible coatings," *Journal of Food Science*, vol. 70, no. 3, pp. S172–S178, 2005.

[11] K. Manning, "Soft fruits," in *Biochemistry of Fruit Ripening*, G. B. Seymour, J. E. Taylor, and G. A. Tucker, Eds., pp. 347–373, Chapman & Hall, London, UK, 1996.

[12] J. K. Fellman, T. W. Miller, D. S. Mattinson, and J. P. Mattheis, "Factors that influence biosynthesis of volatile flavor compounds in apple fruits," *HortScience*, vol. 35, no. 6, pp. 1026–1033, 2000.

[13] G. Lester, "Consumer preference quality attributes of melon fruits," *Acta Horticulturae*, vol. 712, pp. 175–181, 2006.

[14] AOAC, *Official Methods of Analysis*, Association of Official Analytical Chemists, Washington, DC, USA, 17th edition, 2002.

[15] V. L. Singleton, R. Orthofer, and R. M. Lamuela-Raventós, "Analysis of total phenols and other oxidation substrates and antioxidants by means of folin-ciocalteu reagent," *Methods in Enzymology*, vol. 299, pp. 152–178, 1998.

[16] R. E. Wrolstad, R. W. Durst, and J. Lee, "Tracking color and pigment changes in anthocyanin products," *Trends in Food Science and Technology*, vol. 16, no. 9, pp. 423–428, 2005.

[17] R. Apak, K. Güçlü, M. Özyürek, and S. E. Karademir, "Novel total antioxidant capacity index for dietary polyphenols and vitamins C and E, using their cupric ion reducing capability in the presence of neocuproine: CUPRAC method," *Journal of Agricultural and Food Chemistry*, vol. 52, no. 26, pp. 7970–7981, 2004.

[18] B. R. Cordenunsi, J. R. O. Nascimento, and F. M. Lajolo, "Physico-chemical changes related to quality of five strawberry fruit cultivars during cool-storage," *Food Chemistry*, vol. 83, no. 2, pp. 167–173, 2003.

[19] S. K. Lee and A. A. Kader, "Preharvest and postharvest factors influencing vitamin C content of horticultural crops," *Postharvest Biology and Technology*, vol. 20, no. 3, pp. 207–220, 2000.

[20] B. R. Cordenunsi, M. I. Genovese, J. R. Oliveira Do Nascimento, N. M. Aymoto Hassimotto, R. José Dos Santos, and F. M. Lajolo, "Effects of temperature on the chemical composition and antioxidant activity of three strawberry cultivars," *Food Chemistry*, vol. 91, no. 1, pp. 113–121, 2005.

[21] I. Castro, O. Gonçalves, J. A. Teixeira, and A. A. Vicentesc, "Comparative study of Selva and Camarosa strawberries for the commercial market," *Journal of Food Science*, vol. 67, no. 6, pp. 2132–2137, 2002.

[22] W. Kalt and J. E. McDonald, "Chemical composition of lowbush blueberry cultivars," *Journal of the American Society for Horticultural Science*, vol. 121, no. 1, pp. 142–146, 1996.

[23] J. F. Ayala-Zavala, S. Y. Wang, C. Y. Wang, and G. A. González-Aguilar, "Effect of storage temperatures on antioxidant capacity and aroma compounds in strawberry fruit," *LWT-Food Science and Technology*, vol. 37, no. 7, pp. 687–695, 2004.

[24] L. Y. Foo and L. J. Porter, "The structure of tannins of some edible fruits," *Journal of the Science of Food and Agriculture*, vol. 32, pp. 711–716, 1981.

[25] R. L. Prior, X. Wu, and K. Schaich, "Standardized methods for the determination of antioxidant capacity and phenolics in foods and dietary supplements," *Journal of Agricultural and Food Chemistry*, vol. 53, no. 10, pp. 4290–4302, 2005.

[26] A. G. Pérez, C. Sanz, and J. M. Olías, "Partial purification and some properties of alcohol acyltransferase from strawberry fruits," *Journal of Agricultural and Food Chemistry*, vol. 41, no. 9, pp. 1462–1466, 1993.

[27] V. de Boishebert, L. Urruty, J.-L. Giraudel, and M. Montury, "Assessment of Strawberry Aroma through Solid-Phase Microextraction-Gas Chromatography and Artificial Neuron Network Methods. Variety Classification versus Growing Years," *Journal of Agricultural and Food Chemistry*, vol. 52, no. 9, pp. 2472–2478, 2004.

[28] L. Re, B. Maurer, and G. Ohloff, "4-hydroxy-2,5-dimethyl-3(2H)-furanone (furaneol) einem aromabestandteil und erdbeere," *Helvetica Chimica Acta*, vol. 56, pp. 1882–1894, 1973.

[29] G. L. Hunter, W. A. Bucek, and T. Radford, "Volatile components of canned alphonso mango," *Journal of Food Science*, vol. 39, pp. 900–903, 1974.

[30] M. Larsen and L. Poll, "Odour thresholds of some important aroma compounds in strawberries," *Zeitschrift für Lebensmittel-Untersuchung und -Forschung*, vol. 195, no. 2, pp. 120–123, 1992.

26

Protective Role of Catechin and Quercetin in Sodium Benzoate-Induced Lipid Peroxidation and the Antioxidant System in Human Erythrocytes *In Vitro*

Gamze Yetuk, Dilek Pandir, and Hatice Bas

Department of Biology, Faculty of Arts and Science, Bozok University, 66100 Divanli Yolu/Yozgat, Turkey

Correspondence should be addressed to Dilek Pandir; durak77@gmail.com

Academic Editors: K. Ebihara, J. S. Marchini, and H. Zeng

The aim of this study was to evaluate the protective effect of catechin and quercetin in sodium benzoate- (SB-) induced oxidative stress in human erythrocytes *in vitro*. For this, the effects of SB (6.25, 12.5, 25, 50, and 100 μg/mL), catechin (10 μM), and quercetin (10 μM) on lipid peroxidation (LPO) and the activities of SOD, CAT, GPx, and GST were studied. Significantly higher LPO and lower activities of antioxidant enzymes were observed with the increasing concentrations of SB. Catechin or quercetin protected the erythrocytes against SB-induced toxicity only at low concentrations of SB. The presence of catechin or quercetin at 10 μM have no effect on SB-induced toxicity at high concentrations of SB (50 and 100 μg/mL). In conclusion, SB may cause oxidative stress as food additive in human erythrocytes *in vitro*. So, it appears that our findings provide evidence for the protection of erythrocytes from SB that could be considered for further studies.

1. Introduction

Food additives are chemical substances added to foods for various reasons to preserve flavor or enhance its taste and appearance. Various food additives are preservative in character. Preservatives are compounds that delay or prevent microbiological, enzymatic, or chemical changes of foods. They do not only act against visible spoilage by yeasts, molds, and bacteria but also prevent the formation of toxins, especially those produced by bacteria and molds [1]. They play an important role in the safety of food supply; many studies revealed the potential genotoxic and mutagenic effects of the additives [2–5]. Consumption of food additives has caused various diseases such as eczema, urticaria, diarrhea, nausea, migraine, and vomiting [6].

Sodium benzoate is widely used as food preservatives [7] on salad dressings, carbonated drinks, jams, and fruit juices [5]. The acceptable daily intake (ADI) levels recommended by the Joint FAO/WHO Expert Committee on Food Additives (JECFA) for sodium benzoate and potassium benzoate are 0–5 mg/kg body weight [5, 8]. In general the sodium and potassium salts are preferred over the acid form because they are more soluble in water [9].

Flavonoids are polyphenolic compounds found in significant quantities in the human diet [10, 11]. The flavonoids are potent antioxidants *in vitro* [12, 13]. Quercetin, a flavonoid found in fruits and vegetables [14], exerts beneficial effects [15] that contribute to human health. The antioxidant effect by scavenging free radicals and chelating iron ions of quercetin has been extensively studied [12, 16] because free radicals are involved in pathogenesis of many diseases [17]. Catechins are flavonoids that have particularly attracted attention because of their relatively high antioxidant capacity. Green and black tea contain considerable amounts of catechins and several studies have attributed the *in vitro* antioxidant properties of tea extracts to the presence of these flavonoids [18, 19].

According to the literature survey, no study has been conducted on enzyme activities and LPO of sodium benzoate (SB) + catechin and SB + quercetin in human erythrocytes using spectrophotometric analysis *in vitro*. For these reasons, the aim of this study was to investigate the effect of SB in human erythrocytes as *in vitro*; then malondialdehyde

(MDA) levels, SOD, CAT, GPx, and GST activities were assessed and undertaken to determine whether the free radical scavengers catechin or quercetin could inhibit the oxidative destruction of unsaturated fatty acids and alter enzymatic activities.

2. Materials and Methods

2.1. Chemicals. SB (99% purity) was obtained from Merck (Germany). Quercetin and catechin were supplied by Sigma-Aldrich (Germany), and dimethyl sulfoxide (DMSO) was supplied by Merck (Germany). SB was dissolved in distilled water [5] and quercetin and catechin were dissolved in 0.5% DMSO [20]. All other chemicals used were analytical grade and were of obtained from Sigma-Aldrich (Germany).

2.2. Treatment of Erythrocytes. Blood was collected from normal healthy volunteers into tubes containing heparin approximately 20 mL of fresh blood. Erythrocytes were separated from blood plasma by centrifuge and were divided into nontreated control and experimental groups. The control group was incubated in 0.9% NaCl at pH 7.4. Experimental groups were divided into treatment groups: SB ($n = 6$), catechin ($n = 6$), quercetin ($n = 6$), SB + catechin ($n = 6$), and SB + quercetin ($n = 6$) groups. The control group was incubated for 1 h at 37°C in 0.9% NaCl [21–23]. Erythrocytes in the experimental group were treated with 6.25, 12.5, 25, 50, and 100 μg/mL of SB in the presence or absence of catechin (10 μM) and quercetin (10 μM) for 1 hr at 37°C. After incubation, the cell mixtures were stored at −20°C for 24 h. The mixtures were thawed; the erythrocytes were destroyed by osmotic pressure and then subjected to centrifugation. Supernatants were isolated and MDA levels and the activities of SOD, CAT, GPx and GST, were measured by spectrophotometer (Shimadzu UV-1800, Japan). The concentration of hemoglobin was determined using the method of Drabkin [24].

2.3. Lipid Peroxidation in Erythrocytes. LPO was measured in erythrocytes as MDA whose content was assayed by using the thiobarbituric acid test as described by Ohkawa et al. [25]. The absorbance at 532 nm was measured by a spectrophotometer. Specific activity is presented as nmol/mg hemoglobin.

2.4. Antioxidant Enzymes in Erythrocytes. SOD, CAT, GPx, and GST enzyme activities were determined in erythrocytes lysate prepared according to the method of McCord and Fridovich (1969) [26]. SOD was assayed according to the technique of S. Marklund and G. Marklund (1974) [27]. One unit of SOD activity was calculated as the amount of protein causing 50% inhibition of pyrogallol autooxidation. Activity was monitored at 440 nm. Data were expressed as USOD/mg hemoglobin. CAT was estimated according to the method of Aebi (1984) [28] and rate of decomposition of hydrogen peroxide by CAT enzyme at 240 nm was evaluated. CAT activity was read at 240 nm and expressed as UCAT/mg hemoglobin. GPx activity was measured by the method described by Paglia and Valentine (1967) [29]. It catalyses the oxidation of glutathione (GSH) by cumene hydroperoxide. GPx activity was read at 340 nm and expressed as UGPx/mg hemoglobin. GST activity was measured according to the method of Habig et al. (1974) [30]. The principle of the assay is based on the determination of the formation of GSH and the 1-chloro-2,4-dinitrobenzene conjugate. Increases in absorbance were recorded at 340 nm. The specific activity of GST is expressed as UGST/mg hemoglobin.

2.5. Statistical Analysis. The data are expressed as the means ± standard deviation (SD). Differences among experimental groups were analyzed by software program SPSS 11.0 for Windows. Comparison between means was carried out using one-way analysis of variance (ANOVA), followed by Tukey's procedure for multiple comparisons. $P < 0.05$ was taken as statistically significant.

3. Results

There were no statistically significant changes in MDA levels and in SOD, CAT, GPx, and GST activities between the catechin- and quercetin-treated groups compared with the control group ($P > 0.05$, Figures 1–5).

3.1. Measurement of Level of Malondialdehyde (MDA). SB treatment (12.5, 25, 50, and 100 μg/mL) increased significantly the level of MDA compared with control, catechin, and quercetin-treated groups ($P < 0.05$). In contrast, any change of MDA level was not detected at only the lowest dose of SB (6.25 μg/mL). The MDA levels were decreased statistically significantly in the SB + catechin treated group and SB + quercetin-treated group compared to SB-treated group ($P < 0.05$, Figure 1). Decreasing the MDA level of 50 μg/mL of SB incubated with catechin or quercetin group was measured not to be statistically significant ($P > 0.05$). The protective effect of catechin or quercetin was not detected in the 100 μg/mL SB-treated group in human erythrocytes *in vitro*.

3.2. Measurement of Superoxide Dismutase (SOD) Activity. Decreases in SOD activity were found in human erythrocytes in used high four concentrations. No differences in the activity of SOD were observed in treated erythrocytes at the lowest dose of SB-(6.25 μg/mL). The SOD activity was increased statistically significantly in the SB + catechin treated group and SB + quercetin treated group compared to SB (12.5 and 25 μg/mL) treated group ($P < 0.05$, Figure 2). Increasing the SOD activity of 50 μg/mL of SB incubated with catechin or quercetin group was measured not to be statistically significant ($P > 0.05$). The protective effect of catechin or quercetin was not detected in the 100 μg/mL SB-treated group in human erythrocytes *in vitro*.

3.3. Measurement of Catalase (CAT) Activity. Any alternation of CAT activity was not detected in the human erythrocytes in 6.25 μg/mL, decreased significantly in 12.5, 25, 50, and 100 μg/mL compared with control groups ($P < 0.05$). Catechin or quercetin supply combined with SB partially reversed this change only at 12.5 and 25 μg/mL doses of

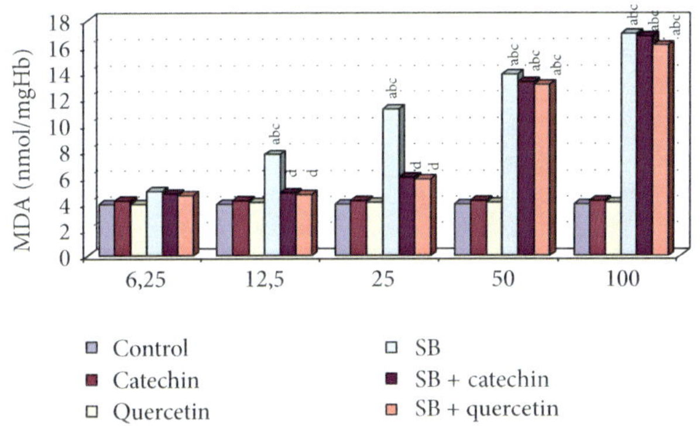

FIGURE 1: MDA level in erythrocytes of control and experimental groups. Different letters above bars indicate significant differences between exposure concentrations; bars with the same letter are not significantly different. Values are mean ± SD in each group. Significance at $P < 0.05$.

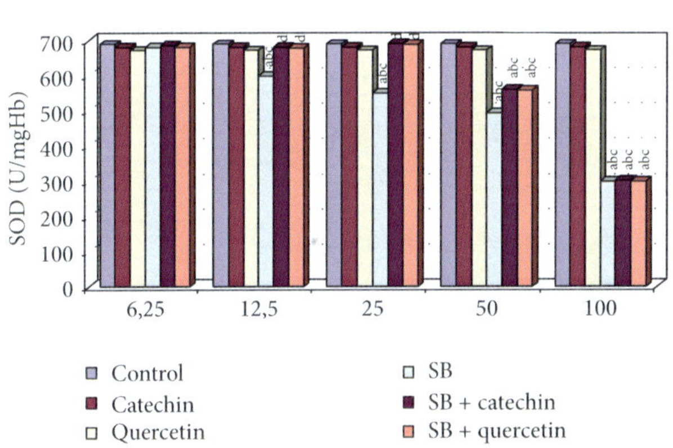

FIGURE 2: SOD activity in erytrocytes of control and experimental groups. Different letters above the bars indicate significant differences between exposure concentrations; bars with the same letter are not significantly different. Values are mean ± SD in each group. Significance at $P < 0.05$.

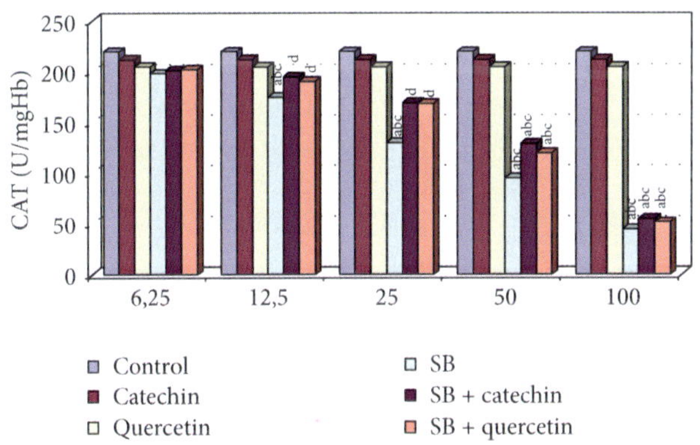

FIGURE 3: CAT activity in erytrocytes of control and experimental groups. Different letters above the bars indicate significant differences between exposure concentrations; bars with the same letter are not significantly different. Values are mean ± SD in each group. Significance at $P < 0.05$.

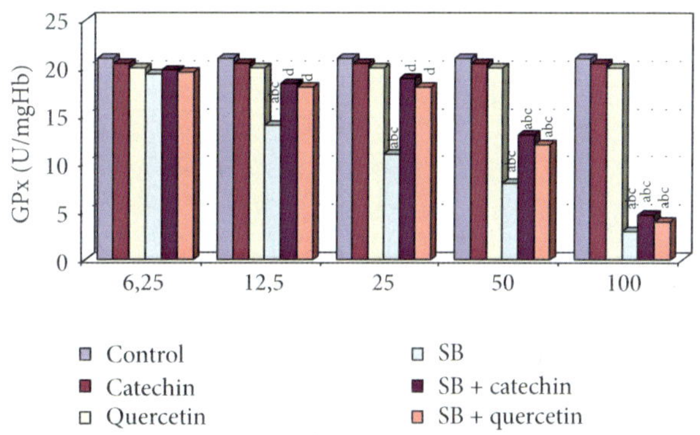

FIGURE 4: GPx activity in erytrocytes of control and experimental groups. Different letters above the bars indicate significant differences between exposure concentrations; bars with the same letter are not significantly different. Values are mean ± SD in each group. Significance at $P < 0.05$.

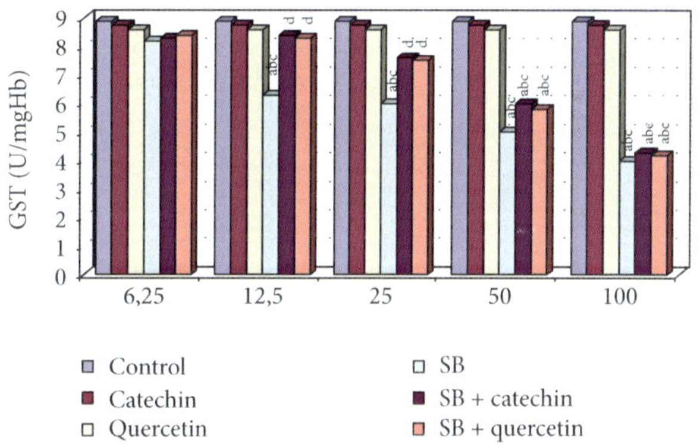

FIGURE 5: GST activity in erytrocytes of control and experimental groups. Different letters above the bars indicate significant differences between exposure concentrations; bars with the same letter are not significantly different. Values are mean ± SD in each group. Significance at $P < 0.05$.

SB. CAT activity in 50 μg/mL SB + catechin and 50 μg/mL SB + quercetin groups was significantly higher than SB-exposed erythrocytes but it was not detected to be statistically significant compared to control, catechin, and quercetin groups ($P > 0.05$, Figure 3). The protective effect of catechin or quercetin was not detected in 100 μg/mL SB-treated group in human erythrocytes *in vitro*.

3.4. Measurement of Glutathione Peroxidase (GPx) Activity. As shown in Figure 4, the GPx activity was significantly decreased in high doses of SB-exposed erythrocytes, whereas 6.25 μg/mL of SB was no change this enzyme activity as compared to control, catechin and quercetin groups. Catechin or quercetin supply in the SB-treated group significantly increased GPx activity in erythrocytes compared to control groups only at 12.5 and 25 μg/mL SB ($P < 0.05$, Figure 4). Catechin or quercetin has no protective effect on SB-induced changes in GPx activity in erythrocytes at 50 and 100 μg/mL doses of SB.

3.5. Measurement of Glutathione-S-Transferase (GST) Activity. The activity of GST was significantly decreased in the SB-treated (12.5, 25, 50, and 100 μg/mL) groups, and, in contrast, no statistically significant changes were observed in the 6.25 μg/mL of SB compared with the control, catechin, and quercetin groups. However, the GST activity was significantly increased in erythrocytes in the SB + catechin and SB + quercetin groups compared with the SB-only group ($P < 0.05$, Figure 5). There were no statistical differences among 50 μg/mL SB + catechin or quercetin-treated erythrocytes compared to only SB-treated cells. Catechin or quercetin has no protective effect on SB-induced changes in GST activity in erythrocytes at 100 μg/mL dose of SB.

4. Discussion

Different increasing doses of SB were tested by using chromosome aberrations, sister-chromatid exchanges, and micronucleus in cultured human lymphocytes and comet assay in isolated human lymphocytes. The results show that SB is genotoxic to the human peripheral blood lymphocytes *in vitro* at the highest concentrations [5]. So, potential genotoxic effects of food preservatives SB was used in the present study same concentrations that by the previous works reported in human blood *in vitro*.

Piper (1999) [31] says that SB can create free radicals and damage cells. SB intoxication showed increased erythrocyte LPO associated with lowered antioxidant enzymes; as the activities of SOD, CAT, GPx, and GST decreased, the MDA level increased. The mechanism of the effect of SB on enzyme activities and MDA level of erythrocytes may be as well as many chemical substances [32]. The decrease in SOD, CAT, GPx, and GST activities in erythrocytes may be due to the inactivation of these enzymes, as superoxide anions have been shown to reduce the activity of these enzymes [33]. The depletion of erythrocyte GSH along with the decrease in SOD and CAT activities may affect the ability of erythrocytes to scavenge superoxide anions and hydroxyl radicals. The decrease of GSH content in erythrocytes by SB intoxication may be due to depletion of GSH, SB-SH binding, or an effect on glutathione reductase activity [32].

The antioxidants protect the erythrocyte membrane from oxidative damage [34, 35] and also prevent oxidative damage as a result of their ability to scavenge reactive oxygen species such as hydroxyl radical and superoxide anion [36]. Studies in animals and humans suggest that flavonoids may reduce the risk of cardiovascular diseases [11, 37, 38], cerebrovascular diseases [39], and cancers [40]. Catechins are flavonoids that are found in green tea, black tea, and other plant foods and they are reported to have various physiological effects in terms of their antioxidative ability [20, 41]. The protective effects of myricetin, quercetin, (+)-catechin, and (−)-epicatechin were investigated against N-nitrosodibutylamine and N-nitrosopiperidine-induced DNA damage in HepG2. (+)-catechin at the lowest concentration (10 μM) showed the maximum reduction of DNA strand breaks [42]. Lotito and Fraga (2000) [43] have shown that (+)-catechin was an effective antioxidant in human blood plasma, delaying the consumption of endogenous lipid soluble antioxidants and inhibiting lipid oxidation. Quercetin, a potent antioxidant, scavenges free radicals directly, inhibits LPO, and alters antioxidant defence pathway *in vivo* and *in vitro* [44]. Quercetin, a naturally occurring flavonoid, is able to protect RPE cells from oxidative damage and cellular senescence *in vitro* dose-dependent manner [45]. (+)-catechin and quercetin at the lowest concentration (10 μM) were used against SB-induced oxidative stress in human erythrocytes *in vitro* in this study. Our results indicated that the presence of (+)-catechin and quercetin at 10 μM concentration could be able to ameliorate SB-induced oxidative stress by decreasing LPO and altering antioxidant defense system in erythrocytes.

In conclusion, the effects of SB, catechin, and quercetin on LPO and the antioxidant enzyme systems were evaluated in human erythrocytes *in vitro* in this study. High concentrations of SB may induce oxidative stress by enhancing LPO and by altering the antioxidant enzyme systems in erythrocytes. We observed that the antioxidant enzyme activities and MDA levels were ameliorated in the catechin or quercetin + SB treated groups. These protective effects may be due to antioxidant effects of catechin and quercetin. So, our findings suggest that using of SB as food preservatives caution be taken and should be preferred lowest concentrations of SB.

Conflict of Interests

There is no conflict of interests.

Acknowledgment

The support for this study was provided by the Bozok University Scientific Research Project Funding Unit thanks were extended to it as well.

References

[1] S. Mamur, D. Yuzbasıoglu, F. Ünal, and H. Aksoy, "Genotoxicity of food preservative sodium sorbate in human lymphocytes *in vitro*," *Cytotechnology*, vol. 64, pp. 553–562, 2012.

[2] S. Yılmaz, F. Unal, D. Yuzbasıoglu, and H. Aksoy, "Clastogenic effects of food additive citric acid in human peripheral lymphocytes," *Cytotechnology*, vol. 56, pp. 137–144, 2008.

[3] S. Yılmaz, F. Unal, and D. Yuzbasıoglu, "The *in vitro* genotoxicity of benzoic acid in human peripheral blood lymphocytes," *Cytotechnology*, vol. 60, pp. 55–61, 2009.

[4] S. Mamur, D. Yuzbasıoglu, F. Ünal, and S. Yılmaz, "Does potassium sorbate induce genotoxic or mutagenic effects in lymphocytes?" *Toxicology in Vitro*, vol. 24, no. 3, pp. 790–794, 2010.

[5] N. Zengin, D. Yüzbaşioğlu, F. Ünal, S. Yılmaz, and H. Aksoy, "The evaluation of the genotoxicity of two food preservatives: sodium benzoate and potassium benzoate," *Food and Chemical Toxicology*, vol. 49, no. 4, pp. 763–769, 2011.

[6] H. Dogruyol, "Gıdalardaki katkı maddeleri ve zararları, çocukluk hiperaktivitesi," *Güncel Pediatri*, vol. 2, pp. 42–48, 2006.

[7] B. Saad, M. F. Bari, M. I. Saleh, K. Ahmad, and M. K. M. Talib, "Simultaneous determination of preservatives (benzoic acid, sorbic acid, methylparaben and propylparaben) in foodstuffs using high-performance liquid chromatography," *Journal of Chromatography A*, vol. 1073, no. 1-2, pp. 393–397, 2005.

[8] WHO, *Principles for the Safety Assessment of Food Additives and Contaminants in Food*, Environmental Health Criteria, 1987.

[9] M. B. Liewen and E. H. Marth, "Growth and inhibition of microorganisms in the presence of sorbic acid: a rewiew," *Journal of Food Protection*, vol. 48, pp. 364–375, 1985.

[10] M. G. L. Hertog, E. J. M. Feskens, P. C. H. Hollman, M. B. Katan, and D. Kromhout, "Dietary antioxidant flavonoids and risk of coronary heart disease: the Zutphen Elderly study," *The Lancet*, vol. 342, no. 8878, pp. 1007–1011, 1993.

[11] M. G. L. Hertog, P. C. H. Hollman, M. B. Katan, and D. Kromhout, "Intake of potentially anticarcinogenic flavonoids and their determinants in adults in The Netherlands," *Nutrition and Cancer*, vol. 20, no. 1, pp. 21–29, 1993.

[12] I. Morel, G. Lescoat, P. Cogrel et al., "Antioxidant and iron-chelating activities of the flavonoids catechin, quercetin and diosmetin on iron-loaded rat hepatocyte cultures," *Biochemical Pharmacology*, vol. 45, no. 1, pp. 13–19, 1993.

[13] N. Cotelle, J. Bernier, J. Catteau, J. Pommery, J. Wallet, and E. M. Gaydou, "Antioxidant properties of hydroxy-flavones," *Free Radical Biology and Medicine*, vol. 20, no. 1, pp. 35–43, 1996.

[14] C. Manach, G. Williamson, C. Morand, A. Scalbert, and C. Rémésy, "Bioavailability and bioefficacy of polyphenols in humans. I. Review of 97 bioavailability studies," *The American Journal of Clinical Nutrition*, vol. 81, pp. 230–242, 2005.

[15] R. J. Williams, J. P. E. Spencer, and C. Rice-Evans, "Flavonoids: antioxidants or signalling molecules?" *Free Radical Biology and Medicine*, vol. 36, no. 7, pp. 838–849, 2004.

[16] M. Leopoldini, N. Russo, S. Chiodo, and M. Toscano, "Iron chelation by the powerful antioxidant flavonoid quercetin," *Journal of Agricultural and Food Chemistry*, vol. 54, no. 17, pp. 6343–6351, 2006.

[17] B. Halliwell, "Role of free radicals in the neurodegenerative diseases: therapeutic implications for antioxidant treatment," *Drugs and Aging*, vol. 18, no. 9, pp. 685–716, 2001.

[18] S. Miura, J. Watanabe, M. Sano et al., "Effects of various natural antioxidants on the Cu^{2+}-mediated oxidative modification of low density lipoprotein," *Biological and Pharmaceutical Bulletin*, vol. 18, no. 1, pp. 1–4, 1995.

[19] J. A. Vinson, Y. A. Dabbagh, M. M. Serry, and J. Jang, "Plant flavonoids, especially tea flavonols, are powerful antioxidants using an *in vitro* oxidation model for heart disease," *Journal of Agricultural and Food Chemistry*, vol. 43, no. 11, pp. 2800–2802, 1995.

[20] Y. Kalender, S. Kaya, D. Durak, F. G. Uzun, and F. Demir, "Protective effects of catechin and quercetin on antioxidant status, lipid peroxidation and testis-histoarchitecture induced by chlorpyrifos in male rats," *Environmental Toxicology and Pharmacology*, vol. 33, no. 2, pp. 141–148, 2012.

[21] D. Durak, S. Kalender, F. G. Uzun, F. Demir, and Y. Kalender, "Mercury chloride-induced oxidative stress in human erythrocytes and the effect of vitamins C and E *in vitro*," *African Journal of Biotechnology*, vol. 9, no. 4, pp. 488–495, 2010.

[22] O. Tezcan, D. Pandır, and H. Bas, "The effects of cadmium on enzymatic antioxidant system and lipid peroxidation of human erythrocytes *in vitro* and the protective role of plasma level of vitamins C and E," *Polish Journal of Environmental Studies*, vol. 21, no. 6, pp. 1849–1854, 2012.

[23] S. Eroglu, D. Pandır, G. F. Uzun, and H. Bas, "Protective role of vitamins C and E in diclorvos-induced oxidative stress in human erythrocytes *in vitro*," *Biological Research*, vol. 46, no. 1, pp. 33–38, 2013.

[24] D. I. Drabkin, "Spectrophotometric studies. XIV. The crystallographic and optical properties of the hemoglobin of man in comparison with those of other species," *The Journal of Biological Chemistry*, vol. 164, pp. 703–723, 1946.

[25] H. Ohkawa, N. Ohishi, and K. Yagi, "Assay for lipid peroxides in animal tissues by thiobarbituric acid reaction," *Analytical Biochemistry*, vol. 95, no. 2, pp. 351–358, 1979.

[26] J. M. McCord and I. Fridovich, "Superoxide dismutase. An enzymic function for erythrocuprein (hemocuprein)," *The Journal of Biological Chemistry*, vol. 244, no. 22, pp. 6049–6055, 1969.

[27] S. Marklund and G. Marklund, "Involvement of the superoxide anion radical in the autoxidation of pyrogallol and a convenient assay for superoxide dismutase," *European Journal of Biochemistry*, vol. 47, no. 3, pp. 469–474, 1974.

[28] H. Aebi, "Catalase *in vitro*," *Methods in Enzymology*, vol. 105, pp. 121–126, 1984.

[29] D. E. Paglia and W. N. Valentine, "Studies on the quantitative and qualitative characterization of erythrocyte glutathione peroxidase," *The Journal of Laboratory and Clinical Medicine*, vol. 70, no. 1, pp. 158–169, 1967.

[30] W. H. Habig, M. J. Pabst, and W. B. Jakoby, "Glutathione S transferases. The first enzymatic step in mercapturic acid formation," *The Journal of Biological Chemistry*, vol. 249, no. 22, pp. 7130–7139, 1974.

[31] P. W. Piper, "Yeast superoxide dismutase mutants reveal a pro-oxidant action of weak organic acid food preservatives," *Free Radical Biology and Medicine*, vol. 27, no. 11-12, pp. 1219–1227, 1999.

[32] S. Sarkar, P. Yadav, and D. Bhatnagar, "Lipid peroxidative damage on cadmium exposure and alterations in antioxidant system in rat erythrocytes: a study with relation to time," *BioMetals*, vol. 11, no. 2, pp. 153–157, 1998.

[33] Y. Kono and I. Fridovich, "Superoxide radical inhibits catalase," *The Journal of Biological Chemistry*, vol. 257, no. 10, pp. 5751–5754, 1982.

[34] S. Sarkar, Y. Poonam, and D. Bhatnagar, "Cadmium-induced lipid peroxidation and the antioxidant enzymes in rat tissues: role of vitamin E and selenium," *Trace Elements and Electrocytes*, vol. 14, no. 1, pp. 41–45, 1997.

[35] S. Sarkar, P. Yadav, and D. Bhatnagar, "Cadmium-induced lipid peroxidation and the antioxidant system in rat erythrocytes the role of antioxidants," *Journal of Trace Elements in Medicine and Biology*, vol. 11, no. 1, pp. 8–13, 1997.

[36] G. Galati, O. Sabzevari, J. X. Wilson, and P. J. O'Brien, "Prooxidant activity and cellular effects of the phenoxyl radicals of dietary flavonoids and other polyphenolics," *Toxicology*, vol. 177, no. 1, pp. 91–104, 2002.

[37] S. Liu, J. E. Manson, I.-M. Lee et al., "Fruit and vegetable intake and risk of cardiovascular disease: the Women's Health study," *American Journal of Clinical Nutrition*, vol. 72, no. 4, pp. 922–928, 2000.

[38] H. D. Sesso, J. M. Gaziano, S. Liu, and J. E. Buring, "Flavonoid intake and the risk of cardiovascular disease in women," *American Journal of Clinical Nutrition*, vol. 77, no. 6, pp. 1400–1408, 2003.

[39] P. Knekt, J. Kumpulainen, R. Järvinen et al., "Flavonoid intake and risk of chronic diseases," *American Journal of Clinical Nutrition*, vol. 76, no. 3, pp. 560–568, 2002.

[40] I. C. Arta, P. C. Hollman, E. J. Feskens, M. H. B. Bueno, and D. Kromhout, "Catechin intake might explain the inverse relation between tea consumption and ischemic heart disease: the Zutphen Elderly study," *American Journal of Clinical Nutrition*, vol. 74, no. 2, pp. 227–232, 2001.

[41] S. Baba, N. Osakabe, M. Natsume, Y. Muto, T. Takizawa, and J. Terao, "In vivo comparison of the bioavailability of (+)-catechin, (−)-epicatechin and their mixture in orally administered rats," *Journal of Nutrition*, vol. 131, no. 11, pp. 2885–2891, 2001.

[42] M. E. Delgado, A. I. Haza, A. García, and P. Morales, "Myricetin, quercetin, (+)-catechin and (−)-epicatechin protect against N-nitrosamines-induced DNA damage in human hepatoma cells," *Toxicology in Vitro*, vol. 23, no. 7, pp. 1292–1297, 2009.

[43] S. B. Lotito and C. G. Fraga, "Catechins delay lipid oxidation and alpha-tocopherol and beta-carotene depletion following ascorbate depletion in human plasma," *Proceedings of the Society for Experimental Biology and Medicine*, vol. 225, pp. 32–38, 2000.

[44] M. Anjaneyulu and K. Chopra, "Quercetin, an anti-oxidant bioflavonoid, attenuates diabetic nephropathy in rats," *Clinical and Experimental Pharmacology and Physiology*, vol. 31, no. 4, pp. 244–248, 2004.

[45] D. Kook, A. H. Wolf, A. L. Yu et al., "The protective effect of quercetin against oxidative stress in the human RPE *in vitro*," *Investigative Ophthalmology and Visual Science*, vol. 49, no. 4, pp. 1712–1720, 2008.

Permissions

The contributors of this book come from diverse backgrounds, making this book a truly international effort. This book will bring forth new frontiers with its revolutionizing research information and detailed analysis of the nascent developments around the world.

We would like to thank all the contributing authors for lending their expertise to make the book truly unique. They have played a crucial role in the development of this book. Without their invaluable contributions this book wouldn't have been possible. They have made vital efforts to compile up to date information on the varied aspects of this subject to make this book a valuable addition to the collection of many professionals and students.

This book was conceptualized with the vision of imparting up-to-date information and advanced data in this field. To ensure the same, a matchless editorial board was set up. Every individual on the board went through rigorous rounds of assessment to prove their worth. After which they invested a large part of their time researching and compiling the most relevant data for our readers. Conferences and sessions were held from time to time between the editorial board and the contributing authors to present the data in the most comprehensible form. The editorial team has worked tirelessly to provide valuable and valid information to help people across the globe.

Every chapter published in this book has been scrutinized by our experts. Their significance has been extensively debated. The topics covered herein carry significant findings which will fuel the growth of the discipline. They may even be implemented as practical applications or may be referred to as a beginning point for another development. Chapters in this book were first published by Hindawi Publishing Corporation; hereby published with permission under the Creative Commons Attribution License or equivalent.

The editorial board has been involved in producing this book since its inception. They have spent rigorous hours researching and exploring the diverse topics which have resulted in the successful publishing of this book. They have passed on their knowledge of decades through this book. To expedite this challenging task, the publisher supported the team at every step. A small team of assistant editors was also appointed to further simplify the editing procedure and attain best results for the readers.

Our editorial team has been hand-picked from every corner of the world. Their multi-ethnicity adds dynamic inputs to the discussions which result in innovative outcomes. These outcomes are then further discussed with the researchers and contributors who give their valuable feedback and opinion regarding the same. The feedback is then collaborated with the researches and they are edited in a comprehensive manner to aid the understanding of the subject.

Apart from the editorial board, the designing team has also invested a significant amount of their time in understanding the subject and creating the most relevant covers. They scrutinized every image to scout for the most suitable representation of the subject and create an appropriate cover for the book.

The publishing team has been involved in this book since its early stages. They were actively engaged in every process, be it collecting the data, connecting with the contributors or procuring relevant information. The team has been an ardent support to the editorial, designing and production team. Their endless efforts to recruit the best for this project, has resulted in the accomplishment of this book. They are a veteran in the field of academics and their pool of knowledge is as vast as their experience in printing. Their expertise and guidance has proved useful at every step. Their uncompromising quality standards have made this book an exceptional effort. Their encouragement from time to time has been an inspiration for everyone.

The publisher and the editorial board hope that this book will prove to be a valuable piece of knowledge for researchers, students, practitioners and scholars across the globe.

List of Contributors

Deanna M. Minich and Jeffrey S. Bland
Personalized Lifestyle Medicine Institute, 800 Fifth Avenue, Suite 4100, Seattle, WA 98104, USA

Natacha Toral
Nutrition Department, Health Sciences School, University of Brasília, Campus Universitário Darcy Ribeiro, Asa Norte, 70910-900 Brasília, DF, Brazil

Betzabeth Slater
Nutrition Department, Public Health School, University of Sao Paulo, Avenida Dr. Arnaldo, 715, 2 No. andar, 01246-904 São Paulo, SP, Brazil

Juliana Rombaldi Bernardi, Renata de Souza Escobar, Charles Francisco Ferreira and Patrícia Pelufo Silveira
Núcleo de Estudos da Saúde da Criança e do Adolescente, Hospital de Clínicas de Porto Alegre (HCPA), Universidade Federal do Rio Grande do Sul, Rua Ramiro Barcelos 2350, 90035-903, Porto Alegre, RS, Brazil

Cihad Dündar
Department of Public Health, Faculty of Medicine, Ondokuz Mayıs University, 55139 Samsun, Turkey

Hatice Öz
Provincial Directorate of Health, 55060 Samsun, Turkey

Azin Pourkhalili and Ebrahim Rahimi
Department of Food Science and Technology, Faculty of Agriculture, Islamic Azad University, Shahrekord Branch, Shahrekord 88137-33395, Iran

Maryam Mirlohi
Food Security Research Center, School of Nutrition and Food Science, Isfahan University of Medical Science, Isfahan 8174-73461, Iran

Brigitta Wichert, Julia Trossen and Marcel Wanner
Institute of Animal Nutrition, Vetsuisse Faculty, University of Zurich, Winterthurerstraße 260, 8057 Zurich, Switzerland

Daniel Uebelhart
Department of Rheumatology and Institute of Physical Medicine, University Hospital Zurich, Gloriastraße 25, 8091 Zurich, Switzerland

Sonja Hartnack
Section of Epidemiology, Vetsuisse Faculty, University of Zurich, Winterthurerstraße 270, 8057 Zurich, Switzerland

Muhammad Nadeem, Mian Anjum Murtaza and Ghulam Mueen-ud-Din
Institute of Food Science and Nutrition, University of Sargodha, Sargodha, Pakistan

Salim-ur-Rehman and Faqir Muhammad Anjum
National Institute of Food Science and Technology, University of Agriculture, Faisalabad, Pakistan

Hamid Abdi
Departments of Acupuncture Therapy, Beijing University of Chinese Medicine, Beijing 100029, China
Biochemistry and Nutrition Research Center, Faculty of Medicine, Mashhad University of Medical Sciences (MUMS), Mashhad, Iran

Baixiao Zhao
Departments of Acupuncture Therapy, Beijing University of Chinese Medicine, Beijing 100029, China

Mahsa Darbandi, Shima Tavallaie, Seyyed Mohammad Reza Parizadeh, Mohammad Safariyan, Mohsen Nemati, MaryamMohammadi, Parisa Abbasi-Parizad, Sara Darbandi and Saeed Akhlaghi
Biochemistry and Nutrition Research Center, Faculty of Medicine, Mashhad University of Medical Sciences (MUMS), Mashhad, Iran

Majid Ghayour-Mobarhan
Biochemistry and Nutrition Research Center, Faculty of Medicine, Mashhad University of Medical Sciences (MUMS), Mashhad, Iran
Cardiovascular Research Center, Faculty of Medicine, Mashhad University of Medical Sciences, Mashhad 9196773117, Iran

Amir Ali Rahsepar
Cardiovascular Research Center, Faculty of Medicine, Mashhad University of Medical Sciences, Mashhad 9196773117, Iran
Young Researchers Club, Mashhad Branch, Islamic Azad University, Mashhad 9187147578, Iran

Gordon A. A. Ferns
Institute for Science and Technology in Medicine, Keele University, Thornburrow Drive, Hartshill, Stoke-on-Trent, ST4 7QB, UK

Teresa Malecka-Massalska
Physiology Department, Medical University of Lublin, Radziwiłłowska 11 Street, 20-080 Lublin, Poland

Agata Smolen
Department of Mathematics and Biostatistics, Medical University of Lublin, Jaczewskiego 4 Street, 20 090 Lubin, Poland

Elzbieta Madro
Institute of Hematology and Transfusiology, Indiry Gandhi 14 Street, 02-776 Warsaw, Poland

Wojciech Surtel
Department of Electronics, University of Technology, Nadbystrzycka 38a Street, 20-618 Lublin, Poland

Chi-Hua Yen
Department of Family and Community Medicine, Chung Shan Medical University Hospital, Taichung 40201, Taiwan
School of Medicine, Chung Shan Medical University, Taichung 40201, Taiwan
Center for Education and Research on Geriatrics and Gerontology, Chung Shan Medical University, Taichung 40201, Taiwan

Nae-Cherng Yang and Ping-Ting Lin
School of Nutrition, Chung Shan Medical University, Taichung 40201, Taiwan
Department of Nutrition, Chung Shan Medical University Hospital, Taichung 40201, Taiwan

Bor-Jen Lee
The Intensive Care Unit, Taichung Veterans General Hospital, Taichung 40705, Taiwan

Jui-Yuan Lin
School of Nutrition, Chung Shan Medical University, Taichung 40201, Taiwan

Simon Hsia
Department of Nutrition and Institute of Biomedical Nutrition, Hungkuang University, Taichung 43346, Taiwan

Ju-Sheng Zheng, Yuan-Qing Fu, Qi Chen, Tao Huang, Jing Yang and Duo Li
Department of Food Science and Nutrition, Zhejiang University, 866 Yuhangtang Road, Hangzhou 310058, China
APCNS Centre of Nutrition and Food Safety, 866 Yuhangtang Road, Hangzhou 315200, China

Hye-Sook Chang, Akira Yabuki and Osamu Yamato
Laboratory of Clinical Pathology, Department of Veterinary Medicine, Kagoshima University, 1-21-24 Kohrimoto, Kagoshima 890-0065, Japan

Daiji Endoh, Yushi Ishida and Masanobu Hayashi
Department of Veterinary Radiology, School of Veterinary Medicine, Rakuno Gakuen University, 582 Midorimachi, Bunkyodai, Hokkaido 069-8501, Ebetsu, Japan

Hiroyuki Takahashi
Information Systems Department, Industrial Research Institute, Hokkaido Research Organization, Kita-19 Nishi-11, Hokkaido 060-0819, Sapporo, Japan

Shuji Ozawa
Laboratory of Natural Products Chemistry, Department of Sustainable Agriculture, Rakuno Gakuen University, 582 Midorimachi, Bunkyodai, Hokkaido 069-8501, Ebetsu, Japan

Fahad Mohammed Al-Jasass
General Directorate of Research Grants, King Abdulaziz City for Science and Technology, P.O. Box 6086, Riyadh 11442, Saudi Arabia

Mohammed Saud Al-Jasser
Department of Food Science and Nutrition, College of Food and Agricultural Sciences, King Saud University, P.O. Box 2460, Riyadh 11451, Saudi Arabia

Elisabeth De Waele, Herbert Spapen, P. M. Honoré, Thomas Rose and Luc Huyghens
Department of Intensive Care Medicine, University Hospital, Vrije Universiteit Brussel, Laarbeeklaan 101, 1090 Brussels, Belgium

Sabrina Mattens
Department of Dietetics, University Hospital, Vrije Universiteit Brussel, 1090 Brussels, Belgium

Tao Huang
Department of Food Science and Nutrition, Zhejiang University, 866 Yu-Hang-Tang Road, Hangzhou 310059, China
APCNS Centre of Nutrition and Food Safety, Hangzhou, China
Department of International Health, Johns Hopkins Bloomberg School of Public Health, Baltimore, MD 21205, USA

Nicholas Khan
Department of International Health, Johns Hopkins Bloomberg School of Public Health, Baltimore, MD 21205, USA

Xiaojie Hu, Jing Yang and Duo Li
Department of Food Science and Nutrition, Zhejiang University, 866 Yu-Hang-Tang Road, Hangzhou 310059, China
APCNS Centre of Nutrition and Food Safety, Hangzhou, China

Qin Tang, Chunfang Wang, Congxin Xie and Jiali Jin
College of Fisheries, Huazhong Agricultural University, Wuhan 430070, China

Yanqing Huang
East China Sea Fisheries Research Institute, Chinese Academy of Fishery Sciences, Shanghai 200090, China

Farokh Kafilzadeh, Habibollah Kheirmanesh, Hamed Karami Shabankareh, Mohhamad Reza Targhibi and Elaheh Maleki
Department of Animal Science, Faculty of Agriculture, Razi University, Kermanshah, Iran

Mahdi Ebrahimi
Department of Veterinary Preclinical Sciences, Faculty of Veterinary Medicine, Universiti Putra Malaysia (UPM), 43400 Serdang, Selangor, Malaysia

Goh Yong Meng
Department of Veterinary Preclinical Sciences, Faculty of Veterinary Medicine, Universiti Putra Malaysia (UPM), 43400 Serdang, Selangor, Malaysia
Institute of Tropical Agriculture, Universiti Putra Malaysia, 43400 Serdang, Selangor, Malaysia

Gita Bisla and Shailza Choudhary
Department of Food Science and Nutrition, Banasthali University, Rajasthan 304022, India

Vijeta Chaudhary
Department of Commerce, V.M.L.G College, Ghaziabad, Uttar Pradesh, India

Leticia Elizondo-Montemayor, Diana Moreno-Sànchez, Norma G. Gutierrez, Fabiola Monsivais-Rodriguez, Ubaldo Martinez and Ana C. Lamadrid-Zertuche
Clinical Nutrition and Obesity Research Center, School of Medicine and Health Sciences, Tecnológico de Monterrey, Avenue Morones Prieto 3000 Pte., Col. Los Doctores, 64710 Monterrey, NL, Mexico

Martin M. Hernandez-Torre
Tecnológico de Monterrey, Avenue Morones Prieto 3000 Pte., Col. Los Doctores, 64710 Monterrey, NL, Mexico

Danijela Ristic-Medic, Marija Takic, Tamara Popovic, Aleksandra Arsic and Marija Glibetic
Centre of Research Excellence in Nutrition and Metabolism, Institute for Medical Research, University of Belgrade, P.O. Box 102, 11000 Belgrade, Serbia

Gordana Perunicic-Pekovic
Department of Nephrology and Dialysis, Clinical Hospital Zemun, University of Belgrade, Belgrade, Serbia

Zorica Rasic-Milutinovic
Department of Endocrinology, Diabetes and Metabolism, Clinical Hospital Zemun, University of Belgrade, Belgrade, Serbia

Kolsoom Parvaneh, Rosita Jamaluddin and Golgis Karimi
Department of Nutrition and Dietetics, Faculty of Medicine and Health Sciences, University Putra Malaysia, 43400 Serdang, Selangor, Malaysia

Reza Erfani
Department of Orthopaedics and Traumatology, Faculty of Medicine, Universiti Kebengsaan Malaysia, 56000 Kuala Lumpur, Malaysia

H. Alemán-Mateo and Roxana E. Ruiz Valenzuela
Coordinación de Nutrición, Centro de Investigación en Alimentación y Desarrollo (CIAD), A.C. Carretera a La Victoria Km. 0.6, 83304 Hermosillo, Sonora, Mexico

Cristina Sánchez-González, Carlos López-Chaves, Pilar Aranda, María López-Jurado and Juan Llopis
Department of Physiology, Faculty of Pharmacy, University of Granada, 18071 Granada, Spain

Cristina E. Trenzado
Department of Cellular Biology, Faculty of Sciences, University of Granada, 18071 Granada, Spain

Jorge Gómez-Aracena
Department of Analytical Chemistry, Faculty of Chemistry, University of Oviedo, 33007 Oviedo, Spain

Alfredo Sanz-Medel and María Montes-Bayón
Department of Preventive Medicine and Public Health, Faculty of Medicine, University of Málaga, 29071 Málaga, Spain

Loredana Salerno, Maria N. Modica, Valeria Pittalà, Giuseppe Romeo, Maria A. Siracusa, Claudia Di Giacomo, Valeria Sorrenti and Rosaria Acquaviva
Dipartimento di Scienze del Farmaco, Universitàdegli Studi di Catania, Viale A. Doria 6, 95125 Catania, Italy

Rachna Mishra and Abhijit Kar
Division of Post Harvest Technology, Indian Agricultural Research Institute, Pusa Campus, New Delhi 110 012, India

Gamze Yetuk, Dilek Pandir and Hatice Bas
Department of Biology, Faculty of Arts and Science, Bozok University, 66100 Divanli Yolu/Yozgat, Turkey